Body Rejuvenation

Murad Alam · Marisa Pongprutthipan

Editors

Body Rejuvenation

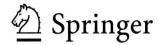 Springer

Editors
Murad Alam, MD, MSCI
Associate Professor, Departments
    of Dermatology, Otolaryngology-Head
    and Neck Surgery, and Surgery
Chief, Section of Cutaneous and Aesthetic
    Surgery
Northwestern University, Feinberg
    School of Medicine
Chicago, IL
USA

Marisa Pongprutthipan, MD
Visiting Instructor,
Department of Dermatology,
Northwestern University, Feinberg
    School of Medicine
Chicago, IL
USA
and
Clinical Instructor, Division of
    Dermatology, Department of Medicine
Chulalongkorn University
Bangkok
Thailand

ISBN 978-1-4419-1092-9   e-ISBN 978-1-4419-1093-6
DOI 10.1007/978-1-4419-1093-6
Springer New York Dordrecht Heidelberg London

Library of Congress Control Number: 2009942274

Printed on acid-free paper

Springer is part of Springer Science+Business Media (www.springer.com)

Contents

Contributors

Murad Alam, MD
Departments of Dermatology, Otolaryngology—Head and Neck Surgery, and
Surgery, Northwestern University, Feinberg School of Medicine, Chicago, IL, USA

Francesca Albani, MD
Gynecological Endocrinology and Menopause Unit, IRCCS Maugeri Foundation,
Pavia, Italy

Macrene Alexiades-Armenakas, MD, PhD
Department of Dermatology, Yale University School of Medicine,
New Haven, CT, USA

Kenneth A. Arndt, MD
Department of Dermatology, Harvard Medical School, Boston, MA, USA
SkinCare Physicians, Chestnut Hill, MA, USA

Kenneth R. Beer, MD
Esthetic, Surgical and General Dermatology Center, West Palm Beach, FL, USA
Department of Dermatology and Cutaneous Surgery, University of Miami, Miller
School of Medicine, Miami, FL, USA

Emil Bisaccia, MD
Department of Dermatology, Columbia University, College of Physicians
and Surgeons, New York, NY, USA

Katherine K. Brown, MD
Department of Dermatology, Northwestern University, Feinberg School
of Medicine, Chicago, IL, USA

Donald W. Buck II, MD
Division of Plastic and Reconstructive Surgery, Northwestern University,
Feinberg School of Medicine, Chicago, IL, USA

Mariano Busso, MD
Department of Dermatology and Cutaneous Surgery, University of Miami, Miller
School of Medicine, Miami, FL, USA
Private Practice, Coconut Grove, FL, USA

Henry H.L. Chan, MD, FRCP
Division of Dermatology, Department of Medicine, University of Hong Kong;
Division of Dermatology, Department of Pediatrics; Department of Medicine
and Therapeutics, Chinese University of Hong Kong, Hong Kong
Department of Dermatology, Fudan University, Shanghai, China

Brenda Chrastil-LaTowsky, MD
North Valley Dermatology, Peoria, AZ, USA

Taciana Dal'Forno, MD, PhD
Research Department, Brazilian Center for Studies in Dermatology, Porto,
Alegre, Brazil

Francesca De Lorenzi, MD
Division of Plastic Surgery, Preventative Gynecology Unit,
European Institute of Oncology, Milan, Italy

Zoe Diana Draelos, MD
Department of Dermatology, Duke University School of Medicine,
Durham, NC, USA

Mohamed Lotfy Elsaie, MD, MBA
Department of Dermatology and Cutaneous Surgery,
National Research Center, Cairo, Egypt
Department of Dermatology and Cutaneous Surgery, University of Miami, Miller
School of Medicine, Miami, FL, USA

Douglas Fife, MD
Surgical Dermatology and Laser Center, Las Vegas, NV, USA

Richard Fitzpatrick, MD
La Jolla Cosmetic Surgery Centre, La Jolla, CA, USA

Paul M. Friedman, MD
DermSurgery Assocaites, Houston, TX, USA

Robert D. Galiano, MD
Division of Plastic Surgery, Department of Surgery, Northwestern University,
Feinberg School of Medicine, Chicago, IL, USA

Hayes B. Gladstone, MD
Department of Dermatology, Stanford University School of Medicine,
Redwood City, CA, USA

David J. Goldberg, MD
Skin Laser & Surgery Specialists of NY/NJ; Department of Dermatology, Mount
Sinai School of Medicine, New York, NY, USA
Sanctuary Medical Aesthetic Center, Boca Raton, FL, USA

Emmy M. Graber, MD
SkinCare Physicians, Chestnut Hill, MA, USA

William Groff, DO
La Jolla Cosmetic Surgery Centre, La Jolla, CA, USA

Elizabeth K. Hale, MD
Ronald O. Perelman Department of Dermatology, New York University
School of Medicine, New York, NY, USA

Camile L. Hexsel, MD
Department of Dermatology, Henry Ford Hospital, Detroit, MI, USA

Doris Hexsel, MD
Department of Dermatology, University of Passo Fundo School of Medicine,
Porto Alegre, Brazil

Jeffrey T.S. Hsu, MD
The Dermatology Institute, Dupage Medical Group, Naperville, IL, USA

Carolyn I. Jacob, MD
Department of Dermatology, Northwestern University, Feinberg School of
Medicine, Chicago, IL, USA

Smita S. Joshi, BAS
Department of Dermatology, Northwestern University, Feinberg
School of Medicine, Chicago, IL, USA

Michael S. Kaminer, MD
SkinCare Physicians, Chestnut Hill, MA, USA

Julie K. Karen, MD
Ronald O. Perelman Department of Dermatology, New York University
School of Medicine, New York, NY, USA

John Y.S. Kim, MD
Division of Plastic and Reconstructive Surgery, Northwestern University,
Feinberg School of Medicine, Chicago, IL, USA

Natalie A. Kim, BA
Department of Dermatology, Northwestern University, Feinberg School of
Medicine, Chicago, IL, USA

Roopal V. Kundu, MD
Department of Dermatology, Northwestern University, Feinberg School of
Medicine, Chicago, IL, USA

Samuel M. Lam, MD, FACS
Lam Facial Plastic Surgery Center, Plano, TX, USA

Vicki J. Levine, MD
Ronald O. Perelman Department of Dermatology, New York University
School of Medicine, New York, NY, USA

Matthew J. Mahlberg, MD
Ronald O. Perelman Department of Dermatology, New York University
School of Medicine, New York, NY, USA

Mary Martini, MD
Department of Dermatology, Northwestern University, Feinberg School of
Medicine, Chicago, IL, USA

Angela C. Martins, MD
Department of Dermatology and Cutaneous Surgery, University of Miami,
Miller School of Medicine, Miami, FL, USA

Elena Mascolo, MD
Preventative Gynecology Unit, European Institute of Oncology, Milan, Italy

Luciana Molina de Medeiros, MD
Department of Dermatology, University of São Paulo, Sao Paulo, Brazil

Girish Munavalli, MD, MHS
Department of Dermatology, Johns Hopkins School of Medicine, Baltimore, MD, USA
Dermatology, Laser and Vein Specialists of the Carolinas, Charlotte, NC, USA

Keyvan Nouri, MD, FAAD
Department of Dermatology and Cutaneous Surgery, and
Department of Otolaryngology, University of Miami,
Miller School of Medicine, Miami, FL, USA

Anthony Petelin, MD
Department of Dermatology, University of California at Irvine,
College of Medicine, Irvine, CA, USA

Marisa Pongprutthipan, MD
Department of Dermatology, Northwestern University,
Feinberg School of Medicine, Chicago, IL, USA
Division of Dermatology, Department of Medicine,
Chulalongkorn University, Bangkok, Thailand

Zakia Rahman, MD
Department of Dermatology, Stanford University School of Medicine,
Redwood City, CA, USA

Adam M. Rotunda, MD
Division of Dermatology, Department of Medicine, University of California
at Los Angeles, David Geffen School of Medicine, Los Angeles, CA, USA

Arlene Ruiz de Luzuriaga, MD, MPH
Department of Dermatology, Cleveland Clinic, Cleveland, OH, USA

Liliana Saap, MD
Department of Dermatology and Skin Surgery, Roger Williams Medical
Center, Providence, RI, USA

Neil S. Sadick, MD
Department of Dermatology, Weill Cornell Medical College, New York, NY, USA

Dwight Scarborough, MD
Division of Dermatology, Department of Medicine, Ohio State University
College of Medicine, Columbus, OH, USA

Sherry Shieh MD
Department of Dermatology, Columbia University College of Physicians
and Surgeons, New York, NY, USA

Mario Sideri, MD
Preventative Gynecology Unit, European Institute of Oncology, Milano, Italy

Kevin C. Smith, MD
Niagara Falls Dermatology & Skin Care Centre, Niagara Falls, ON, Canada

Mariana Soirefmann, MD, MPH
Research Department, Brazilian Center for Studies in Dermatology, Porto, Alegre, Brazil

John M. Strasswimmer, MD, PhD
Dermatology Associates of the Palm Beaches, Delray Beach, FL, USA

Amy Forman Taub, MD
Advanced Dermatology, SkinQRI and Skinfo, Lincolnshire, IL, USA
Department of Dermatology, Northwestern University, Feinberg School of Medicine, Chicago, IL, USA

Rebecca Tung, MD
Department of Dermatology, Case Western Reserve University, Cleveland, OH, USA

Voraphol Vejjabhinanta, MD
Department of Dermatology and Cutaneous Surgery, University of Miami, Miller School of Medicine, Miami, FL, USA
Department of Dermatology, Mahidol University, Bankok, Thailand

Mark Villa, MD
Department of Plastic Surgery, University of Texas, M.D. Anderson Cancer Center, Houston, TX, USA

William Philip Werschler, MD
Department of Dermatology, University of Washington School of Medicine, Seattle, WA, USA
Spokane Dermatology Clinic, Spokane, WA, USA

Lucile E. White, MD
Pearland Dermatology, Pearland, TX, USA

Simon Yoo, MD
Department of Dermatology, Northwestern University, Feinberg School of Medicine, Chicago, IL, USA

Part I
Neck and Upper Chest

Chapter 1
Treatment of Platysmal Bands with Botulinum Toxin

Kenneth R. Beer

Introduction

The use of Botulinum toxins for the upper third of the face has been a well-ensconced facet of dermatologic surgery for over a decade. With greater experience with this toxin, additional areas have been treated with varying degrees of success. The middle third of the face as well as the lower thirds of the face may be injected by physicians with advanced technical abilities and knowledge of the relevant anatomy. Within the lower third of the face, the mentalis and platysma are easily treated with Botulinum toxins. Despite the fact that the platysma is not technically part of the lower third of the face, the muscle functions as a depressor of this region and its treatment greatly impacts the overall aesthetic of the entire face. Its treatment with Botulinum toxins is a relatively simple technique that can be mastered by those with experience in the upper third of the face and it can be extremely rewarding for both patient and physician. Newer modalities of radiofrequency, fractional resurfacing, and laser are able to change the texture and color of the neck. Combining these with injections of botulinum toxins offers the opportunity to dramatically improve an area that has traditionally been recalcitrant to rejuvenation.

Clinical Examination

The lower third of the face has several depressors that serve to pull it in a caudal direction. These include the depressor anguli oris, depressor labii, the mentalis and, to an extent, the platysma. Inactivation of the depressors will tend to enable the elevator muscles to lift the lower third of the face. When used in conjunction with fillers for this area, the results of these treatments can be dramatic and synergistic. Injections of the platysma

tend to neutralize the downward pull from this muscle and also to affect the appearance of the muscle, which has a dramatic result in many individuals.

As with the rest of the body, platysmal bands change over time. During the first few decades of life, the platysma is camouflaged by a thin layer of subcutaneous fat. In addition, the anatomy of the muscle is that of a diffuse band rather than a group of strings. With age, the layer of fat disappears and there is no barrier between the muscle and the skin. Thus, each string of the muscle can be visualized. Concurrently, the muscle becomes a series of fibrous bands rather than a homogenous layer. The combination of the loss of a barrier layer and development of discrete bands lends itself to treatment with Botulinum toxins.

The platysma is a superficial and diffuse muscle. Its insertion is onto the chin and its origin is on the sternum. It may be best visualized by asking the patient to grimace or make a monster face (Fig. 1.1). Variations in individual anatomy are common and each patient should be assessed and treated according to their anatomy.

One caveat that bears mention is that injections into patients without dynamic contributions from the platysma (e.g., those with flaccid necks that require liposuction or that have redundant skin for which surgery is the only solution) will result in patients who are dissatisfied. As with other Botulinum toxin treatments, proper patient selection is important when injecting the neck.

Treatment Indications

Setting Selection

In comparison with upper facial injections, the dilution of Botulinum toxin for this area may be more diffuse as the muscle itself is diffuse rather than discrete.

M. Alam and M. Pongprutthipan (eds.), *Body Rejuvenation*,
DOI 10.1007/978-1-4419-1093-6_1, © Springer Science+Business Media, LLC 2010

Fig. 1.1 Well defined platysma bands are evident in this 6-year-old girl

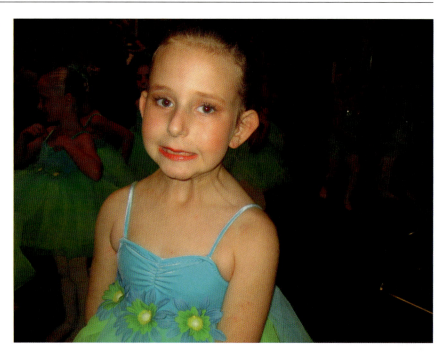

When injecting Botox, dilutions between 2 and 4 mL per 100 units, is appropriate. For Dysport, the dilution should be between 2 and 4 mL per 300 units. Dilution with more saline than these amounts may be beneficial for this area since diffusion may help to deactivate this diffuse muscle.

Treatment Technique

Anatomic considerations when injecting the neck are paramount to patient safety. The strap muscles of the neck are adjacent to the thyroid cartilage and errant injection of toxin may potentially interfere with their functions. This may impair the ability to swallow and, in rare instances, necessitate a feeding tube (a suboptimal outcome for a cosmetic patient). If a patient treated in the neck with Botulinum toxin reports difficulty swallowing, immediate consultation with an otorhinolaryngologist for a swallowing study is indicated. Fortunately, this complication is extremely rare.

Injection techniques depend on the anatomy being treated. To visualize the platysma and observe the function of the muscle, one needs to activate it by asking the patient to grimace or to show you their lower teeth. In some individuals, the platysma muscle is broad and drapes out over the span of the neck. Other individuals have vertical muscles that are typically 2–4 bands that can be easily grasped.

For patients with broad diffuse muscles of the neck, injections should be diffuse and should be spaced out across the area that moves with contraction (Fig. 1.2). Each injection should be approximately 1.5–2 cm apart and it is helpful to inject in a horizontal manner. Subcutaneous injections should be made with the needle in the superficial dermis. Raising a bleb, each area should be injected with about 2.5 units of toxin for Botox or 7.5 units for Dysport. When beginning to treat this area, women may be treated with between 25 and 50 units of Botox or 50-120 units of Dysport depending on their muscle mass. Men require more than this and may be treated with between 30 and 75 units of Botox or 60-180 units of Dysport.

Discrete muscle bands are best injected by grabbing the band and injecting it by putting the needle into the muscle (in contrast with the subcutaneous injections for diffuse platysma) (Fig. 1.3). Injections of 2.5 units of Botox or about 6-8 units of Dysport are made about 1–1.5 cm apart. Total amount of Botox or Dysport injected into patients with discrete bands is about what is used for patients with diffuse bands but many injectors find it helpful to use slightly higher doses directly into the muscles.

Fig. 1.2 Injection pattern for patients with broad diffuse muscle patterns. Courtesy of Sarah Weitzul, MD

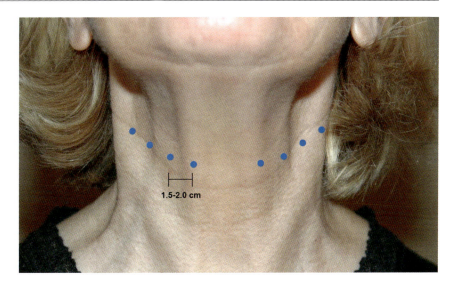

Fig. 1.3 Injection pattern for patients with discrete muscle bands. Courtesy of Sarah Weitzul, MD

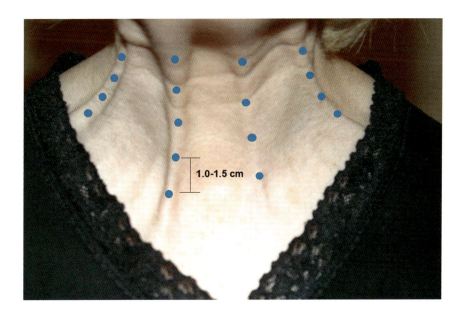

Carruthers and Carruthers have provided an excellent description for the treatment of the platysmal area with Botulinum toxins.[1] They describe the horizontal neck lines that may be seen in younger patients with thick necks. These, they believe, are caused by the superficial musculoaponeurotic bands. In their article, they recommend "dancing" along the neck, injecting 1–2 units of Botox in the deep dermis at intervals of about 1 cm apart. This technique has significant

appeal for patients with this type of anatomy and the referenced article recommends injecting no more than 15–20 units.

The platysma, as it invests the inferior sternum, also gives rise to wrinkles of the décolleté. This area is one of the most frequently cited for cosmetic enhancement. Botulinum toxins have been successfully used to smooth this area.[2] As with other areas, patient selection is paramount. For patients who have significant rippling when asked to show their lower teeth or to grimace, the activity of the inferior platysma may be dampened with injections of Botulinum toxins. Suggested doses range from 25 to 75 units, depending on the length and breadth of the muscle. Injections should be made approximately 1–1.5 cm apart (Fig. 1.4). The décolleté, when combined with modalities such as fractional resurfacing and photodynamic light treatment, can produce dramatic and gratifying results.

There are several caveats about Botulinum toxin treatments of the platysma. Obviously, there are numerous vascular structures in this area and they should be avoided.

Straying superior or diffusion into the musculature of the lower third of the face can cause asymmetry of the mouth.

Alternative Treatment Methods

Alternatives to Botulinum treatments for the neck include minimally invasive surgical approaches, traditional surgery, and laser treatments. Perhaps the treatment best suited for those who are not candidates for treatment with toxin because they have loose bands

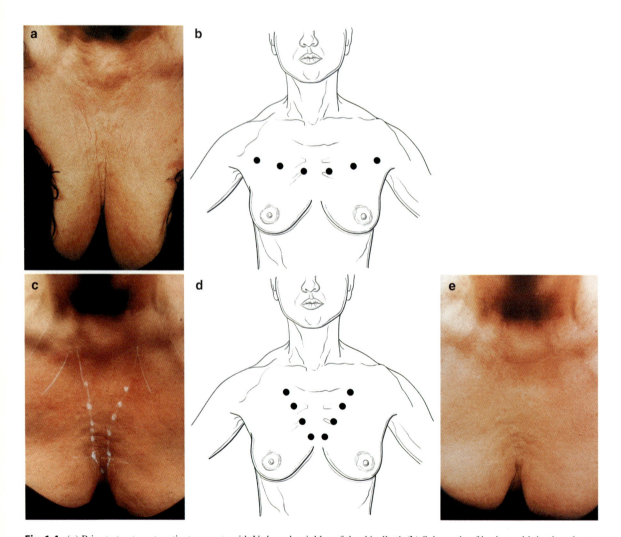

Fig. 1.4 (**a**) Prior to treatment, patient presents with V-shaped wrinkles of the décolleté. (**b**) Schematic of horizontal injection sites to treat vertical wrinkles. (**c**) Patient 1 week after horizontal injections. However, patient still presents with horizontal wrinkles of the décolleté. (**d**) Schematic of vertical injection sites to treat horizontal wrinkles. (**e**) Patient 1 week after vertical injections

that no longer contract is a modified platysma banding such as that described by Kaminer et al. If this minimally invasive technique is not adequate, traditional rhytidectomy may be performed.

Combinations of Botulinum Toxins with Other Modalities

Treatment of the platysma area may obtain optimal results when combined with other modalities. As lasers and other energy devices become more effective, they may be used to enhance patient outcomes. Among the devices that are potential, synergistic opportunities for treatment with Botulinum toxins are radiofrequency, fractional resurfacing, infrared, and liposuction.

Radiofrequency has been utilized for cosmetic enhancement of the neck with varying degrees of success. Recent advances in the settings used for this treatment and improvements in the tips have enhanced the ability of these devices to treat the neck successfully. When used in conjunction with Botulinum toxins, they may help to create a smoother contour of the neck as the toxins reduce the bands formed by the platysma. This area seems ripe for further exploration as the radiofrequency technology improves and controlled trials in this area would be worthwhile.

A second energy device used in conjunction with Botulinum toxins in the neck is fractional resurfacing. There are several variations of this technology (discussed elsewhere in the book) but each removes small areas of the skin and stimulates collagen formation. They may enhance the appearance of the neck by removing many of the signs of aging from the skin. In conjunction with toxins, this affords the neck a more youthful appearance and the synergy between these techniques is likely to result in increased patient satisfaction. There is documentation that treatments with

Botulinum toxins improves the results from laser resurfacing and it is likely that it will also enhance the outcomes from fractional resurfacing since the mechanism of action is similar.[3]

Liposuction is a minimally invasive technique to reduce the fat in the neck. Following this procedure, the muscular bands may become more prominent. Botulinum toxin may be injected in this scenario to minimize the appearance of these bands, which may have been camouflaged by the adipose. It is likely that many patients undergoing liposuction of the neck will want to have this area treated with Botulinum toxins for optimal outcomes.

Conclusion

Treatments of the lower third of the face and neck with Botulinum toxins may produce significant cosmetic improvements in these areas. Injections of Botulinum toxins into the platysma bands are relatively simple from a technical perspective. Newer modalities, such as radiofrequency and fractional resurfacing, may be used with these injections to produce a more comprehensive rejuvenation of the neck. For patients with dynamic platysmal bands and physicians with experience, injections of Botulinum toxins into the lower face and neck can be one of the most gratifying treatments performed.

References

1. Carruthers A, Carruthers J. Aesthetic Botulinum toxin in the mid and lower face and neck. *Dermatol Surg.* 2003;29:468-476.
2. Becker-Wegerich PM, Rauch L, Ruzicka T. Botulinum toxin A: Successful décolleté rejuvenation. *Dermatol Surg.* 2002;28(2):168-171.
3. West T, Alster T. Effect of Botulinum toxin on following resurfacing. *Dermatol Surg.* 1999;25(4):259-261.

Chapter 2
Treatment of Neck Laxity with Radiofrequency and Infrared Light

Macrene Alexiades-Armenakas

Introduction

Neck rejuvenation predominantly targets skin laxity, with a lesser emphasis on rhytides and photoaging. Neck laxity may increase with age due to progressive prominence of platysmal bands, loss of bony mass along the mandible and mental region, increased subcutaneous fat, and loosening of the connective tissue framework. Additionally, photoaging may result in progressive solar elastosis, which may contribute to rhytides, laxity, and poor texture. Important limitations to treatment include the anterior location of the thyroid and parathyroid glands, which must be shielded from deeply penetrating wavelengths. The increased scarring risk on chest secondary to pulsed light indicates a potential increased scarring risk on the inferior aspect of the neck as compared to face, thus necessitating greater care and lower fluences in this region. Overall, neck rejuvenation targets skin laxity bringing skin tightening technologies to the forefront in this category.

Clinical Examination and Patient History

The classification of neck laxity, rhytides, and photoaging into quantitative grades has been previously published and evaluated in clinical trials of laser and light-based treatments of laxity and rhytides (Table 2.1). A patient presenting with a grading score of two or higher may experience less utility from treatment of neck laxity with radiofrequency and infrared light. Patients aged over 65 are less likely to respond to radiofrequency treatment for reasons that remain to be elucidated and therefore, should be strongly discouraged from this form of treatment. Patients with a history of thyroid or parathyroid disease or neoplasia are contraindicated. In addition, patients with rheumatologic or connective tissue diseases, such as fibromyalgia rheumatica, lupus erythematosus, scleroderma, dermatomyositis, or other autoimmune skin diseases, are also contraindicated. Baseline and follow-up photography from both sides is exceedingly important, as the degree of improvement in neck laxity is often best appreciated by side views. It is recommended that the baseline and first set of follow-up photographs be reviewed with the patient if the level of efficacy is in question. Patients are cautioned that in the vast majority of cases, a minimum of three treatments are required to achieve significant tightening, though some patients opt to pursue as many as five treatment sessions. Managing patient expectations at the outset are very important: it is best to explicitly elicit from the patient that they have ruled out the option of a neck lift and are willing to invest the time, effort, and funds toward three tightening sessions before determining whether the treatment was a success. The level of patient satisfaction has varied depending on the technology and protocol used between 30 and 70%.

Method of Device or Treatment Application

Radiofrequency

Dose/Settings

1. *Monopolar RF (Thermage, ThermaCool system, Solta Medical Inc., Hayward, CA)*: The manufacturer suggests avoiding the use of topical anesthetics whenever possible, as it may mask discomfort and

M. Alam and M. Pongprutthipan (eds.), *Body Rejuvenation*,
DOI 10.1007/978-1-4419-1093-6_2, © Springer Science+Business Media, LLC 2010

Table 2.1 Quantitative grading and classification system of laxity, rhytides, and photoaging

Grading Scale	Descriptive parameter	Categories of skin aging and photodamage							Overall score	Patient satisfaction (Y/N)
		Rhytides	Laxity	Elastosis	Dyschromia	Erythema-Telangiectasia (E-T)	Keratoses	Texture		
0	None	None	None	None	None	None	None	None		
1	Mild	Wrinkles in motion, few, superficial	Localized to nasolabial (nl) folds	Early, minimal yellow hue	Few (1–3) discrete small (<5 mm) lentigines	Pink E or few T, localized to single site	Few	Subtle irregularity		
1.5	Mild	Wrinkles in motion, multiple, superficial	Localized, nl and early melolabial (ml) folds	Yellow hue or early, localized periorbital (po) elastotic beads (eb)	Several (3–6), discrete small lentigines	Pink E or several T localized two sites	Several	Mild irregularity in few areas		
2	Moderate	Wrinkles at rest, few, localized, superficial	Localized, nl/ml folds, early jowls, early submental/submandibular (sm)	Yellow hue, localized po eb	Multiple (7–10), small lentigines	Red E or multiple T localized to two sites	Multiple, small	Rough in few, localized sites		
2.5	Moderate	Wrinkles at rest, multiple, localized, superficial	Localized, prominent nl/ml folds, jowls and sm	Yellow hue, po and malar eb	Multiple, small and few large lentigines	Red E or multiple T, localized to three sites	Multiple, large	Rough in several, localized areas		
3	Advanced	Wrinkles at rest, multiple, forehead, periorbital and perioral sites, superficial	Prominent nl/ml folds, jowls and sm, early neck strands	Yellow hue, eb involving po, malar and other sites	Many (10–20) small and large lentigines	Violaceous E or many T, multiple sites	Many	Rough in multiple, localized sites		
3.5	Advanced	Wrinkles at rest, multiple, generalized, superficial; few, deep	Deep nl/ml folds, prominent jowls and sm, prominent neck strands	Deep yellow hue, extensive eb with little uninvolved skin	Numerous (>20) or multiple large with little uninvolved skin	Violaceous E, numerous T little uninvolved skin	Little uninvolved skin	Mostly rough, little uninvolved skin		
4	Severe	Wrinkles throughout, numerous, extensively distributed, deep	Marked nl/ml folds, jowls and sm, neck redundancy and strands	Deep yellow hue, eb throughout, comedones	Numerous, extensive, no uninvolved skin	Deep, violaceous E, numerous T throughout	No uninvolved skin	Rough throughout		

result in local adverse events. However, for patient comfort, some practitioners do use topical anesthetics in concert with a safe low energy multi-pass treatment approach. Moisten skin with alcohol. Apply the 3.0-cm² skin marking paper to the neck. Dab with alcohol then remove the marking paper. Commence initial treatment level at 362.0 for the 3.0-cm² ThermaTip TC. Apply coupling fluid and deliver application of energy to assess pain tolerance. Titrate the setting based on patient's heat sensation feedback. Continue to titrate setting until patient reports heat sensation feedback of 2–2.5 based on a 0–4 point scale. Current recommendations are to perform several (4–6) passes at lower settings (352.0–354.0) within each treatment area before treating the next area. See Fig. 2.1 for photographic example of reduction of neck laxity with monopolar RF (Table 2.2).

2. *Bipolar RF combined with diode (900 nm) laser (Polaris and Galaxy, Syneron Inc.)*: Anesthesia in the form of topical EMLA is applied for 1 h. No grounding pad is necessary. Aqueous gel is applied in a thin 2–3 mm layer. For neck, commence the RF fluence at 80 J/cm². Increase by 10 J/cm² as tolerated to 100 J/cm² maximum. For the initial treatment, employ moderate laser fluence, commencing at 20–22 J/cm² and increasing by 2–4 J/cm² per treatment session to a maximum of 36 J/cm² in type I skin. Multiple passes of 6–10 are administered with each treatment session. The clinical endpoint is diffuse erythema and immediate tightening. Key pearls during treatment include maintaining good contact with adequate aqueous gel to avoid arcing, and not stacking pulses to avoid ischemia.

3. *Bipolar RF (ST ReFirme, Syneron Inc.)*: No topical anesthetic is necessary. Aqueous gel is applied in a

Monopolar RF (Thermage)

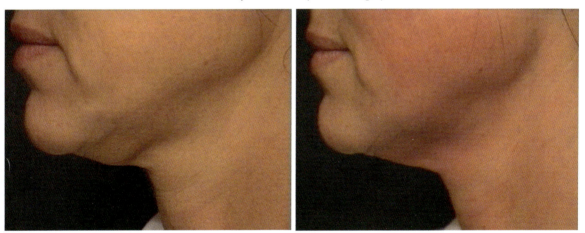

Courtesy Tina Alster MD

Fig. 2.1 Treatment zones of the neck for radiofrequency protocols

Table 2.2 Treatment protocols of neck laxity with radiofrequency technologies. All technologies should be applied to submental, submandibular, and lateral neck regions, strictly avoiding thyroid region

Device	Fluence J/cm²	Pulses/Passes	Target temp (Celcius)	Rx # interval
Monopolar (thermage 3.0 cm² tip, Solta Medical Inc.)	20–162 (352–364 treatment level)	4–6 passes	NA	3–5 q month
Bipolar with diode 900 nm laser (Polaris and Galaxy, Syneron Inc.)	90–100	6–10 passes	NA	3–5 q month
Bipolar with Infrared light (ST ReFirme, Syneron Inc.)	100–120	200 pulses per target zone	39	3–6 q 1–4 wk
Bipolar (Accent, Alma)	70, 60, 50, 40	1-3,1,1,1 (30-s) passes	40–43	3–5 q 1–4 wk
Unipolar (Accent, Alma)	90, 80, 70, 60	1-3,1,1,1 (30-s) passes	40–43	3–5 q 1–4 wk

2–3 mm film. RF fluence should be commenced at 100 J/cm^2 increasing to 120 J/cm^2 as tolerated at normal cooling. Apply a series of pulses numbering 100–250 to each treatment zone, commencing with each temporomandibular junction, followed by the lateral submandibular and upper neck region, and the submental region. If an infrared thermometer is employed, a peak temperature of 40°C is the desired endpoint. A total of 750–1,000 pulses should be administered to the neck.

4. *Unipolar and Bipolar RF (Accent, Alma)*: No topical anesthetic is necessary. Mineral oil is applied to the skin. All passes with the unipolar followed by bipolar handpiece should be administered to one side of the neck followed by the other, avoiding the thyroid region. Unipolar RF is applied first with a starting fluence of 90–100 J/cm^2 for 1–2 20-second passes. Once a target temperature of 40°C is achieved, three maintenance passes should be delivered at decrements of 10 J/cm^2 per pass. Bipolar RF is then administered with a starting fluence of 68–70 J/cm^2 for 1–2 20-second passes followed by three maintenance passes at decrements of 10 J/cm^2. Treatments may be administered weekly to monthly, totaling 3–5 treatment sessions. The key pearls include applying adequate mineral oil so that the handpiece is kept mobile and applied in a circular fashion, while avoiding the large superficial and vascular structures of the carotid system, which are present at the far lateral edges of the anterior neck. Figure 2.2 demonstrates the degree of efficacy of unipolar and bipolar RF on reduction of neck laxity, which is notable immediately postoperatively.

Postoperative Care

None of the skin tightening technologies require postoperative care. Postoperative erythema is expected and typically dissipates over minutes to hours.

Management of Adverse Events

In the case of monopolar radiofrequency, rare cases of superficial burns, erythematous nodules, and atrophy have been reported. Nodules are best treated with intralesional corticosteroids. Superficial burns are treated with topical silver sulfadiazine (e.g., Silvadene) or other wound dressing protocols. With the bipolar RF device Polaris, vascular necrosis is possible if pulses are stacked and crusting is produced by inadvertent arcing of the device if inadequate contact is made. These should be treated with silvadene or other wound care protocols. Rarely, superficial crusting may be observed with the ST as well. No adverse events were

Laser Skin Tightening
Unipolar and Bipolar RF

Pre   Immediately Post 1 Rx

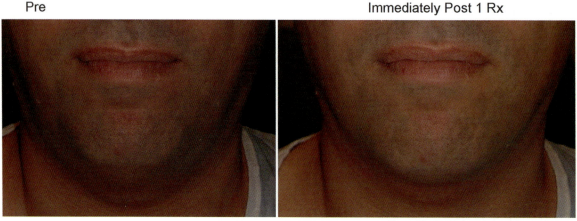

From M. Alexiades-Armenakas MD PhD

Fig. 2.2 Degree of efficacy of unipolar and bipolar RF on reduction of neck laxity, which is notable immediately postoperatively

observed during the author's experience with the Accent device, though the handpiece was kept mobile to avoid potential burns.

Infrared Wavelengths

Infrared Light (1,100–1,800 nm, Titan, Cutera)

1. *Dose/Settings*: No topical anesthetic is needed for the procedure. A thin 1-mm layer of cold 4°C aqueous ultrasound gel is applied. The treatment area on the neck is confined to midway up the neck to the mandible, excluding the thyroid region. Energy may be delivered in a stationary manner, applying adjacent pulses without moving the handpiece, or in a mobile manner, making circular movements. The fluence is commenced at 32 J/cm^2 for the stationary protocol and 40 J/cm^2 for the mobile protocol and titrated as tolerated to a maximum of 36 J/cm^2 for the majority of stationary pulses and 44 J/cm^2 for mobile administration, while adjusting based on patient comfort (range: 30–36 J/cm^2 stationary; 40–44 J/cm^2 mobile). Three passes of adjacent nonoverlapping pulses are administered, each covering an area of 1.5 cm^2. The clinical endpoints are warmth but no discomfort following the first pass, followed by pain tolerance to the end of the second "vector" or focused pass that is applied to a targeted region. The pulses over bony areas (e.g., mandible) should be administered with a reduced fluence of 30–32 J/cm^2. The target number of pulses applied to the anterior neck should number 100 following a total of two passes. Pre-, parallel, and post-cooling of the epidermis is applied to under 40°C through continuous contact with a sapphire tip.

2. *Treatment technique*: A minimum of two passes are required in order to achieve demonstrable results and three passes are typically recommended. The pulses should be administered in a linear fashion along the jawline, along the upper neck and in the submental area. Three passes are administered in succession to each linear area before commencing in a new area. A total of 3 monthly treatment sessions are recommended. Figure 2.3 demonstrates reduction of laxity and rhytides on the anterior neck through application of passes to the lateral and submental regions.

3. *Postoperative Care*: Postoperative erythema resolves within minutes to hours and no postoperative care is needed.

4. *Management of Adverse Events*: Vesiculation or blistering have been reported infrequent complications. During the procedure, this may be averted by utilizing the mobile technique and discontinuing administration of a pulse when discomfort is heightened. Wound care such as topical silvadene cream should be applied to facilitate healing. Post-

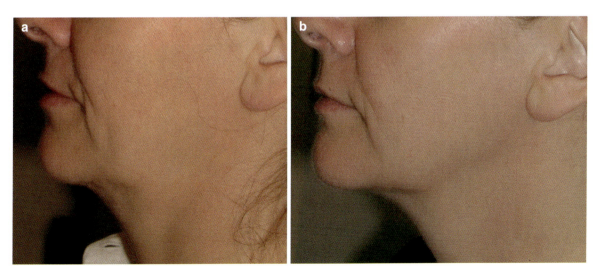

Fig. 2.3 Treatment of neck laxity with a broadband 1,100–1,800 nm infrared device. Patient prior to treatment (**a**) and 1 month following two treatments (**b**)

inflammatory hyperpigmentation may be observed following healing which gradually fades.

1,310 nm Diode Laser (Candela)

1. *Dose/Settings*: No anesthesia is required for this device. Aqueous ultrasound gel is applied in a thin 1–2 mm film. The variable depth device allows for targeting of different depths (Table 2.3).
2. *Treatment Technique*: A total of three passes are administered in succession. Pressure needs to be applied when delivering the pulses to the submandibular region in order to maintain good contact. The aqueous gel should be removed for the superficial targeting pass. The different depth targeting parameters may be combined in a single treatment, delivering one pass at deep, one pass at a medium depth setting, and a final pass at the superficial setting. Power may be titrated upward as tolerated, not to exceed 30 W. In Fig. 2.4, the mandibular defini-

tion is improved with a reduction of joweling and mandibular laxity following three treatments with the 1,310 nm laser to the lower face and neck.

3. *Postoperative Care*: Minimal erythema lasting several minutes to one hour is expected. No postoperative care is required.
4. *Management of Adverse Events*: In clinical trials, rare instances of superficial burns were reported, which healed with silver sulfadiazine cream topically twice daily.

Minimally-Invasive Radiofrequency (Miratone System, Primaeva Medical, Inc., Pleasanton, CA)

1. *Dose/Settings*: Prior to treatment, the patient's skin was cleansed with Betadine® and treatments were delivered medial to lateral in rows following anatomical margins. Topical (EMLA) and/or local anesthesia with dilute lidocaine (¼ % with 1:400,000 epinephrine) is administered. A local anesthetic

Table 2.3 Variable depth 1310 nm laser parameters for treatment of facial and neck laxity

Targeting	Spot size (mm)	Starting power (W)	Precool (s)	Laser pulse duration (s)	Postcool (s)	Cooling temp
Deep Dermis	12	24	1	1	1–3	2°C
Mid Dermis I	18	24	1	3	1	2°C
Mid Dermis II	18	17	1	5	1	2°C
Superficial Dermis	18	20	0.1	1	0.1	No cooling

1310nm laser Candela

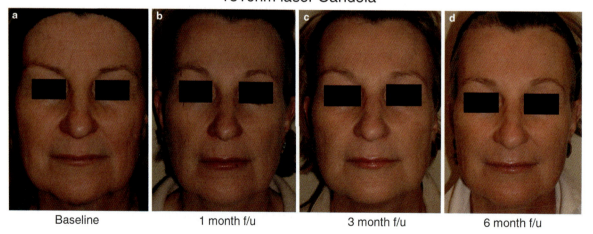

| Baseline | 1 month f/u | 3 month f/u | 6 month f/u |

Fig. 2.4 Treatment of neck laxity with a variable depth heating 1,310 nm laser. A patient prior to (**a**) and at 1 month (**b**), 3 months (**c**), and 6 months (**d**) following 3 monthly treatments. Note the progressive improvement in facial and neck laxity from 1 to 6 months follow-up

quantity of 18 cc of ¼ % lidocaine is used to infiltrate both cheeks, submental and lateral neck regions per patient. Fractional radiofrequency (FRF) energy is delivered through five micro-needle electrode pairs deployed into the reticular dermis at an angle of 20° to the skin surface with the exposed electrode length extending from 0.75 to 2 mm below the skin surface. The intra-dermal location of the electrode tips is determined by real-time impedance measurements, such that impedance measurements of between 300 and 2000 Ohms are used to define ideal intra-dermal placement. Software built into the device preclude energy delivery if impedance between an electrode pair measured below 300 or over 3000 Ohms, thereby restricting energy delivery to proper intra-dermally placed electrodes. Software is programmed to delivery energy until a pre-selected intradermal target temperature is attained, and for a specified duration in seconds.

2. *Treatment Technique*: Conservative treatment parameters of 62°C and 3 seconds may be selected for initial cases. More aggressive treatment parameters of 68-75°C and 5 seconds may be selected. Epidermal cooling is achieved by positioning a cooling device maintained at a temperature of 15°C, directly on the skin surface above the exposed electrode length. The spacing of the bipolar needle pairs and the spacing of successive applications of the device are selected to give 15% to 35% fractional skin coverage by surface projection.

3. *Post-operative Care*: The patient's skin is cleansed with normal saline, and a thin coat of white petrolatum is applied. Patients are allowed to resume normal activities immediately, and instructed to wash the skin with mild cleansers, to avoid makeup for 24 hours, and to minimize sun exposure for 14 days.

4. *Management of Adverse Events*: Superficial placement of electrodes may result in superficial thermal burns and pinpoint scar-formation in rare instances. Application of silver sulfadiazidine cream twice daily topically will facilitate healing.

Conclusion

Radiofrequency therapy applied to the skin is limited by penetration depth and protection of epidermis from thermal injury by surface cooling. Infrared lasers provide the option of variable depth targeting, which will require further investigation to determine the optimal depth or range of depths needed in order to achieve demonstrable tightening. It is not possible to definitively distinguish between these tightening modalities regarding degree of treatment efficacy. The impact of differences in treatment parameters and patient-specific anatomic features can outweigh the impact of mechanical differences across devices. Overall, efficiency may vary from 0 to approaching 50% improvement in skin laxity.

Most recently, a minimally-invasive fractional radiofrequency device completed FDA trials and has been FDA-approved for the treatment of rhytides. Efficacy rates determined by blinded, randomized grading using the validated laxity grading scale demonstrated higher efficacy rates that skin surface technologies.

Future aims include improving the degree of contracture and degree of accuracy of targeting to various depths of the tissue. It will be determined whether different penetration depths are needed for different body sites and tissues. Newer devices are being developed, which will greatly improve the level of targeting and temperature regulation at these depths.

Chapter 3
Treatment of Neck Laxity with Therapeutic Ultrasound

Lucile E. White, Mark Villa, and Natalie A. Kim

Introduction

Ultrasound represents sound waves above the capacity for human hearing (16 kHz). Generally, the ultrasound used in clinical practice utilizes a spectrum of frequencies between 1 and 20 MHz. When applied diffusely, these waves have broad applicability as a diagnostic imaging modality.

Ultrasound may also be applied by a variety of means including curved transducers or phased arrays that enable focusing of the waves. This method of application is known as High Intensity Focused Ultrasound (HIFU). Depending on how these waves are focused, small, high-energy foci can be created at variable depths within tissues that result in coagulative necrosis and cavitation (Fig. 3.1). This technique was first described in the mid 20th century and has subsequently been used clinically for the ablation of various types of tumors, including those of the liver, the uterus, and the prostate.

As high-energy sound waves propagate through tissues, a certain amount is absorbed by the tissue. This mechanical energy is converted into thermal energy causing selective tissue necrosis in a well-defined area, at a specified distance from the transducer. This depth depends on the size of the transducer, the frequency of the waves, and their angle of incidence. The ability to tailor the depth at which this coagulation occurs establishes the basis for HIFU as a potential means of non-invasive skin tightening. HIFU has been shown to elevate the brow and cause clinically appreciable results for facial rejuvenation.[1]

Generally, higher frequencies are used for more superficial effects compared to lower frequencies, which may penetrate tissues more deeply.[2] One device, the Ulthera System (Ulthera Inc., Mesa, AZ), can administer ultrasound at 7 MHz on the neck to target the mid-to-deep reticular layer of dermis and subdermis, sparing the overlying papillary dermis and epidermis. This device is specifically designed for the treatment of the dermis in comparison to previously available HIFU devices, which facilitates fat reduction. Based on the biophysical properties of the skin tissue, rapid heating of this focal zone to greater than 60°C results in rapid denaturation of collagen, producing controlled regions of coagulative necrosis with an approximate volume of 1 mm^3.[3,4] The ensuing wound healing process will promote new collagen production. This chapter will focus on transcutaneous devices and not on ultrasound-assisted liposuction, which is outside the scope of this chapter.

Patient History and Clinical Examination

Candidates for therapeutic ultrasound to the neck are patients who do not have active systemic or local infections including labial HSV or folliculitis. Additionally, patients should not be on anticoagulants and should have not taken isotretinoin within past 6 months. If patients report a past surgical history of carotid endarterectomy or surgery to other anatomical structures of the neck, inquire about the possible presence of surgical clips or prosthetic materials in the neck, which could interfere with treatment.

As is standard practice with any elective, aesthetic procedure, patient's expectations must be addressed. The ideal candidates for this procedure are those with mild jowling, neck sagging, and rhytides (Fig. 3.2). Given our clinical experience thus far, patients with

M. Alam and M. Pongprutthipan (eds.), *Body Rejuvenation*,
DOI 10.1007/978-1-4419-1093-6_3, © Springer Science+Business Media, LLC 2010

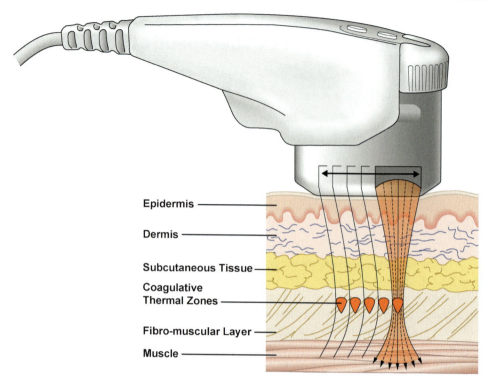

Epidermis

Dermis

Subcutaneous Tissue

Coagulative
Thermal Zones

Fibro-muscular Layer

Muscle

Fig. 3.1 The effect of High Intensity Focused Ultrasound (HIFU) on subcutaneous tissues. Note: during skin tightening treatments, the coagulative thermal zone are placed in the reticular dermis. However, since the underlying ultrasound technology permits these to be placed arbitrarily deeply into tissues, for illustrative purposes, the above diagram shows these zones within the fibromuscular layer.

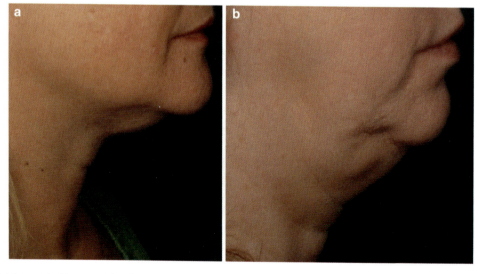

Fig. 3.2 (**a**) Lax neck skin appropriate for treatment and (**b**) a neck with a significant amount of subdermal fat

severe neck laxity should be counseled that the desired effect may be beyond the capacity of this modality and offered full disclosure of surgical and nonsurgical options. Patients with obvious submental fat pads should be considered for liposuction before undergoing ultrasound therapy.

Method of Device or Treatment Application

Dose/Setting Selection

The Ulthera System has adjustable parameters including depth and amount of energy delivered. The device energy can vary from 0.25 J up to 0.9 J. When used on the neck, the device is typically used at energies lower than those used on the face due to the often thinner dermis on the neck and the dense anatomy of the underlying structures. Also, the device is used with the more superficial probes that penetrate to a depth of 3 or 4.5 mm. It is recommended that the neck be treated with a first pass using the 4.5-mm transducer, followed by a second pass using the 3-mm transducer, both at the highest energy setting as tolerated by the patient. For each transducer, three energy levels can be chosen. When delivering the first line, the highest energy setting is used (for the 3-mm transducer, 0.45 J and for the 4.5-mm transducer, 0.9 J). With the recommended settings, the patient may feel tolerable pain. While the highest energy setting has been shown to be safe, if a patient's pain score is a 7 or above, on a scale of 1–10, the energy setting should be adjusted.

Treatment Technique

Because the zones of thermal injury are delivered to the mid-to-deep reticular dermis, patients are usually treated without any topical anesthetic prior to performing the procedure. Oral premedication with pain medications or benzodiazepines is seldom necessary.

The patient should be in supine position to enable access to the neck and submental regions. Cool ultrasound gel is applied onto the transducer hand piece.

Then the transducer is placed firmly on the targeted skin surface, and pressed firmly to the skin surface. The therapeutic ultrasound function is used to image the skin and confirm that the transducer base is in full contact with the skin without any air bubbles in the underlying gel. The image also is used to confirm that the predicted target depth is in the mid-to-deep reticular dermis.

Firing is then initiated. The device applies a 1-mm linear array of 17 coagulative zones over 2.5 cm. It is important to maintain full contact with the skin during energy delivery to avoid the formation of whitish wheal-like striations from superficial coagulation. With the more superficial transducer, more erythema will be observed in comparison to the deeper transducers. However, much of this resolves in 20–40 min after the procedure. The handpiece is moved approximately 2–3 mm up the neck before firing it again. This is repeated until the entire neck and submental areas have been treated. Typically, two passes on either side of the trachea is sufficient. The submental area can be treated with one pass over the center of the submental area or bilateral passes that merge as you move the hand piece anteriorly (Fig. 3.3). If the external jugular vein is appreciated, this area is avoided. Patients report most sensitivity when treating the mandible and when

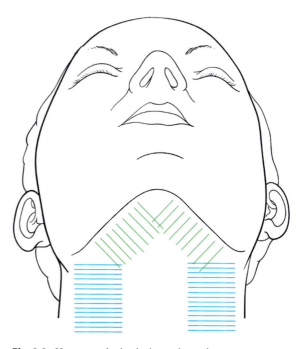

Fig. 3.3 How to apply the device to the neck

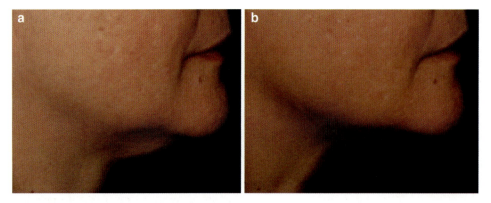

Fig. 3.4 (**a**) Before and (**b**) after treatment of the neck

treating more laterally on the neck. It is important to document how many lines were applied to each side of the neck to ensure an even application of the device and prevent asymmetry.

This ultrasound device therapy can be repeated every 30–45 days for up to three treatments. However, to obtain optimal results from subsequent treatments, patients may be recommended to wait at least 90 days for new collagen to be formed.

Alternative Treatment Methods

Other options to maximize neck rejuvenation include pretreatment liposuction of any focal fat pads that may be contributing to the appearance of neck laxity. A variety of other modalities for treating neck laxity include radiofrequency, infrared, and fractional resurfacing. About 2 weeks after ultrasound device therapy, one of these modalities can be used to supplement the treatment of neck laxity.

Postoperative Care

After treatment, patients should wash the treated area. The area may feel as if it has been sunburned. Thus, patients should be told to practice gentle skin care. Patients should be contacted one day posttreatment to assess for any skin changes that may not

have been present in the office after their treatment. Patients may follow-up for additional treatments if they are desired.

As with other noninvasive devices that cause collagen remodeling, the patient should be counseled that changes to the collagen, and thus, clinical improvement in neck laxity may take up to 3 months to observe (Fig. 3.4). This improvement may persist for up to 10 months.

Management of Adverse Events

Ultrasound can cause dermal and subdermal zones of necrosis; however, these zones of necrosis may rarely occur closer to the epidermis. In these rare instances, erythematous lines may occur on the neck immediately after treatment (Fig. 3.5). The linear arrays of pink papules likely represent superficial changes of necrosis. When these occur, a high potency topical steroid such as clobetasol propionate can be prescribed twice a day for 5 days and complete resolution usually occurs within 4 weeks. In early clinical trials, these linear arrays have not resulted in skin sloughing, hyperpigmentation, scarring, or any other permanent adverse effects. There has also been one reported case of folliculitis that may or may not have been a result of the treatment. These patients can be treated with a 2-week course of oral doxycycline and topical clindamycin solution. The folliculitis usually resolves within 2 weeks.

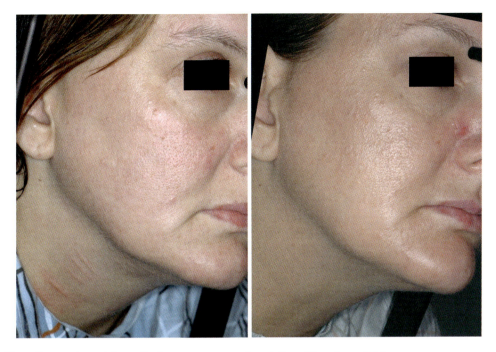

Fig. 3.5 Linear lines on the neck immediately posttreatment and resolution of lines 1 month later

Conclusion

The early experience looks promising for nonsurgical neck rejuvenation. The treatment is well-tolerated with mild intraprocedural pain, and transient redness and swelling. Ultrasound can be used to penetrate deeper into the skin without significantly injuring superficial skin layers. The safe and effective treatment settings have been defined, but certainly are not yet maximized. Further clinical experience will work to optimize treatment parameters including intervals between treatments, optimal number of treatments, and optimal numbers of passes with this device.

References

1. Alam M, White LE, Miller N, et al. Safety and efficacy of a novel ultrasound device for skin tightening on the face and neck. American Society for Dermatologic Surgery Meeting 2007, Oct. 11–14, 2007
2. Kennedy JE, Ter Haar GR, Cranston D. High intensity focused ultrasound: surgery of the future? *Br J Radiol.* 2003;76:590-599
3. Laubach H-J, Makin IRS, Slayton MH, et al. Intense Ultrasound (IUS) in Dermatology: An in-vitro evaluation of a new approach for precise microsurgery of the skin. American Society for Dermatologic Surgery Meeting 2005, Oct. 27–30, 2005
4. White WM, Laubauch H-J, Makin IRS, et al. Selective transcutaneous delivery of energy to facial subdermal tissue using the ultrasound therapy system. American Society for Lasers in Med. and Surgery Meeting 2006, April 5–9, 2006

Chapter 4
Treatment of Neck Fat with Injectable Adipolytic Therapy

Adam M. Rotunda

Introduction

Adipolytic therapy is a novel technique that uses subcutaneous injections of pharmacologically active, natural detergents to chemically ablate adipose tissue. The technique has been notoriously described as *meso-therapy* or *Lipodissolve*®, and its popularity can be attributed due in large part to direct consumer advertising and controversy rather than rigorous scientific investigation. However, the following chapter describes what is perhaps best described as *adipolytic therapy* or *lipodissolution*, which is increasingly recognized in the literature as a novel method to treat fat, using injections rather than surgery or energy devices. Phosphatidylcholine (PC), a phospholipid derived from lecithin, has been historically incorporated with its solvent, the ionic detergent sodium deoxycholate (DC), as the two primary injected medications. Recently, numerous reports attribute the fat ablation effects of this treatment to DC, which is a bile salt possessing potent cell lytic activity, and so this chapter will describe primarily the author's experience with this compound. It is imperative to note that as of this writing, DC is not approved by any regulatory authority and therefore must be obtained from compounding pharmacies. Physicians are advised to inquire about the status of this procedure with their malpractice carrier, and become informed (and likewise appropriately consent patients) of the literature, risks, benefits, and alternatives of this technique.

Clinical Examination and Patient History

Ideal candidates for the procedure have relatively small, localized fat deposits on the submental region, mandible, and jowls. Numerous reports and expert experiences describe the use of adipolytic therapy on the trunk and/or extremities. It is the author's opinion that these areas are generally too large to be effectively treated with injections, leaving the patient and physician unsatisfied with the number of treatments and medication volume required for an adequate outcome. Furthermore, adverse effects (systemic and local) from the injected medication are more probable and pronounced when dosage is increased in order to accommodate large areas. Therefore, fat on the trunk and extremities are best treated with liposuction unless they are postliposuction contour defects or *very* modest fat collections too small for liposuction (i.e., bra-strap fat, posterior arm, small collection on the anterior abdomen), which both can be adequately treated with injections. Patients considered candidates for submental liposuction are *not* candidates for adipolytic therapy unless they have adamantly expressed interest in a noninvasive option.

The treatment area should be approximately one inch in subcutaneous fat thickness upon pinching. Patients should not have any significant skin laxity, platysmal banding, significant photodamage, or history of keloid formation. Patients at least 18 years of age to approximately 50 years of age are generally best candidates. The patient should have maintained a stable body weight for the last 6 months (i.e., plus or minus 5% of initial consultation weight) and generally be in good physical conditioning.

Female patients who are pregnant, breast-feeding, or those of childbearing potential who are not observing adequate contraceptive precautions should not receive treatment. Laboratory studies are generally not necessary unless during the initial screening the patient reports a co-morbid medical condition on history. Patients should therefore have normal blood counts, serum lipids, liver and renal function. Darkly pigmented patients

M. Alam and M. Pongprutthipan (eds.), *Body Rejuvenation*,
DOI 10.1007/978-1-4419-1093-6_4, © Springer Science+Business Media, LLC 2010

(skin types Fitzpatrick IV–VI) are at increased risk for postinflammatory hyperpigmentation.

At the initial consultation, the patient must comprehend that swelling, local tenderness and nodularity are anticipated and necessary for efficacy. Further, the patient is explained that multiple treatments (three to four) are necessary to appreciate changes in fat volume. Patients often inquire whether the effects are "permanent." Just as liposuction aspirated fat will not recur, "chemically ablated" fat cells will not reappear. Yet, both of these techniques do not eliminate completely all the subcutaneous fat in the target areas, therefore fat may return with added bodyweight.

Pre- and post-treatment photography, examination, and subjective feedback are used to assess results, as photography cannot convey the "firmer, tighter" sensation most patients experience after treatment. Comparing standardized photographs of pre- and post-treatment profiles with patients is a useful and gratifying exercise (Figs. 4.1 and 4.2). Selecting the correct patient, those who have the most suitable fat collections and correct expectations, will lead to a satisfied patient, physician, and staff.

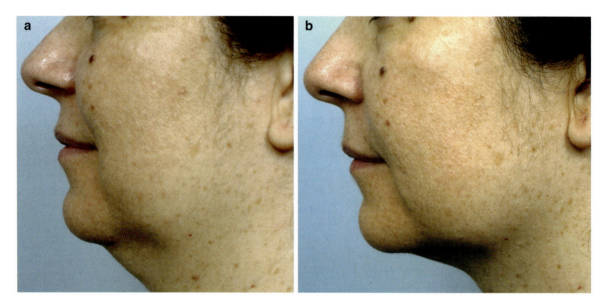

Fig. 4.1 (a) Profile of patient at baseline. (b) Same patient 2 months after 5 monthly, 1 mL subcutaneous injections of 1% DC into the submental fat

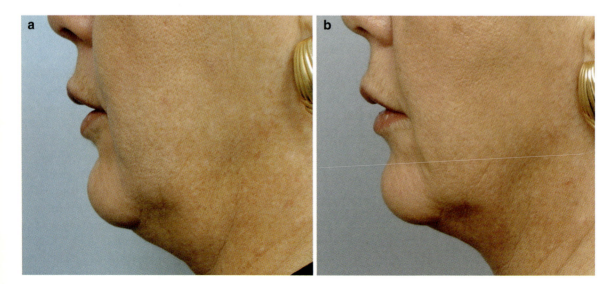

Fig. 4.2 (a) Profile of patient at baseline. (b) Same patient 2 months after 5 monthly, 1 mL subcutaneous injections of 1% DC into the submental fat

Method of Treatment Application

Treatment can be limited to the submental fat or rather, extended to the mandible and jowls (Fig. 4.3). Treatment along the mandible can yield a pleasing contour and enhance jawline definition. Combination treatment using adipolytic therapy to the face and neck along with botulinum toxin to the masseter muscle can provide dramatic facial contouring. Treatment on the lower face should be restricted to lateral to the depressor anguli oris (DAO) muscle. "When treating submental (under the chin) area, inject only the subcutaneous fat by pinching and elevating the skin prior to injection. Confine the submental treatment to the area bordered laterally by sternocleidomastoid muscles and inferiorly by the hyoid cartilage."

Generally, pretreatment is not necessary, yet some patients may benefit from Arnica several days prior to the procedure. Some clinicians prescribe a Medrol dose pack started 2 days prior to the procedure to reduce swelling. Materials required:

(a) 30-gauge, 0.5-inch needles for injection and 18-gauge, 1-inch needles for withdrawing medication.
(b) Depending on the total volume, several 1, 3, or 5 mL syringe(s) will suffice.
(c) Surgical marking or eyeliner pen for mapping of injection sites
(d) Isopropyl alcohol with cotton/gauze
(e) Sodium deoxycholate (DC) at 1% (10 mg/mL) in sterile water (i.e., water for injection with 0.9% benzyl alcohol) obtained from a compounding pharmacy
(f) Lidocaine (1%) without epinephrine

The DC and lidocaine are mixed prior to injecting. A 3:1 ratio of DC and lidocaine are drawn into the same syringe (i.e., 3.75 mL of DC is mixed with 1.25 mL of lidocaine for a total volume 5.0 mL). A white precipitate may become evident transiently as DC is mixed with lidocaine, but it should resolubilize instantly or with a gentle mix of the syringe. It is unadvisable to order premixed lidocaine and DC; the stability and these solutions are not known.

Patients are made comfortable either sitting upright or lying down and the treatment site is exposed, cleansed, and marked in a grid-like fashion, placing the points in a staggered manner 1.5 cm apart. Refer to Fig. 4.4 for additional detail of sequence of treatment events, which are represented grossly and microsopically in Fig. 4.5. Topical anesthetic is usually not used, but this can be offered. Injections of 0.25–0.33 mL are made into the *mid-subcutaneous fat* to circumvent migration of the solution into the dermis above and the fascia below. Apply no pressure on the syringe plunger as the needle is withdrawn, as this may lead to leakage of the detergent into the dermis, causing necrosis. The skin is generally pinched for more accurate and safer placement.

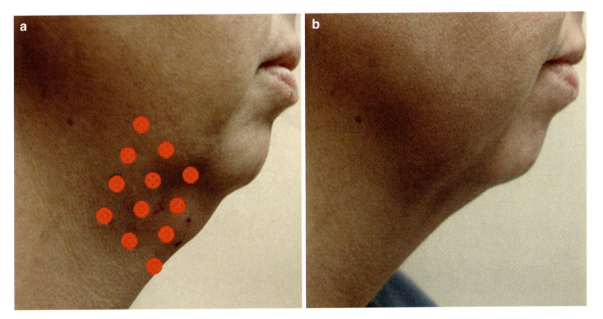

Fig. 4.3 (a) Injection grid before treatment demonstrating injection sites placed 1.5 cm apart on the submental anterior neck. (b) Patient 1 month after three injection sessions using 5 mL per session of 1% DC

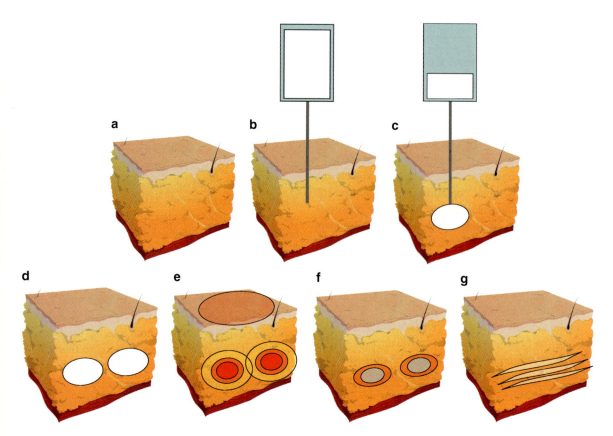

Fig. 4.4 Summary of adipolytic therapy treatment. (**a**) Cross-section of skin and subcutaneous tissue. (**b**) 30 g ½ inch needle is inserted directly into subcutaneous fat. (**c**) 0.25–0.33 mL solution is injected. (**d**) An adjacent injection is made at the same depth 1.5 cm apart provides an even plane of treatment. (**e**) Detergent effects of the solution induce a rapid localized response, including overlying erythema and subcutaneous edema. (**f**) Throughout days to weeks, the localized reaction significantly resolves, but the ablated fat tissue remains surrounded by inflammation histologically and may be apparent as subcutaneous nodules. These mildly tender to nontender nodules, if recognized, resolve over several weeks (commonly) to months (rarely). (**g**) The injected site eventually heals with fibrosis (not apparent cutaneously) with associated reduction of subcutaneous fat thickness

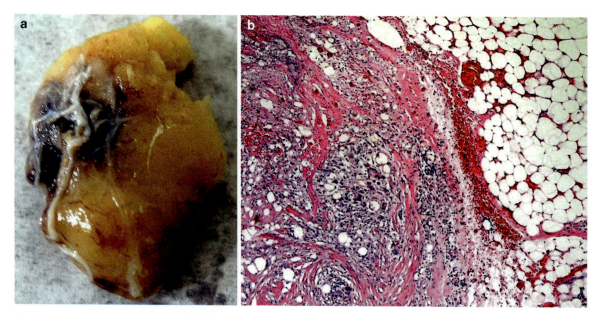

Fig. 4.5 (**a**) Excised lipoma 48 h after 1% DC injection, revealing gross evidence of hemorrhage and inflammation. (**b**) Microscopic findings (H&E,10×) revealing relatively normal appearing fat (*right*) immediately adjacent to necrosis and significant inflammation

The total volume injected per session is site dependent; it varies according to the area injected, typically between 2 mL for relatively small submental fat collections to upwards of 20 mL should submental, mandible, and jowl regions be treated together.

Immediately after the procedure, the skin should be cleansed with water or alcohol (to remove blood, pen marks) and patients can be offered a cold pack for immediate comfort. Extra-strength acetaminophen (no NSAIDS) is recommended the day of treatment and over the next several days as needed. Some clinicians recommend gentle pressure garments similar to those worn after submental liposuction, worn for 3–5 days.

Patients are treated typically every 4 weeks, although some authors recommend as short as 2 and as long as 8 weeks between sessions. A standard treatment regimen is four to six consecutive sessions (or less, depending upon patient's response) and final evaluation is performed 2–3 months after the last session. In general three treatments are required before results are seen or felt by the patient; the risk of not explaining this to the patient is noncompliance, disappointment, and lack of follow-up.

Adverse Effects

Local Effects

Immediately After Injection – Day 1

Some patients experience mild tenderness, burning, or itching. Erythema and moderate edema will persist.

Days 2–3

Edema will be moderate to significant, as will focal tenderness, although erythema will have resolved (Fig. 4.6). Swelling is often described as "jelly-like" by patients. A majority of swelling subsides after 3 days. Cutaneous anesthesia may begin and persist for 1–2 weeks. Some patients may experience ecchymoses, which will fade over the week. First treatments are best performed immediately prior to a weekend of social inactivity. After the initial treatment, patients will anticipate their reaction and adjust their social schedule accordingly; however, most patients are pleasantly surprised to experience less florid swelling and tenderness after subsequent treatmen (even with similar volumes).

Day 3 to 1 Week

Tenderness and edema gradually resolve, but may persist to a milder degree, along with superficial paresthesia (most often mild numbness, not tingling), beyond this period.

Weeks 2–4

Most anticipated adverse events have passed at this point, although firm, minimally tender, subcutaneous nodules may be felt at the injection site. Patients should be reassured that the nodule is ablated fat, is a good effect (a sign that "it is working"), and will disappear

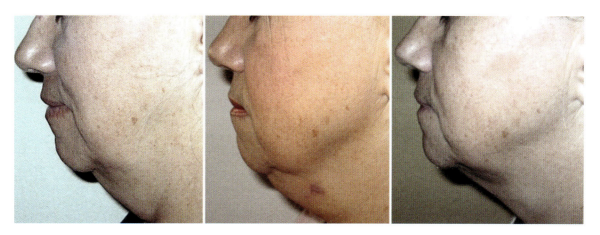

Fig. 4.6   Patient before (*left image*), 24 h after (*middle image*), and 2 months after four injection sessions (*right image*) using 7.5 mL of 1% DC combined with lidocaine. Note significant swelling and ecchymoses

slowly as the site recovers. Nodules present at follow-up should not be re-injected directly at the follow-up treatment, lending additional support for pinching the skin prior to injection

Weeks 4+

Rarely, localized nodularity persists beyond 4–6 weeks.

Systemic Effects

Gastrointestinal effects (such as nausea and diarrhea) have been described by some authors who use Lipodissolve® (PC in combination with DC). It is therefore prudent to limit total volume to 20 mL per session. Published and ongoing studies with DC reveal no systemic alterations in serum chemistries, lipids, or blood counts at conservative doses.

The adverse events described above are *expected* and should be explained as such to the patient. A call of reassurance the next day to treated patients is good medicine in general, as these treatments are unlike the relatively benign reactions experienced after other injectables (fillers and botulinum toxin), to which patients have become accustomed. It may be that the vigorous inflammatory reaction can wholly be attributed to the detergent (necrotic) effects of DC upon the adipose tissue, release of cellular debris, influx of inflammatory cell and mediators.

More serious, potential adverse effects should be noted:

Skin necrosis: This is a very rare but probable event should the detergent solution be inadvertently injected superficially. Conservative wound care (occlusion with emollients) is advised.

Hyperpigmentation: The brisk inflammatory reaction may lead to postinflammatory pigmentation in darker skin types.

Significant ecchymoses: More likely to occur in patients on blood thinners of any type (prescription or over the counter). Pretreatment with Arnica is advised for those patients at higher risk.

Persistent nodularity (>2 months): More likely to occur in patients receiving multiple high volume injections at the same location. At the time of this writing (with 5 years of follow-up), the author has not witnessed any patient with permanent nodularity (or any untoward reaction, for that matter). Patience, reassurance, and regular follow-up visits until disappearance of the nodules have been the rule.

Persistent paresthesias: Rarely, patients may experience numbness at the injection site at follow-up (i.e., 4 weeks). A significant number of more patients will have anesthesia of the skin overlying the treatment site with shorter treatment cycles (i.e., 2 weeks). Paresthesias likely represents persistent subcutaneous reaction rather than overt nerve necrosis, which has not been recorded in the literature, nor reported anecdotally. Reinjection into a site with paresthesia depends on whether the area is still significantly sore to touch and swollen on examination. It is prudent to avoid reinjection at that time and have the patient return in several weeks for a reevaluation.

Conclusion

Despite the controversy and skepticism, injectable adipolytic treatments are here to stay. With additional rigorous, controlled data in the literature, we will have a deeper understanding of its potential and limitations. Mandatory and extensive safety testing and numerous clinical trials will be required for regulatory authority approval. Until then, physicians interested in the technique should seek training and become very familiar with the literature in order to deliver a relatively safe, effective, and gratifying procedure to their properly selected patients.

Suggested Reading

Duncan D, Hasengschwandtner F. Lipodissolve for subcutaneous fat reduction and skin retraction. *Aesthetic Surg J.* 2005; 25:530-543.

Odo MEY, Cuce LC, Odo LM, Natrielli A. Action of sodium deoxycholate on subcutaneous human tissue: local and systemic effects. *Dermatol Surg.* 2007;33:178-189.

Rittes PG. The use of phosphatidylcholine for correction of localized fat deposits. *Aesthetic Plast Surg.* 2003;27:315-318.

Rotunda AM, Ablon G, Kolodney MS. Lipomas treated with subcutaneous deoxycholate injections. *J Am Acad Dermatol.* 2005;53:973-978.

Rotunda AM, Kolodney MS. Mesotherapy and phosphatidyl-choline injections: historical clarification and review. *Dermatol Surg*. 2006;32:465-480.

Rotunda AM, Suzuki H, Moy RL, Kolodney MS. Detergent effects of sodium deoxycholate are a major feature of an injectable phosphatidylcholine formulation used for localized fat dissolution. *Dermatol Surg*. 2004;30: 1001-1008.

Salti G, Ghersetich I, Tantussi F, Bovani B, Lotti T. Phosphatidylcholine and sodium deoxycholate in the treatment of localized fat: a double-blind, randomized study. *Dermatol Surg*. 2008;34:60-6.

Schuller-Petrovic S, Wölkart G, Neuhold N, Freisinger F, Brunner F. Tissue toxic effects of Lipostabil after subcutaneous injection for fat dissolution in rats and a human volunteer. *Dermatol Surg*. 2008;34:529-42.

Chapter 5
Treatment of Poikiloderma with Fractional Resurfacing

Zakia Rahman

Introduction

Poikiloderma, by definition, occurs in the setting of hyperpigmentation, hypopigmentation, atrophy, and telangiectasias. There are numerous entities where poikiloderma is present, the most common being a result of chronic photodamage and is termed poikiloderma of Civatte (PC). PC was initially described by Civatte in 1923. Recently, histologic evaluation has confirmed the aforementioned characteristics, in addition to degeneration of collagen bundles and solar elastosis.[1]

When PC is present on the neck and chest, it often displays a geometric V-shaped pattern that appears unnatural and can draw unwanted attention to the area. There are numerous modalities that have been used in the treatment of PC. Given the heterogeneity of signs, the condition is difficult to completely eradicate with one single treatment modality. The ideal modality would repigment skin, eliminate excess pigmentation, regenerate damaged collagen and elastic fibers as well as normalize the dilated dermal blood vessels (Fig. 5.1).

Fractional resurfacing has been used extensively for resurfacing on and off the face since it was first introduced in 2004.[2] Various modalities are available on the market that utilize the concept of fractional treatment, either in the nonablative or ablative mode.

Wanner et al. reported safe and efficacious treatment of nonfacial photodamage with the 1,550 nm erbium fiber laser (Fraxel™, Solta Medical Inc., Hayward, CA).[3] Recently, Behroozan et al. reported successful use of a fractional scanned erbium fiber laser at 1,550 nm (Fraxel™ SR, Solta Medical Inc., Hayward, CA) for the treatment of PC.[4] The authors reported one patient who received a single treatment

and was noted to have improvement of erythema, dyschromia, and overall texture for up to 2 months. Successful treatment of hypopigmentation with nonablative fractional resurfacing has been reported in six patients as well.[5] Recently, the first report of successful treatment of PC with ablative fractional lasers was published. The authors noted ten patients with PC who underwent one to three treatments with the Dermal Optical Thermolysis (DOT) laser (Eclipse Med, Ltd. Dallas, TX) and had significant improvement of erythema, pigmentation, and texture.[6]

Clinical Examination and Patient History

Treatment of nonfacial areas should be approached with greater caution because of the paucity of pilosebaceous units in comparison to the face. Most reports of nonfacial treatments have been done with nonablative fractional lasers. Lines of demarcation, prolonged erythema, and risk of scarring are greater for nonfacial ablative treatments. Nonablative fractional treatments are characterized by rapid wound healing and a low side effect risk profile. For this reason, nonablative fractional treatments are recommended for the treatment of photodamage and PC of the neck and chest. When ablative fractional modalities are utilized, treating less than 30% of the skin is recommended to reduce the likelihood of prolonged healing and subsequent scarring.

Patient history and physical examination should be performed with emphasis on a history of delayed or altered wound healing and retinoid use. Blood thinners, such as aspirin, NSAIDs, and vitamin E, can predispose the patient for development of petechiae

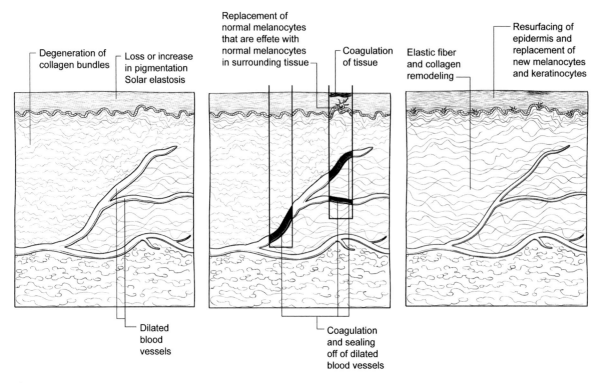

Fig. 5.1 Possible mechanisms of action for fractional laser improvement of PC (Illustration by Alice Y. Chen)

and pinpoint bleeding following fractional laser treatment. Contraindications to treatment include active infection, breakdown of skin barrier function, history of oral retinoid use in the previous 6 months, and a poor physician–patient relationship. Standardized patient photographs are critical to monitoring treatment success.

The most important preoperative wash-out for fractional treatments is topical retinoids. Upregulation of heat shock proteins (HSP) following fractional laser treatment leads to TGF-β expression and the wound healing cascade. Tosi et al. reported that retinoids blunt heat shock response, with the greatest decrease noted with all-trans retinoid acid and minimal response with 13-cis retinoic acid.[7] A 2-week washout for topical retinoids prevents alteration of cellular response to laser thermal injury.

Sun protection and sun avoidance should be stressed as the salient part of every patient's skin care regimen. In addition to preventing melanocyte stimulation following ultraviolet light exposure, sunscreens prevent long-term effects of solar elastosis, rhytides, and pigment alteration as manifested in PC.

Method of Device or Treatment Application

Stumpp et al. reported the wound healing process following fractional nonablative treatments through confocal evaluation.[8] Rapid wound healing, as demonstrated by repair of the dermal–epidermal junction and replacement of coagulated epidermis, of less than 24 h is achieved when the width of the microthermal zone (MTZ) is less than 500 μm. Fractional technology selection should take into account devices that offer truly microscopic (less than 500 μm wide) microthermal zones to prevent negative sequelae. Width of thermal injury, depth of penetration, method of delivery, and ablative versus nonablative laser tissue interaction are the major differences in the available fractional technologies (Table 5.1).

1. Dose/setting selection: Treatment energies and coverages are patient Fitzpatrick skin type independent when treating neck and chest photodamage. Considerations for nonfacial treatments include lowering total area of skin treated at one time to less

Table 5.1 Nonablative fractional devices

Device	Wavelength	Energy settings	Treatment level/ coverages	Method of delivery, device specifications
Affirm 1,440™ Laser (Cynosure)	1,440 nm/ 1,320 nm	8 J/cm², 3 ms	3 ms pulse duration	Combined Apex Pulse™ (CAP) technology, Stamping, Smart-Cool air cooling device.[10]
Affirm™ (Cynosure)	560–950 nm Intense Pulsed Light	20 J/cm²	5–35 ms pulse duration	Combined Apex Pulse™ (CAP) technology, Stamping, Smart-Cool air cooling device
Fraxel Re:fine™ (Solta Medical Inc.)	1,410 nm	1–10 mJ/cm²	5–20% coverage	Intelligent Optical Tracking System™ (IOTS), Scanning
Fraxel Re:store™ (Solta Medical Inc.)	1,550 nm	4–70 mJ/cm²	4–48% coverage	Intelligent Optical Tracking System™ (IOTS), Scanning
Lux 1,540™ (Palomar)	1,540 nm	Up to 70 mJ per microbeam, 10 mm and 15 mm handpieces	100 mbs/pulse for 10 mm handpiece (14–100 mJ)	Stamping. Contact cooling on tip
			320 mbs/pulse for 15 mm handpiece (3–15 mJ), Approximately 4% coverage with each pulse	
Mosaic (Lutronic)	1,550 nm	5–40 mJ	Dynamic Mode: Normal speed, Half speed, One third speed Static Mode: 50–500 spots/cm²	Multiple treatment tips, Dual operating modes: stamping and CCT (Controlled Chaos Technology)

than 40% of the skin to prevent bulk heating. If ablative modalities are utilized, total area should be less than 30% of the skin's surface. Treatment energies used for PC of the neck and chest are usually 8–10 mJ/cm². Higher energies of 40–50 mJ/cm², can be employed for patients with severe PC. A typical treatment covers 20–40% of the skin at each session. Treatment coverage can be reduced in darker skin patients if there is a concern for postinflammatory pigmentary alteration. Treatment intervals should also be spaced out every 6 weeks for such patients. Sessions are spaced 2–4 weeks apart and a series of four to six treatments are required to resurface the entire skin.

2. Treatment techniques: The majority of patients treated with nonablative fractional lasers require topical anesthetic. The type of anesthetic used varies from topical 5% Lidocaine, 2.5% Lidocaine/2.5% Prilocaine in a Eutectic Mixture (EMLA) to 7% Lidocaine/7% Tetracaine that is either compounded (Compounded by Central Avenue Pharmacy 133

15th Street Pacific Grove, CA 93950, www.caprx.com, 831-373-1225) or available as Pliaglis™ (Galderma Laboratories 14501 North Freeway Ft. Worth, TX 76177, www.pliaglis.com). While the majority of patients require some topical anesthetic, approximately 10–20% of patients can be treated with forced air cooling or contact cooling alone. Topical anesthetic can be applied to the area to be treated for 45–60 min. Toxicity of anesthetics should be well understood by the treating physician. Limiting the surface area to less than 10% of total body surface area per session can limit transcutaneous absorption of anesthetic. Anesthetic should always be applied in a supervised medical setting and the patient should be monitored frequently for signs of toxicity or allergy.

Cooling of the skin reduces the risk of bulk heating and also increases patient comfort. The most commonly used device for cooling employs a forced air chiller (Zimmer Medizine Systeme, Neu-Ulm, Germany) that can be used as a stand-alone device

(Fraxel™ or Mosaic) or incorporated in the handpiece (Affirm™). Although contact cooling is employed in the Lux 1540™ system, additional use of forced air cooling can increase patient comfort during treatment.

Treatment techniques vary based on the fractional technology used. Currently, the Affirm™ and Mosaic lasers and the Lux 1540™ handpiece employ a stamping technique. Circular or rectangular patterns of MTZs are laid down at a certain repetition rate. These technologies are more operator dependent in the pattern of microthermal injury that is laid down. The Fraxel™ laser employs a rectangular pattern with Intelligent Optical Tracking System™ (IOTS), which lays down an even density of MTZs independent of operator velocity.

Figure 5.2 depicts the unidirectional and bidirectional treatment techniques that can be employed on the neck and chest. The unidirectional technique works best on the neck and perpendicular passes with a bidirectional technique work best on the chest. The laser tip should always remain normal to the skin surface during treatment. Certain bony prominences can present challenges in maintaining a perpendicular position of the laser tip. These are highlighted in Fig. 5.3.

3. Alternative treatment methods: Treatment of PC usually employs several different modalities. Fractional lasers have variable success in treating the telangiectatic component of PC. Modalities that are selective for hemoglobin can be considered if a patient fails to respond completely to fractional resurfacing. Vascular Lasers and IPLs are modalities with a successful track record in the treatment of PC.[9] When they are used in conjunction with fractional photothermolysis, a 1-month interval is recommended before initiating these adjunctive modalities.

4. Postoperative care: A significant advantage of nonablative fractional technology is the limited

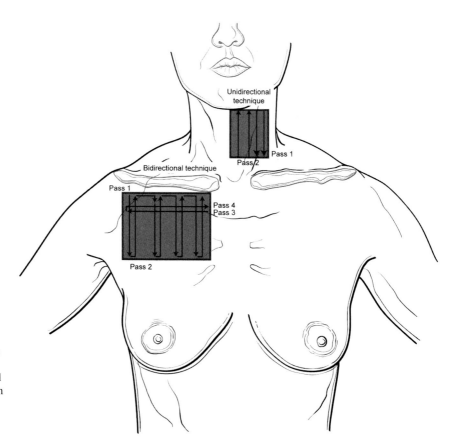

Fig. 5.2 Multiple nonoverlapping passes as performed to achieve a uniform treatment. Four to eight passes usually required. Unidirectional and bidirectional techniques can be employed to suit operator and patient preference. (Illustration by Alice Y. Chen)

Fig. 5.3 Areas of specific consideration on the neck and chest. (Illustration by Alice Y. Chen)

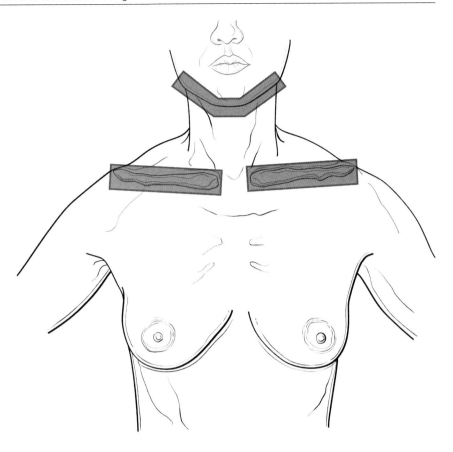

postoperative care required. The most common side effect noted is erythema. This can range from mild to moderate and is directly correlated with the treatment level. Erythema is directly correlated to the percentage of skin treated at each session (treatment level). Erythema duration ranges from 1 to 3 days on average, but can persist up to 2 weeks. Erythema can persist longer on the chest as compared to the face and neck. Edema is the second most common side effect, which seems to be more patient-dependent than erythema. Higher energy treatments usually elicit greater edema. Patients who are on blood thinners may not some petechiae after treatment. This usually resolves within 2 to 5 days.

Immediately after treatment, the neck and chest should be cleansed gently to remove any remaining topical anesthetic. A moisturizing sunscreen can be applied followed by ice packs for 10-min intervals for the first 24 h post-op. Complex aftercare is not required with nonablative fractional treatments.

5. Management of Adverse Events: The safety profile of nonablative fractional treatments is high. Common, transient side effects include erythema, edema, and petechiae. When performed properly, the risk of bulk heating at densities of less than 40% total coverage is extremely low. If bulk heating is encountered, there is a risk of blistering of the skin and scarring. Improper treatment technique that involves treatment of a small area of the skin in a short time interval or repeat firing in the same area with a stamping laser can also lead to bulk heating.

Direction for the Future and Conclusions

Nonablative fractional technology offers a relatively safe and efficacious treatment for PC and photodamage of the neck and chest. The significant safety profile, lack of lines of demarcation, low risk of hypopigmentation, and scarring make this modality preferable

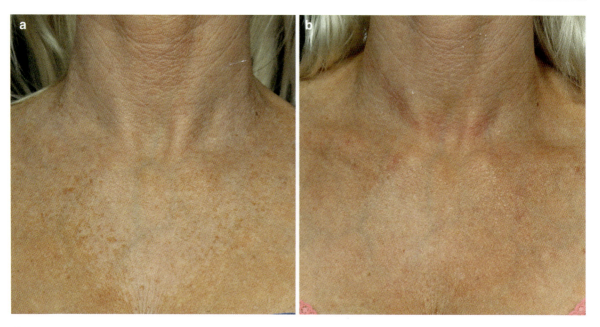

Fig. 5.4 Forty-eight-years-old (**a**) female patient treated on the neck and chest. Baseline and 1 month after three treatments on the chest and four treatments on the neck (**b**). Chest treated at 6–9 mJ, treatment levels 4–6, every 2 weeks. Neck treated at 15–20 mJ, treatment level 6–7 every two weeks. Note significant improvement of PC

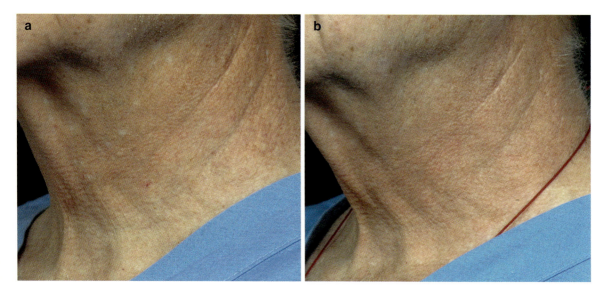

Fig. 5.5 Sixty-three-year-old male treated for PC on the neck treated with the Fraxel SR 750 laser at 8 mJ, 2,000 MTZ/cm² every 2 weeks for a total of four treatments. Baseline (**a**) and one month after four treatments (**b**). Note significant improvement of hypopigmentation

for nonfacial treatments. Fractional lasers offer the greatest improvement of hypopigmentation, hyperpigmentation, and skin atrophy associated with PC. The results on telangiectasias are variable and can sometimes require adjunctive treatment with a vascular specific light device for optimal treatment (Fig. 5.4 and 5.5).

References

1. Katoulis AC, Stavrianeas NG, Panayiotides JG, et al. Poikiloderma of civatte: a histopathological and ultrastructural study. *Dermatology*. 2007;214:177-182.
2. Manstein D, Herron GS, Skin RK, et al. Fractional photothermolysis: a new concept for cutaneous remodeling using microscopic patterns of thermal injury. *Laser Surg Med*. 2004;34:426-438.
3. Wanner M, Tanzi EL, Alster TS. Fractional photothermolysis: treatment of facial and nonfacial cutaneous photodamage with a 1,500 nm erbium-doped fiber laser. *Dermatol Surg*. 2007;33:23-28.
4. Behroozan DS, Goldberg LH, Glaich AS, et al. Fractional photothermolysis for treatment of poikiloderma of civatte. *Dermatol Surg*. 2006;32:298-301.
5. Glaich AS, Rahman Z, Goldberg LH, et al. Fractional resurfacing for the treatment of hypopigmented scars. *Dermatol Surg*. 2007;33(3):289-294.
6. Tierney EP, Hanke CW. Treatment of poikiloderma of civatte with ablative fractional laser resurfacing: a prospective study and review of literature. *J Drugs Dermatol*. 2009;8(6):527-533.
7. Tosi P, Visani G, Ottaviani E, et al. Reduction of heat shock protein-70 after prolonged treatment with retinoids: biological and clinical implications. *Am J Hematol*. 1997;56(3):143-150.
8. Stumpp OF, Rahman Z, Jiang K. In-vivo confocal imaging of epidermal cell migration and dermal changes post non-ablative fractional resurfacing. *Lasers Surg Med*. 2007;23(Suppl):8.
9. Rusciani A, Motta A, Fino P, et al. Treatment of poikiloderma of civatte using intense pulsed light source: seven years of experience. *Dermatol Surg*. 2008;34(3):314-319.
10. Gold MH. Fractional technology: a review and clinical approaches. *J Drugs Dermatol*. 2007;6(8):849-852.

Chapter 6
Treatment of Poikiloderma with Chemical Peeling

Luciana Molina de Medeiros, Arlene Ruiz de Luzuriaga, and Rebecca Tung

Introduction

Poikiloderma of Civatte (POC) is a common skin disorder characterized by reticular hyperpigmentation with telangiectasia and slight atrophy involving sun-exposed areas especially of the neck and upper chest. There is usually a sparing of the submental area. It occurs most commonly in middle aged fair-skinned women, but is also seen in men.

Treatment of POC is challenging and involves the elimination of both vascular and pigmented components simultaneously. Although various modalities have been used, complete clearing is often difficult to achieve. Monotherapy can be disappointing while combination therapy has proven to be more effective in clinical practice.

Laser and light systems can be primarily employed to address the vascular features.[1-3] Intense pulsed light (IPL) sessions have been shown to be beneficial in the treatment of POC. Goldman and Weiss demonstrated improvement in the extent of both telangiectasias and hyperpigmentation.[1] The parameters used to treat most patients included initial use of 515–570 nm filters and pulse durations of 2–4 ms, separated by a 10 ms delay. On average, patients in this study required 2.8 treatments. IPL was found to be a versatile device that ameliorates both pigmentation and telangiectasia-associated erythema, with minimal side effects.[1] Vascular lasers such as the V Beam Perfecta (Candela Corp., Wayland, MA, 595 nm) offer an improved safety profile compared to earlier pulsed dye laser technology due to the addition of a dynamic cooling device (DCD) and adjustable pulse duration that minimize the risk of postprocedural purpura and depigmentation. Typical settings of the 595 nm pulsed dye laser when treating poikiloderma of the neck and chest are of a 10 ms pulse duration, an adjustable spot size 7–10 mm, energy

settings of 5.0–6.5 J/cm^2, and the DCD (spray of 30 ms and a delay of 20–30 ms). Meijs et al. treated POC with a 585 nm pulsed dye laser. They found that by using lower fluences (5.0 J/cm^2 or less) at a fixed pulse duration of 450 μs and a larger spot sizes (10 mm), the risk of unwanted pigmentation effects (hypopigmentation) could be reduced.

Generally, a series of laser or IPL sessions are needed. However, these treatments can be costly and may not consistently treat the hyperpigmentation and textural aspect of POC.

Recently, the use of fractional photothermolysis (laser technology which generates microthermal treatment zones (MTZ) and spares surrounding skin) has had promising results in the treatment of POC. Behroozan et al. reported successful clearing with a single treatment using, 1550 nm wavelength Fraxel SR laser (Solta Medical Inc., Hayward, CA) at pulse energy of 8 mJ and a final density of 2,000 MTZ/cm^2.[4]

In our practices, chemical peels play a vital role in the therapy of POC. Peels can specifically improve underlying photodamage, including textural irregularity and dyschromia. Superficial or medium depth peels may be selected depending on the degree of sun damage. Studies from the literature, report improvement in mild to moderate photodamage on the neck and chest with chemical peeling. Cook et al. popularized the "Cook Body Peel," a procedure for rejuvenating non-facial skin, using glycolic acid gel combined with 40% trichloroacetic acid (TCA).[5] Gladstone et al. demonstrated that the combination of topical glycolic acid with a series of salicylic acid peels was safe and an effective way to rejuvenate photodamaged skin on the neck and upper chest.[6] Cuce et al. reported improvement in the appearance of photodamaged skin, melasma, and acne following series of 1–5% tretinoin peels.[7] Hexsel et al. also demonstrated that retinoic acid 5%

M. Alam and M. Pongprutthipan (eds.), *Body Rejuvenation*,
DOI 10.1007/978-1-4419-1093-6_6, © Springer Science+Business Media, LLC 2010

peels with and without microdermabrasion were effective in the treatment of signs of photoaging.[8]

Clinical Examination and Patient History

Preoperative Evaluation

Preoperative evaluation is essential to identify cosmetic concerns, set realistic goals, review downtime issues, and discuss costs with patients. A written overview of the proposed peeling procedure, listing indications and frequently asked questions, allows a patient to plan and prepare with greater understanding. A signed informed consent form should outline the risks, benefits, alternatives, and limitations associated with chemical peels. (Table 6.1).

Additionally, patients need to be informed that chemical peels alone may not completely be able to treat POC. At this point, explanation of how other procedures may be used in combination with peels for further improvement may be appropriate.

Careful analysis of the patient's skin can be standardized and may be done using the Fitzpatrick classification and Glogau system that stratify individuals by skin type (amount of baseline pigmentation and ability to tan) and extent of photodamage (Glogau stage). While superficial peels are considered safe in all skin types, pigmentary complications can be significant in darker skin types. In most patients with POC, we begin with a series of superficial peels. However, if patients have had recalcitrant POC or present with advanced sun damage, medium depth peels may be indicated at the onset of treatment. In these predisposed patients, using topical bleaching agents both in the preoperative and postoperative period may prevent postinflammatory hyperpigmentation.

Patient Evaluation

It is critical to identify any factors that may result in suboptimal results and complications (Table 6.2).

A time interval of 12 months after isotretinoin therapy is recommended prior to medium depth peeling because this medication produces atrophy of the pilosebaceous units which can result in delayed wound healing and abnormal scarring. Since light chemical peels target the epidermis to papillary dermis, patients need to wait only 3 months after treatment with isotretinoin.

Oral contraceptives, hormone supplementation or minocycline can lead to increased sun sensitivity and predispose to the development of postinflammatory hyperpigmentation.

Similarly, significant undermining of the underlying soft tissues that is commonly performed during flap reconstruction and invasive cosmetic facial and neck surgery can temporarily compromise the blood supply and lead to impaired wound healing. Any history of abnormal scar formation, keloids also warrant extra caution. Past exposure to radiation of the head or neck is also relevant. Therapeutic radiation diminishes the number of pilosebaceous units in treated areas and places these patients at an increased risk for the development of postoperative scarring.

Patients should also be questioned about active or previous bacterial, fungal, and viral infections, including herpes simplex viral infections. Current infection is an absolute contraindication to all types of chemical peeling. If a medium depth peel needs to be performed on the face, a patient should be given prophylaxis (regardless of herpetic history) with an antiviral medication provided there are no contraindications to such treatment.

A history of human immunodeficiency (HIV), hepatitis or immunosuppression due to systemic disease or medications should also be identified as there is a

---

Table 6.1 Preoperative evaluation

Evaluation of patient's cosmetic concerns and goals

Discussion of downtime and budget

Informed consent (risks, benefits, alternatives, and limitations associated with peeling) outlining the details of the procedure, common side effects, recovery time, and wound care

Assessment of skin type (Fitzpatrick classification) and degree of photodamage (Glogau classification)

Table 6.2 Patient evaluation

Complete medical, surgical, and psychosocial history: medications (isotretinoin, minocycline), active infection, history of infections (herpes simplex virus), history of radiation to head and neck, history of keloid formation, history of immunosuppression (disease or medication), and recent neck or upper chest surgery

Skin examination

Photography, including consent for pre and post photos

greater risk of infection and its untoward effects in these patients.

Before and after sequential photographs underscore any temporary lifestyle modifications that they may need to make. Detailed written postoperative instructions can maximize cosmetic outcome and avoid any potential side effects. This regimen includes proper wound care, sun avoidance, and compliance with postoperative medications.

Treatment Application

Preoperative Patient Preparation

Preoperative patient preparation can maximize cosmetic results and minimize complications of chemical peels (Table 6.3).

The American Academy of Dermatology (AAD) has developed Guidelines of Care for chemical peeling. They recommend pretreatment of the skin with topical tretinoin as well as postoperative topical tretinoin to promote wound healing faster and maintain cosmetic benefits of chemical peels.[9] Patients should start using topical tretinoin or another tolerated topical retinoid nightly at least 6 weeks prior to the chemical peel and should discontinue the use of topical treatment at least 48 h prior to a peel to ensure an intact epidermal surface. In darker-skinned patients, tretinoin increases the depth of peeling agents and the possibility of postinflammatory hyperpigmentation. For this reason, topical retinoids may be discontinued as soon as 2–4 weeks before a series of chemical peels in at-risk patients. Topical retinoids can be restarted in the postoperative period when erythema has subsided, and a complete re-epithelialization has occurred.

Table 6.3 Preoperative patient preparation

Prepeel regimen can maximize cosmetic results and minimize complications:
- – Topical retinoids: tretinoin, tazarotene, adapalene, or retinol
- – Alpha Hydroxy Acids (AHAs)
- – Hydroquinones may reduce the incidence of post-inflammatory hyperpigmentation

Sun avoidance and broadspectrum sunscreens with sun protection factor (SPF) 30 plus

Antiviral prophylaxis for all patients before a medium depth peel

Table 6.4 Commonly used concentrations on the neck

Glycolic acid (50–70%)
Trichloroacetic acid (10–25%)
Jessner's solution
Tretinoin (1–5%)
Salicylic acid (20–30%)

Since hyperpigmentation is a hallmark of POC, pre and posttreatment with topical bleaching agents is recommended. Topical hydroquinone is most commonly used. Other non-hydroquinone containing bleaching agents include azelaic acid, aloesin, vitamin C, arbutin, glabridin (licorice extract), mequinol (4-Hydroxyanisol), melatonin, niacinamide, paper mulberry, soy, vitamin E, kojic acid, alpha and beta hydroxy acids, and their retinoids. A combination of hydroquinone products such as Tri-Luma® cream (Galderma Laboratories, Fort Worth, TX) and Glyquin-XM™ can also be used.

Regular application of sunscreen is an integral part of preparing the skin for peels. The main purpose is to reduce baseline hyperpigmentation. All skin types require broad-spectrum sunscreens pre and postpeeling to reduce the risk of pigmentation complications. Extra protection in the ultraviolet A (UVA) range is important to reduce baseline hyperpigmentation and prevent postinflammatory dyschromias. Ingredients such as ecamsule (Mexoryl®SX), stabilized avobenzone (Helioplex®), and physical agents (titanium dioxide and zinc oxide) provide more complete protection against UVA.

Antiviral prophylaxis is not usually necessary for superficial peels or medium depth peels for the body, however, it is strongly recommended for all patients prior to perioral or full face medium depth peels. A commonly used regimen is valacyclovir, 500 mg twice daily or famciclovir 250 mg twice daily starting one day before the procedure and continuing for 12–14 days afterwards.

Chemical Peels

Superficial chemical peels (Table 6.4), when used in the treatment of POC, disrupt and exfoliate all or part of the epidermis. They have also been shown to have dermal effects, including stimulation of collagen and glycosaminoglycan production. Given the limited nature of the injury induced by these peels, patients often need multiple treatments on a weekly or monthly basis to reach the desired result.

1. *Glycolic acid* is an alpha-hydroxy acid (AHA), usually in concentrations up to 70%, that has been used to treat photoaging via stimulation of new collagen synthesis, as well as hyperpigmentation by removing melanin from the epidermis.[10] It is available prepackaged as a preprepared pad, in a gel or liquid formulation, or can be compounded (Table 6.5).

Treatment technique. The area to be peeled is first mildly cleansed and then degreased with alcohol with or without acetone. Rapid application of glycolic acid to clean the entire affected area, for a period of 2–3 min on the neck and 3–5 min on the chest. After this duration, the solution is neutralized with sodium bicarbonate or plain water. Physical signs such as intense erythema or pinpoint frosting can be used as end points. No anesthesia is required for AHA peels since they cause only a slight stinging sensation during application.

Since the skin of the neck is thinner and sensitive, we suggest starting concentrations at 50% and advancing as tolerated to 70%.

2. *Trichloroacetic acid* (TCA) in concentrations of 10–25% is used extensively as a light peel. The depth of cutaneous penetration varies with concentration. In these lower concentrations, it will produce necrosis of superficial layers by precipitation of epidermal proteins, clinically causing a mild epidermal slough (Table 6.6).

As a rule, non-facial skin takes much longer to heal and is at much greater risk of scarring than when using a similar concentration on the face. This is due to the higher concentration of pilosebaceous units on the face compared with non-facial sites. These units play a

critical role in re-epithelialization. As a result, if a peel is performed on non-facial skin such as upper chest and lower neck, one should proceed cautiously and concentrations of greater than 25% TCA ought to be avoided. We also suggest starting with lower concentrations for patients with skin types III or higher.

Treatment technique. The skin is prepared similarly as with other peels. Using a lower concentration TCA, erythema and a white speckled frost are noted within 1 min. A stinging sensation during peel solution application will be felt by the patient, but it should be transient. Multiple coats of the peeling agent can be used to achieve a uniform frosting and deeper peel. TCA does not require neutralization after application. Anesthesia is not required because the chemical solution acts as an anesthetic; but in some patients, topical anesthetic creams may be applied before the peel.

The level of frost is divided into four groups.

- Level 0: No frost. There is minimal to no erythema. It is a fairly superficial peel, that in most cases affects only the stratum corneum.
- Level I: Irregular light frost. The skin shows some erythema and areas of the white frost are disseminated. It is a superficial epidermal peel.
- Level II: White frost with pink showing through. Skin has uniform white color, but with a pink background. It is considered a full thickness epidermal peel.
- Level III: Solid white frost. Skin has solid and an intense white frost with no pink background.

On the neck and chest, a level I to II frost is appropriate. Cold wet compresses should be applied immediately after the peel. The white frosting resolves within 2 h. It may take 7–10 days for the skin to heal.

3. *Jessner's solution* also has been introduced as a treatment option for POC (Figs. 6.1 and 6.2), usually associated with other methods. It combines resorcinol, salicylic acid, and lactic acid in ethanol (Table 6.7). This superficial peel has keratolytic activity.

Treatment technique. Jessner's solution is applied to prepped skin and rubbed or painted on, depending on the degree of penetration desired. It is self neutralizing and multiple applications can be performed to obtain a deeper penetration. There is usually no frosting, only erythema and white speckling.

Table 6.5 Glycolic acid peel formulation

Glycolic acid	70%
Gel	Sufficient quantity to make 100 g

Table 6.6 TCA peel formulation (25%)

Trichloroacetic acid	25 g
Distilled water	100 mL

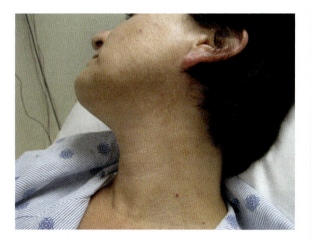

Fig. 6.1 Poikiloderma of Civatte prior to Jessner's solution treatment

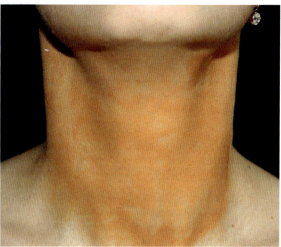

Fig. 6.3 Appearance of tretinoin peel for treatment of poikiloderma

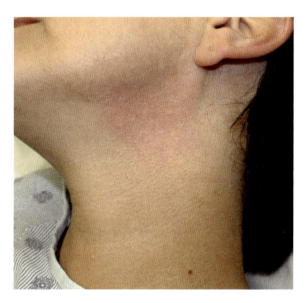

Fig. 6.2 Poikiloderma of Civatte after Jessner's Solution treatment

Table 6.7 Jessner's solution

Resorcinol	14 g
Salicylic acid	14 g
85% Lactic acid	14 g
95% Ethanol	Sufficient quantity to make 100 mL

4. *Tretinoin* peeling can be an excellent choice for improvement of photodamaged skin. Different concentrations from 1% to 5% can be applied depending on the particular skin condition. Four to six sessions are usually needed and are spaced about 1–2 weeks apart.

Treatment technique. Tretinoin peels impart a yellowish coloration upon application (Fig. 6.3) making it easy to identify any untreated areas after cleansing the area with a gentle cleanser followed by alcohol. The peel (which most often comes as a cream or gel) is applied and left in contact with the skin for 4–6 h. To improve efficacy and penetration, a plastic film may be used for occlusion. After the prescribed exposure period, the patient is instructed to wash the treated area with plain water at home.

As the yellowish hue of the tretinoin peel may not be cosmetically appealing, a foundation color is often added at the time of compounding. Tretinoin peels can be safely used in all skin types but care should be taken to avoid excess irritation. To treat areas of excess erythema, 1% topical hydrocortisone cream can be applied after the peel. In patients who have more advanced photodamage, the effects of retinoic acid peels can be increased by preapplication of one coat of either Jessner's solution or a glycolic acid (50–70%) solution. If glycolic acid is chosen, the area must be neutralized with water or sodium bicarbonate after 3 min prior to the application of the tretinoin peel (Table 6.8).

5. *Salicylic acid,* a beta hydroxy acid, has been proven to be safe and effective for acne, melasma, and photoaging in all skin types, including Fitzpatrick types IV and higher.[11]

Treatment technique. Salicylic acid peels offer the opportunity to visualize immediately any skipped areas because white precipitation of salicylic acid crystals occurs at the site of application. A neutralizing agent is not required since the vehicle volatilizes in 2–3 min and very little of the active agent continues to penetrate. Salicylic acid has been attributed with anesthetic properties and is lipophilic, making it well-suited to treat patients who may have oily or acne-prone skin.

6. *Combination peels in non-facial skin*

The Cook Body Peel[5] is a technique for non-facial skin using 70% glycolic acid gel (which acts as a partial barrier to TCA penetration) followed by application with 40% TCA. The treated skin is monitored to the endpoint desired is characterized by erythema with scattered white speckles which usually occurs within 3 min. At this point, neutralization with 10% sodium bicarbonate solution is performed.

Pretreatment with topical tretinoin followed by a methyl salicylate buffered croton oil containing 50% salicylic acid ointment peel, and localized 20% TCA for actinic keratoses or seborrheic keratoses has been shown to be effective to improve photodamaged skin on the body (Table 6.9).[12]

Monheit introduced Jessner's + TCA combination peel of 35% as an effective medium depth peeling procedure that produces a medium-depth peel for photoaging skin, actinic keratoses, and rhytides on the face.[13] For our patients with recalcitrant POC, we have seen good results with a lower concentration combination TCA peel. After standard preparation, the skin of the neck and chest is initially painted with one coat of Jessner's solution followed by the application of 25% TCA. Treated areas develop a light level I to II frosting. Light sedation may be used before and during the procedure to reduce anxiety and keep the patient more comfortable.

Postoperative Care

Postoperative care for superficial peels is minimal and simple. Immediately following the peel, a thin

Table 6.8 Retinoic acid peel formulation (5%)

Retinoic acid	5%
Gel or cream	Sufficient quantity to make 30 g

Table 6.9 Salicylic acid formulation 20 or 30% available prepackaged or compounded

Salicylic acid	20–30 g
95% Ethyl alcohol	Sufficient quantity to make 100 mL

coat of petrolatum ointment or bland moisturizer is applied. Topical hydrocortisone may be substituted if there is an increased degree of erythema or, in individuals with darker skin types, to reduce the recovery time and minimize the chance of postinflammatory hyperpigmentation.

Topical retinoids or AHA products should be avoided until the skin returns to normal, typically within 2–3 days when patient may return to the regular maintenance regimen. Sun block and sun avoidance should also be emphasized. Routine prophylactic or postpeel antiviral or antibiotic treatments are usually not required with superficial peels. For the regimen with the combination of TCA, patients – wound care is slightly more involved. Patients apply dilute 0.025% acetic acid (1 pint warm water with 1 tsp. white vinegar) 3–4 times per day followed by petrolatum ointment applications.

Conclusion

A conservative approach should be followed when treating POC given the risk of uneven removal of pigmentation and erythema resulting in a "footprint" like appearance (which can represent incipient scarring and potential for scarring on the neck and chest). Any patchy erythema should be aggressively treated with hydrocortisone cream 1% 2–3 times daily for 1 week with or without the addition of low energy pulsed dye laser treatments.

Chemical peels are an effective technique to improve photodamaged skin associated with POC. When peeling is combined with laser or light treatments, overall results can be improved. Patients should understand that multiple sessions are usually needed to reach a satisfactory endpoint.

Developing a consistent technique and acquiring a complete understanding of the limitations and complications associated with all chemical peels used in the treatment of POC will permit you to be able to select and safely perform the most appropriate peeling procedure(s) to accommodate the individual needs of your patients.

References

1. Goldman MP, Weiss RA. Treatment of poikiloderma of Civatte on the neck with an intense pulsed-light source. *Plast Reconstr Surg*. 2001;107:1376-1381.
2. Wheeland AR, Applebaum J. Flashlamp-pumped pulsed dye laser therapy for poikiloderma of Civatte. *J Dermatol Surg Oncol*. 1990;16:12-16.
3. Meijs MM, Blok FA, de Rie MA. Treatment of poikiloderma of Civatte with the pulsed dye laser: a series of patients with severe depigmentation. *J Eur Acad Dermatol Venereol*. 2006;20(10):1248-1251.
4. Behroozan DS, Goldberg LH, Glaich AS, Dai T, Friedman PM. Fractional photothermolysis for treatment of poikiloderma of civatte. *Dermatol Surg*. 2006;32(2):298-301.
5. Cook KK, Cook WR Jr. Chemical peel of nonfacial skin using glycolic acid gel augmented with TCA and neutralized based on visual staging. *Dermatol Surg*. 2000;26(11):994-999.
6. Gladstone HB, Nguyen SL, Williams R, et al. Efficacy of hydroquinone cream (USP 4%) used alone or in combination with salicylic acid peels in improving photodamage on the neck and upper chest. *Dermatol Surg*. 2000;26(4):333-337.
7. Cuce L, Bertino M, Scattone L, et al. Tretinoin peeling. *Dermatol Surg*. 2001;27:12-14.
8. Hexsel D, Mazzuco R, Dalforno T, Zechmeisler D. Microdermabrasion followed by a 5% retinoic acid chemical peel vs. a 5% retinoic acid chemical peel for the treatment of photoaging-a pilot study. *J Cosmet Dermatol*. 2005;4: 111-116.
9. Drake LA, Dinehart SM, Goltz RW, et al. Guidelines/outcomes committee: American Academy of Dermatology. *J AM Acad Dermatol*. 1995;33:497-503.
10. Usuki A, Ohashi A, Sato H, Ochiai Y, Ichihashi M, Funasaka Y. The inhibitory effect of glycolic acid and lactic acid on melanin synthesis in melanoma cells. *Exp Dermatol*. 2003;12:43-50.
11. Grimes PE. The safety and efficacy of salicylic acid chemical peels in darker racial-ethnic types. *Dermatol Surg*. 1999;25:18-22.
12. Swineheart J. Salycilic acid ointment peeling of the hands and forearms. *J Dermatol Surg Oncol*. 1992;18:495-498.
13. Monheit GD. The Jessner's + TCA peel: a medium-depth chemical peel. *J Dermatol Surg Oncol*. 1989;15(9):945-950.

Chapter 7
Treatment of Poikiloderma by Pigment and Vascular Lasers

Mohamed Lotfy Elsaie, Voraphol Vejjabhinanta, Angela C. Martins, and Keyvan Nouri

Introduction

Poikiloderma of Civatte (PC) is a condition of the middle aged fair-skinned women and men. It is characterized by a triad of superficial skin atrophy, telangiectasia, and reticulate pattern of pigmentary alterations (both hyperpigmentation and hypopigmentation). Discoloration is usually profound at the lateral aspects of the cheeks, the lower anterior and lateral aspects of the neck, and V shape of the upper chest. The submental area, shaded by the shin, is spared (Fig. 7.1).[1–14] Lesions are usually asymptomatic, although patients occasionally report itching, mild burning, and flushing.

The incidence of the condition is unknown; however, one study in Greece estimated the incidence of PC among dermatologic conditions to be 1.4%.[3] The true incidence appears to be higher, especially among fair skinned females in perimenopausal ages with a past history of chronic sun exposure. Apparently, PC has more predilection to females. Despite the fact that PC runs a chronic, irreversible but benign course, yet the physical disfigurement and self-consciousness about the lesions lead to social withdrawal and has much cosmetic implications on the population affected.[4]

PC is a rather common condition of obscure causes. Several theories and hypothesis have been interpreted as either possible pathologies or exacerbating factors. The exact etiology and pathogenesis of PC is not fully understood. It is believed that it is the sum of genetic predisposition in middle aged fair-skinned women added to an exaggerated exposure to sunlight and tendency to use fragrances that results on the development of Poikiloderma. The distribution of the lesions on sun exposed areas and the characteristic sparing of shaded parts of the skin suggests and dictates a role of solar radiation in the development of this dermatitis.

In addition, solar elastosis is another histopathological feature associated with PC, confirming the implication of sun exposure on the pathogenesis of PC.

A Summary of inducing and perpetuating factors is identified in Table 7.1.[15,16]

Method of Device on Treatment Application

Of all methods used, laser remains to be the most significant effective treatment and will be discussed in more detail as follows.

Based on the theory of selective photothermolysis, a number of laser modalities have been used for targeting the vascular and pigmented components of PC. Although complete clearance cannot be completely achieved and a number of adverse effects were reported, laser therapy remains the most efficient convenient modality for PC. Some laser can target both hemoglobin and melanin, and selecting appropriate wavelengths results in favorable outcomes.

The first laser system used for PC was the blue–green argon laser and it had significant scarring side effects, the most prominent of them was scarring. The 532 nm KTP laser was introduced shortly afterwards, representing an improvement for PC treatment although marked hypopigmentary adverse effect has been reported. The introduction of PDL significantly improved the treatment of PC, however, the first generation of PDL has not been frequently used and a few results were recorded regarding its effectiveness. Newer PDL devices served as a better modality with even greater results reported so far. Intense pulsed light (IPL) sources with a broad wavelength spectrum have

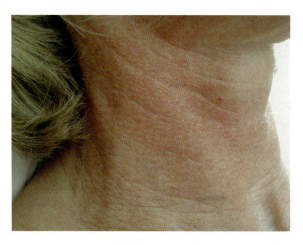

Fig. 7.1 Poikiloderma of Civatte: Ill-defined patches of bilateral symmetrical reddish-brownish reticulate dyspigmentation with atrophy and telangiectasia. This figure illustrates a lesion on the side of the neck with sparing submental area

Table 7.1 Factors contributing to the onset and development of Poikiloderma of Civatte

- Sun exposure
- Genetic predisposition
- Lighter skinned population of females in perimenopausal age group
- Hypersensitivity type of reaction involved with exposure to phototoxic allergens (Kathon CG, which is a mixture of methylchloroisothiazonilone and methylisothiazonilone, was determined to initiate or accentuate the lesions of PC.)

lately been used with reports of initial success and better results.[8,17,18] Fractional photothermolysis represents a more recent modality. The most commonly used laser therapy modalities for the treatment of PC will be discussed in this chapter.

Argon Laser

The argon laser is a nonpulsed, continuous wave laser emitting blue–green visible light. The peak wavelength emissions of this laser are 488 and 514 nm. These bands coincide with the first absorption peak of oxyhemoglobin. The blue–green argon laser was the first laser system to be used in treating PC. It offered improvement despite many of its adverse events, mainly scarring. The laser targeted the erythematous component of PC and despite its effectiveness to a

certain extent, it often led to pitted, atrophic, and hypopigmented scars. Although oxyhemoglobin is the chromophore of target for this laser, the surrounding epidermis, dermis, and melanocytes are also subject to thermal photodamage by the continuous beam of the argon laser.[19,20]

Potassium-titanyl-phosphate Laser

The potassium-titanyl-phosphate (KTP) laser uses a neodymium/YAG laser source emitting at 1,064 nm in the infrared portion of the electromagnetic radiation spectrum. The beam of infrared light is then passed through a crystal made of potassium titanyl phosphate. The frequency is doubled and the wavelength is halved so that the KTP laser emits light at a 532 nm length. At this wavelength, oxyhemoglobin is at a close peak of absorption. In addition, melanin in lesions of Poikiloderma absorbs light at this wavelength as well. The advantage of this laser is targeting both hemoglobin and melanin at the same time. To our knowledge, only one study exists in the literature reporting the use of KTP in PC. Batta and coworkers reported using KTP at 532 nm, 1 msec pulse duration, and a repetition rate of 10 pulses per second at energy fluencies of 10–15 J/cm^2. The study reported very good cosmetic improvement in reducing both the telangiectasia and pigmentation.[6]

Pulsed Dye Laser

The pulsed dye laser (PDL) has been significantly designed for vascular lesions of the skin. According to selective photothermolysis guidelines, this laser targets hemoglobin as its main chromophore. Injury can be induced to a depth of 1.2 mm with minimal destruction to the surrounding structures. First generation of PDL at 585 nm was not much assessed in the treatment of PC due to the paucity of published studies. Still, it had shown good results at fluencies of 6–7 J/cm^2 with a 5 mm spot size (Fig. 7.2). Adverse effects in the form of purpura, hyperpigmentation, or hypopigmentation were reported. With newer PDL devices (595 nm), many reported studies had been encountered in literature, however, no guidelines were exactly specified for

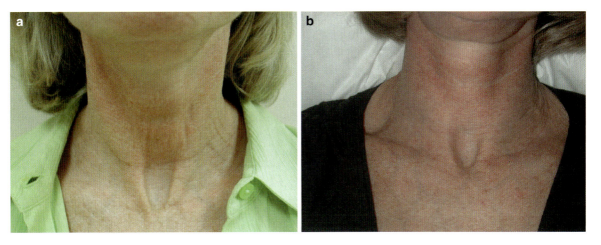

Fig. 7.2 Poikiloderma of Civatte: Before treatment (**a**), and two months after one treatment with the pulsed dye laser (wavelength 585 nm, pulse duration 450 μs, spot size 10 mm, and fluence 3.5 J/cm^2 (**b**)

Table 7.2 A summary of documented studies on PDL treatment of PC

Study	Number of patients	Parameters used	Efficacy and adverse effects
Haywood and Monk (1999)[8]	7	5 J/cm^2 with 10 mm spot and 7 J/cm^2 with 7 mm spot	Five cases of excellent response, one good and one poor and complicated with hypopigmentation in the setting of 7 J/cm^2 and 7 mm spot size
Clark (1994)[9]	1		80% clinical improvement with no side effects
Meijs et al. (2006)[10]	8	3.5–7 J/cm^2, using a 7 or 10 mm spot size	Poor results with high fluencies resulting in hypopigmentation of six out of the eight patients

the ideal usage of the PDL for an optimal effect or results.[8] A small number of published studies targeted PDL treatment of PC and results were variable. The vascular element of PC responded the best, while the hyperpigmentation was not affected or responded poorly. A number of adverse events were also noted within the context of these studies. Haywood and Monk reported scarring and hypopigmentation in one patient treated with 7 J/cm^2 using a 7 mm spot.[8]

In another study, Meijs and coworkers reported hypopigmentation in 6 out of 8 patients treated with variable fluencies ranging between 3.5 and 7 J/cm^2 using 7 and 10 mm spot sizes. They concluded that lower fluencies produce less adverse events. Table 7.2 shows a summary of some of the documented studies on PDL treatment of PC. Despite the side effects, PDL remains a very safe, effective, and efficient modality for the treatment of PC.[10]

Despite the excellent response derived from using PDL in PC, care should be taken when using it on different skin types for risk of complications. It is advisable to use low fluencies and not exceed an upper limit of 5 J/cm^2. Furthermore, the use of sun protection, following the procedure, is of outmost importance for maximum and optimal skin protection.

Intense Pulsed Light

Poikiloderma of Civatte treatment should always address both components, namely the pigmented and vascular lesions at the same time. As mentioned above, many treatments had been used without reaching an optimal treatment effect and with variable degrees of lesion clearance. One of the modalities applied is IPL.[17]

IPL is a broad spectrum, noncoherent, laser-like device that uses a flash lamp to produce a light source in a broad wavelength spectrum of 515–1200 nm. The pulse duration, number of pulses, delay between pulses and fluencies can all be adjusted and varied according to the requirements. This flexible property allows IPL to be used for different skin types with different skin conditions and for many indications such as vascular lesions, pigmented lesion removal, and photoepilation. Owing to its nature and its ability with a wide broad band wavelength spectrum to target both pigmented and vascular lesions, IPL as a source had been used to target lesions of PC. IPL utilizes the theory of selective photothermolysis and targets both chromophores, oxyhemoglobin and melanin. The peaks of oxyhemoglobin absorption are at 418, 542, and 577 nm, whereas melanin absorbs light in the entire UV radiation to near infrared spectral range. For PC, the choice of cut-off filter to be used depends on the pigmentary and the vascular components of the lesion.[17]

More than one major study had targeted the lesions of PC with IPL devices, and their results showed an overall good response with varying degree of improvements. Both the vascular and pigmentary changes of Poikiloderma were targeted. Weiss and coworkers[12] reported earlier a 5-year experience with IPL in the treatment of PC of the neck and chest in 135 patients. They reported a significant improvement of 82%, making the IPL source an effective therapeutic option for PC and allowing a marked improvement of vascular and pigmented lesions with minimal side effects. They used parameters starting with a 515 nm cut-off filter and a fluence of 20–24 J/cm^2 delivered in a single or double pulse duration of 2–4 msec, and using 550 or 570 nm cut-off filters for treatment of larger and deeper telangiectasias. The side effects included pain, erythema, purpura, crusting, and hypopigmentation. The incidence of purpura and hypopigmentation is 5%.

Another major study by Goldman and coworkers included 66 patients with typical changes of PC on the neck whom were treated with various IPL settings until the desired improvement occurred. They reported an efficacy of 50–75% after an average of 2.8 treatments and only with an incidence of 5% complications.[13] A summary of major studies utilizing IPL as a source of PC treatment is summarized in Table 7.3. Given the wide range of potential wave lengths and pulse durations, it is very reliable to use the IPL devices for treatment of PC minimizing the side effects and the risk of scarring and downtime. Caution should be taken into consideration when treating darker skin for the risk of atrophy or depigmentation. Test spots using lower fluencies are advisable before engaging in treatment protocol.

Alternative Treatment of Poikiloderma of Civatte

Offering a therapeutic venue for the treatment of PC is a difficult task. Poikiloderma represents a dermatological condition that represents a cosmetic inconvenience to patients whom often seeks medical attention for the removal of the erythematous and pigmented components of the lesions. Self-consciousness about the lesions can produce a state of social withdrawal and loss of confidence. Moreover, a number of patients experience other symptoms such as burning or itching that must be considered within the scope of treatment.

Many remedies were utilized to treat mostly the cosmetic part associated with PC, but they were proved to be ineffective and inefficient in improving the condition. No specific treatment exists for achieving an optimal result in PC, but there are various treatment modalities with variables outcomes.

Table 7.3 A summary of major studies utilizing IPL as a source of PC treatment

Study (number of patients)	Parameters used	Efficacy	Side effects
Weiss et al. 2000 (135)[12]	515, 550, 570 nm filters, pulse duration of 2–4 msec	82%	5% in terms of purpura, and hypopigmentation
Goldman et al. 2001 (66)[13]	515 nm filter, 2–4 msec pulse duration separated by 10 msec delay	50–75% after an average of 2.8 treatments	5% incidence of purpura, erythema, and hypopigmentation
Rusciani et al. 2007 (175)[17]	550 nm cut-off filter, 2.5–3.5 msec pulse duration with a delay of 10–20 msec, fluence ranging between 32–36 J/cm^2	84% efficacy with 75–100% of lesions completely cleared	Minimal transient effects in 5% of patients with no hypopigmentation

Bleaching treatments using hydroquinone, electro-coagulation, cryotherapy, retinoids, and chemical peels were all used despite of having poor results.

Conclusion

In summary, PC remains a condition that has no specific cause, despite its vast association with a number of factors. Discoveries in the field of genetics raised the possibility of the linkage between PC and a genetically transmitted autosomal dominant trait. No single effective treatment has yet been devised for the condition despite the fact that a number of different treatments have been used. Electrocautery, cryotherapy, bleaching agents, and chemical peels were all offered as a therapeutic modality, but many resulted in adverse events, making them not the best choice to target PC. Lasers targeting the vascular and pigmentary components of the condition by using selective photothermolysis properties are the best choice for treatment despite the variability of the results with the different treatment guidelines. The blue–green argon laser was the first system used for treating PC, and although offered some improvement, it had a significant scarring effect. Afterwards, KTP lasers served as a better choice but hypopigmentation, especially with darker skin types, remained a problem. Pulsed dye lasers emitting 585–595 nm produced even a more pronounced effect and significant clearance of the lesions, targeting mainly oxyhemoglobin as a main chromophore, but still targeting melanin as a part of its absorption spectrum. PDL produces posttreatment purpura which might withstand for several days.

Although no single guideline is available, a test spot using lower fluence is advised before treatment for a more optimal and safer response. IPL with a broad wave length spectrum of 515–1200 nm has most recently been successfully utilized for the treatment of PC despite some of the side effects, which were noted in the form of purpura, erythema, and crustation. Fractional photothermolysis is the latest of all laser advances described in the management of PC. Paucity of data regarding Fraxel necessitates further studying and researching in order to analyze optimization of the technique for safer and more effective results. Above all appropriate discussion of risks, benefits, and patients' expectations are essential in treating the targeted population.

References

1. Graham R. What is Poikiloderma of Civatte? *Practitioner.* 1989;233:1210.
2. Katoulis AC, Stavrianeas NG, Georgala S, et al. Poikiloderma of Civatte: a clinical and epidemiological study. *J Eur Acad Dermatol Venereol.* 2005;19:444.
3. Katoulis AC, Stavrianeas NG, Georgala S, et al. Familial cases of Poikiloderma of Civatte: genetic implications in its pathogenesis? *Clin Exp Dermatol.* 1999;24:385-387.
4. Katoulis AC, Stavrianeas NG, Katsarou A, et al. Evaluation of the role of contact sensitization and photosensitivity in the pathogenesis of Poikiloderma of Civatte. *Br J Dermatol.* 2002;147:493-497.
5. Goldman MP, Fitzpatrick RE. Laser treatment of vascular lesions. In: Goldman MP, Fitzpatrick RE, eds. *Cutaneous laser surgery.* St Louis: Mosby; 1999:19-178.
6. Batta K, Hindson C, Cotterill JA, et al. Treatment of Poikiloderma of Civatte with the potassium titanyl phosphate (KTP) laser. *Br J Dermatol.* 1999;140:1191-1192.
7. Wheeland RG, Applebaum J. Flashlamp-pumped pulsed dye laser therapy for Poikiloderma of Civatte. *J Dermatol Surg Oncol.* 1990;16:12-16.
8. Haywood RM, Monk BE. Treatment of Poikiloderma of Civatte with the pulsed dye laser: a series of seven cases. *J Cutan Laser Ther.* 1999;1:45-48.
9. Clark RE, Jimenez-Acosta F. Poikiloderma of Civatte. Resolution after treatment with the pulsed dye laser. *NC Med J.* 1994;55:234-235.
10. Meijs M, Blok F, de Rie M. Treatment of Poikiloderma of Civatte with the pulsed dye laser: a series of patients with severe depigmentation. *J Eur Acad Dermatol Venereol.* 2006;20:1248-1251.
11. Raulin C, Greve B, Grema H. IPL technology: a review. *Lasers Surg Med.* 2003;32:78-87.
12. Weiss RA, Goldmann MP, Weiss MA. Treatment of Poikiloderma of Civatte with an intense pulsed light source. *Dermatol Surg.* 2000;26:283-828.
13. Goldman MP, Weiss RA. Treatment of Poikiloderma of Civatte on the neck with an intense pulsed light source. *Plast Reconstr Surg.* 2001;107:1376-1381.
14. Anderson RR, Parrish JA. Selective photothermolysis: precise microsurgery by selective absorption of pulsed radiation. *Science.* 1983;220:524.
15. Sahoo B, Kumar B. Role of mehylchloroisothiazolinone/methylisothiazolinone (Kathon® CG) in Poikiloderma of Civatte. *Contact Dermatitis.* 2001;44:249.
16. Lee TY, Lam TH. Allergic contact dermatitis due to Kathon CG in Hong Kong. *Contact Dermatitis.* 1999;41:41-42.
17. Rusciani A, Motta A, Fino P, et al. Treatment of poikiloderma of Civatte using intense pulsed light source: 7 years of experience. *Dermatol Surg.* 2008;34(3):314-319.
18. Behroozan DS, Goldberg LH, Glaich AS, et al. Fractional photothermolysis for treatment of Poikiloderma of Civatte. *Dermatol Surg.* 2006;32(2):298-301.
19. Goldberg DJ. Laser treatment for vascular lesions. *Clinics in plast surg.* 2000;27:173-180.
20. Goldman L, Bauman WE. Laser test treatment for postsolar poikiolderma. *Arch Dermatol.* 1984;120:578-579.

Chapter 8
Treatment of Truncal Acne Scarring

Emmy M. Graber and Kenneth A. Arndt

Introduction

Acne vulgaris is a common condition with a lifetime incidence of over 80%. Acne scarring is an unfortunate, yet, frequent sequela of acne. Any type of acneiform lesion, including comedones, papules, pustules, or nodulocystic lesions, may result in scarring. Although it is impossible to pinpoint exactly which patients with acne will develop scarring, there are some factors that put a patient at higher risk. Acneiform lesions that have been manipulated are more likely to result in scarring. Truncal acne scarring is more common in males than females, and Asian and Black patients are especially prone to keloidal scarring. More severe acne and especially acne conglobata, (Fig. 8.1) has a higher risk of leading to scarring.

Several factors may predispose a patient to acne scarring. Prolonged angiogenesis is seen in lesions that proceed to scarring compared to lesions that resolve without scarring. An excess of metalloproteinases, such as collagenases, may also play a role in scar formation.[1] One study showed that nonscarring patients developed peak inflammation 48 h after an acneiform lesion had arisen. Patients with acne scars developed an inflammatory response later in the acne lesion's evolution and the inflammation was slower to resolve[2] (Fig. 8.2).

Patient History and Clinical Examination

Evaluation of a patient with truncal acne scarring requires consideration of several issues. The age of the scars should be determined since scars continue to evolve over 12 months and some treatment modalities (such as the pulsed dye laser) work best for newer scars. The distribution of the scars should be noted as certain treatments are best utilized for scattered individual scars, while other treatments may be needed for widespread scars. It is also important to identify the acne scar morphology, as different treatment modalities are preferable for particular types of scars. Previous use of isotretinoin should be known, since recent use of isotretinoin (within the last year) may preclude some procedures due to the potential increased risk of scarring.

Facial acne scars have been classified into three primary morphologic types: icepick, boxcar, and rolling scars. While these scar morphologies can also be seen on the trunk, acne scars on the chest and back are usually either: (1) hypertrophic/keloidal (Figs. 8.3–8.5), or (2) atrophic (Figs. 8.6 and 8.7). Some therapies may be directed to both types of scarring, while other therapies are specific to either hypertrophic/keloidal scars or atrophic scars.

Therapeutic Considerations and Applications

The best treatment for scars on the trunk is prevention. Patients who delay starting antiacne medications for at least 3 years from acne onset, have a greater degree of scarring than those who start acne treatment earlier.[3] Isotretinoin therapy is the only proven cure of acne and should be instituted early in the course of severe acne in order to prevent scarring.

Excision

If scarring does occur, either type of acne scars on the trunk may be treated by surgical excision. Given the high tension of the truncal skin, patients should be warned of the high likelihood that the surgical scar

Fig. 8.1 Acne conglobata on the chest of a male patient

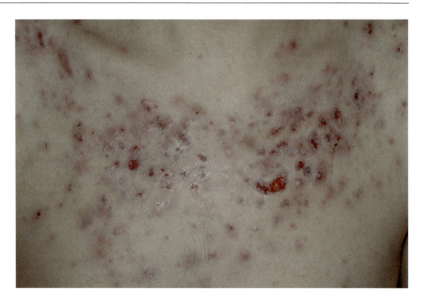

Fig. 8.2 Non-scarrers tend to have an earlier inflammatory response than acne patients that scar. (From: Holland DB et al Inflammation in acne scarring: a comparison of the responses in lesions from patients prone and not prone to scar. *Br J Dermatol.* 2004;150:72-81)

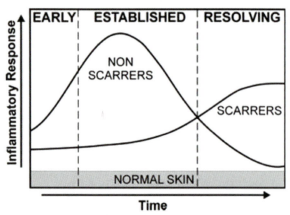

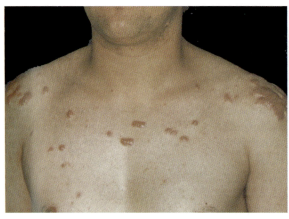
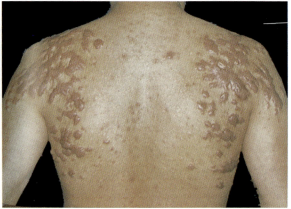

Fig. 8.3 Hypertrophic and keloidal acne scars

might expand or become hypertrophic, resulting in a sub-optimal cosmetic outcome. Surgical excision should be contemplated on the trunk only when the surgeon thinks that the replacement scar will be preferable to the original scar. If a hypertrophic scar is excised, ionizing radiotherapy administered within 24–48 h may inhibit fibroblast proliferation and prevent recurrence of the hypertrophic scar.[4]

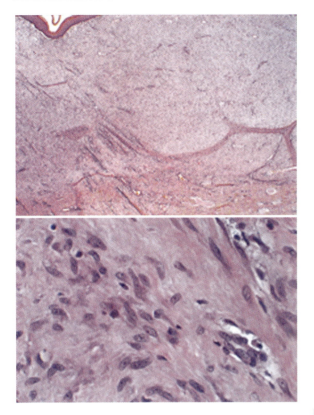

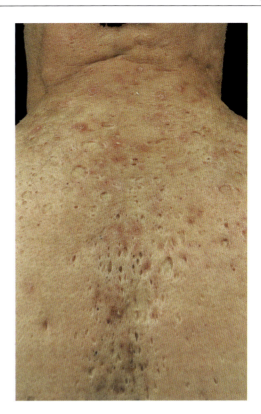

Fig. 8.6 Atrophic scars

Fig. 8.4 Hypertrophic scar. Note the well-circumscribed nodular morphology and marked collagen deposition

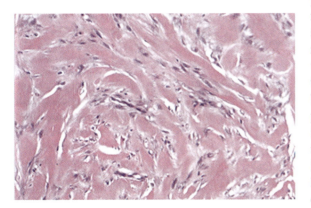

Fig. 8.5 Keloid. This type of scar differs from a hypertrophic scar in that the scarring extends beyond the site of initial injury. Histologically, it is characterized by broad, haphazard bundles of eosinophilic collagen

Pulsed Dye Laser

Both atrophic and hypertrophic/keloidal scars may have a red color, especially early in their evolution, due to microvasculature in the scar. The use of the 585 nm

pulsed dye laser to lessen scar erythema was first recognized in 1993. Alster and colleagues demonstrated a reduction in scar erythema as well as the return of normal skin markings and flattening of elevated scars.[5] Several studies thereafter have confirmed these results and also demonstrated that increasing benefit can be seen with multiple treatments. The pulsed dye laser's exact mechanism of action for scar improvement is not known, but is most likely multifactorial. Damaging the microvasculature may cause ischemia and collagen degradation, thereby, clinically lessening erythema and flattening scars. Thermal damage may also cause dissolution of collagen by breaking down collagen disulfide bonds. Other studies have demonstrated that use of the pulsed dye laser on atrophic scars can actually induce collagen formation and elevate these depressed scars.[6] It is hypothesized that inflammation that follows microvascular damage may trigger fibroblast activity and lead to new collagen formation.[7] When using the pulsed dye laser (595 nm, Vbeam, Candela, Wayland, MA) for scars, purpuric settings should be utilized by delivering energy (6–7.5 mJ/cm^2) over a short pulse duration (1.5–6 ms)

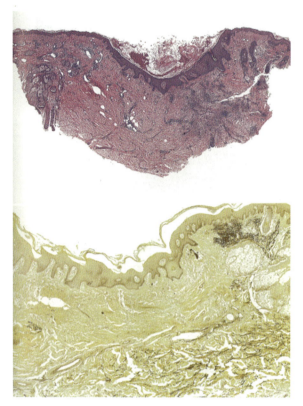

Fig. 8.7 Histopathology of atrophic scars demonstrating diminished collagen and elastic fibers

to have the greatest efficacy. Multiple (4–8) treatments at 4–6 week intervals are needed to maximize the benefits of the pulsed dye laser.

Ablative Lasers

The use of ablative lasers for improving acne scarring on the trunk is limited. Ablative systems (such as the CO_2 and erbium:YAG) that are helpful in improving acne scars on the face are not suitable for use on the chest and back. The lack of adnexal skin appendages on the trunk makes ablative treatments unlikely to re-epithelialize. However, new fractional ablative technologies, such as ActiveFX (10,600 nm CO_2 laser, Lumenis, Santa Clara, CA), Fraxel re:pair (10,600 nm CO_2 laser, Solta Medical, Inc. Hayward, CA), and the ProFractional (2,940 nm Erbium laser, Sciton, Palo Alto, CA), are being used by some to treat truncal acne scarring without prolonged healing. The Fraxel re:pair has been used at 35–50% coverage at 50–70 mJ/cm^2

with good short-term results (personal communication). Although there are no studies currently available to demonstrate this, fractionated ablative CO_2 and erbium technologies may have a future role in treating truncal acne scarring.

Semi-ablative Lasers

Nonablative systems, such as the fractionated 1,550 nm erbium-doped fiber laser (Fraxel, Solta Medical, Inc. Hayward, CA), can be safely used off the face. The Fraxel laser induces collagenesis underneath atrophic scars. Multiple treatments (at least four) are needed to treat atrophic scars, and patients are counseled that about 50% improvement in scars can be seen after several treatments. We usually start treating at 40 mJ with a treatment density level of 6 (20% coverage) and over several treatments increase to 70 mJ at a density of 8 (26% coverage). Fractional resurfacing has been used to improve the clinical appearance of hypertrophic scars. However, an adverse event of this treatment is hypertrophic scarring, particularly when used off the face.[8]

Nonablative Lasers

Other nonablative lasers in the infrared range, such as 1,320 nm (CoolTouch, Cool Touch Corp., Roseville, CA), 1,450 nm (Smoothbeam, Candela, Wayland, MA), and 1,540 nm (Aramis, Quantel Medical, France), also can help to improve atrophic scars. These lasers work by causing thermal injury in the dermis while sparring the epidermis with cooling. The infrared lasers are absorbed by dermal water, and the scattering of thermal energy damages dermal collagen, incites an inflammatory response that activates fibroblasts and stimulates collagen remodeling.[9] Multiple treatments are needed to elevate facial atrophic scars with these laser treatments. In our opinion, these devices have minimal efficacy for acne scars on the trunk. With the exception of the 1,540 nm laser (Aramis), the utility of these devices is limited due to patient discomfort during the procedure. The Aramis delivers a series of stacked micropulses (one to four micropulses) with each micropulse delivering 10–12 J/cm^2.

Intralesional Corticosteroids

Individual hypertrophic and keloidal scars may be treated with intralesional corticosteroids to soften and shrink scars as well as to decrease associated pruritus. Multiple treatments of intralesional triamcinolone acetonide in concentrations ranging from 2.5 to 20 mg/mL are needed depending on the thickness of the scar. To reduce patient discomfort, we use the smallest gauge needle (27G–30G) possible without getting corticosteroid blockage. A Luer lock syringe is safest to prevent a clogged needle from dislodging from the syringe. One-inch needles are preferable to ½ in. needles to minimize needle sticks. Concomitant administration of intralesional corticosteroids and pulsed dye laser treatment has been shown to have greater resolution of scars than pulsed dye laser treatment alone.[10] Intralesional steroid injection tends to be easier and less painful when administered after pulsed dye laser therapy than prior to laser therapy (personal observation). This may be due to laser-induced edema that lessens the resistance of the injection.

Fillers

Individual atrophic scars can be improved by elevating the depression with a filler substance. This may not be a realistic approach in a patient who has copious confluent atrophic scars, but better suited for a patient with fewer individual well-demarcated atrophic scars. Scars may be augmented with substances of varying duration. Some short-lived fillers, such as the collagens (Zyderm, Zyplast, Cosmoderm, and Cosmoplast, Inamed Aesthetics, Santa Barbara, CA), will only last for 3–4 months. Although the longevity of collagen augmentation is limited, it may be beneficial for patients who want to undergo a non-permanent trial before embarking on a more permanent substance. The most commonly used fillers for atrophic scars are those with a somewhat longer lifespan. Hyaluronic acid fillers (Restylane, Medicis, Scottsdale, AZ; and Juvederm, Inamed Aesthetics) last about 6 months when injected into rhytides. When injected into atrophic scars, hyaluronic acid has been observed to last significantly longer than in non-scarred skin (personal observation). Other substances can be used to augment scars and last years or even indefinitely. Liquid silicone (Silikon, Alcon Labs, Fort Worth, TX, USA) fills atrophic scars

permanently due to the formation of collagen around silicone microdroplets. Silicone should be placed into each scar using multiple injection points and administering very small amounts of silicone with each injection (0.01–0.02 cc per puncture). Other injectable materials, such as calcium hydroxyappetite, poly-L lactic acid, and polymethylmethacrylate, may yield more permanent results, but with the risk of an uneven texture due to granuloma formation.

Conclusion

Due to the location and widespread distribution of truncal acne scarring, treatment options are more limited than for facial acne scarring. Similar to many disease states, the best treatment is prevention. Early control of acne, especially severe nodulocystic acne, can prevent permanent sequela. There is currently no treatment for truncal acne scarring that will give perfect results. Therapies that are helpful require multiple treatment sessions. Often, using more than one therapy in combination can optimize results.

References

1. Goodman GJ, Baron JA. The management of postacne scarring. *Dermatol Surg.* 2007;33(10):1175-1188.
2. Holland DB, Jeremy AH. The role of inflammation in the pathogenesis of acne and acne scarring. *Semin Cutan Med Surg.* 2005;24(2):79-83
3. Layton AM, Henderson CA, Cunliffe WJ. A clinical evaluation of acne scarring and its incidence. *Med Exp Dermatol.* 1994; 19:303-308.
4. Decker RH, Wilson LD. Effect of radiation on wound healing and the treatment of scarring. In: Arndt KA, ed. *Scar Revision.* Amsterdam: Elsevier Saunders; 2006:89-104.
5. Alster TS, et al. Alteration of argon laser-induced scars by the pulsed dye laser. *Lasers Surg Med.* 1993;13(3):368-373.
6. Patel N, Clement M. Selective nonablative treatment of acne scarring with 585 nm flashlamp pulsed dye laser. *Dermatol Surg.* 2002;28(10):942-945; discussion 945.
7. Bjerring P, Clement M, Heickendorff L. Selective non-ablative wrinkle reduction by laser. *J Cutan Laser Ther.* 2000;2:9-15.
8. Avram MM, Tope WD, Yu T, Szachowicz E, Nelson JS. Hypertrophic scarring of the neck following ablative fractional carbon dioxide laser resurfacing. *Lasers Surg Med.* 2009;41: 185-188.
9. Lupton JR, Williams CM, Alster TS. Nonablative laser skin resurfacing using a 1,540 nm erbium glass laser: a clinical and histologic analysis. *Dermatol Surg.* 2002;28(9):833-835.
10. Goldman MP, Fitzpatrick RE. Laser treatment of scars. [see comment]. *Dermatol Surg.* 1995;21(8):685-687.

Chapter 9
Truncal Hair Removal

David J. Goldberg

Introduction

Excess or unwanted hair is a common problem affecting both genders. Over time, this problem has been dealt with in various ways, including plucking, threading, shaving, waxing, and electrolysis. Although effective for short-term control of hair growth, most of these methods are associated with significant pain and prolonged treatment times, making them fairly impractical for larger areas such as the human trunk.

Clinical Examination

The majority of laser procedures aimed at truncal hair removal in both genders are not performed for medically excessive hair growth but rather for unwanted hair. Patient preferences may be influenced by social or personal perceptions of normal hair distribution and density. Thus, a clear understanding of the patient's specific expectations and of the actual capabilities of laser hair removal is a must for anyone undertaking such procedures.

Treatment Application

First introduced in the mid-1990s, laser hair removal has become an accepted treatment modality for patients seeking to reduce unwanted hair and has been found to improve quality of life for many patients.[1] Lasers currently in use for hair removal include the normal-mode ruby, normal-mode alexandrite, diode, and neodymium: yttrium-aluminum-garnet (Nd:YAG) lasers as well as intense pulsed light devices.

Excess hair can be classified as either hypertrichosis or hirsutism. Hypertrichosis occurs in all genders and may be present at any body site. It can be further subdivided into acquired and congenital as well as localized and generalized forms.

Hirsutism is the presence of excess terminal hairs in women in androgen-dependent locations, most commonly on the face. Excess endogenous androgen may be released either by the ovaries or the adrenal glands, most commonly in the setting of polycystic ovarian syndrome, congenital adrenal hyperplasia, or adrenal tumors. Exogenous androgens may also cause this condition, whereas most other medications cause hypertrichosis rather than hirsutism. Genetic predisposition may also play a role, as some ethnic groups have relatively more facial hair than others. Excess truncal hair may be seen with both hypertrichosis and hirsuitism.

Generally, three types of hair are recognized: lanugo, vellus, and terminal. Lanugo is fetal-type soft, fine hair. Vellus hairs are nonpigmented, superficially located, and are typically under 30 μm in cross-sectional diameter. Terminal hairs are usually thicker than 40 μm, but may vary widely in their thickness, depending on the size of the hair bulb.[2]

Anatomically, a terminal hair follicle can be subdivided into the inferior segment, the isthmus, and the infundibulum. The inferior segment extends from the deepest portion of the hair follicle to the bulge and contains the hair bulb with germinative matrix cells and melanocytes. It also envelops dermal papilla, a highly vascularized connective tissue. The isthmus includes the portion of the hair follicle from the bulge, where the arrector pili muscle attaches, to the opening of the sebaceous duct. The infundibulum then extends from the sebaceous duct opening to the surface of the epidermis. Of note, hair follicles are angled so that the bulge lies on the deeper aspect of the follicle.

From the outside in, a hair follicle is composed of the outer root sheath, the inner root sheath, and the hair shaft, with further subdivisions within each structure. The inner root sheath provides a rigid support for the growing hair shaft and disintegrates above the level of the bulge in the isthmus. The slippage plane between thus encased hair shaft and the remainder of the hair follicle is at the companion layer of the outer root sheath.[i] In its turn, the outer root sheath becomes continuous with the epidermis at the level of the infundibulum. In addition to epithelial cells, the outer root sheath contains melanocytes, Langerhans' cells, mast cells, Merkel cells, and neuronal stem cells, all of which function within the hair follicle itself and may serve as a reservoir for repopulation of epidermis following injury.

Hair undergoes asynchronous cycling between periods of active synthesis (anagen), regression (catagen), rest (telogen), and shedding (exogen). Hair shaft growth and pigmentation takes place only during anagen, which starts with the secondary hair germ at the level of the bulge, about 1.5 mm below the surface of the skin. As the anagen phase continues, the hair bulb moves deeper into the dermis and reaches its deepest position within the subcutaneous fat, about 2–7 mm below the surface of the skin, depending on the location. Transition from anagen to catagen, an important process in hair removal, appears to be regulated by changes in the expression of multiple growth factors, such as transforming growth factor-beta 2 and fibroblast growth factor 5.

During catagen, controlled involution results from massive apoptosis of follicular epithelial cells in the inferior segment. By the end of this phase, the dermal papilla condenses and moves up to the level of the bulge, while the involuting epithelial column is reduced to a secondary germ. This is accompanied by cessation of melanin production and apoptosis of some follicular melanocytes, eventually resulting in depigmented club hairs during telogen. Telogen is characterized by relative proliferative rest. The mechanism of transition back to the active anagen phase is not completely worked out, but likely involves interactions between the secondary germ, the bulge, dermal papilla, and various signal molecules.

The duration of anagen determines the length of the hair shaft. Catagen phase is relatively constant throughout different locations and usually lasts around 3 weeks. On the other hand, telogen and, especially, anagen phases vary significantly between different body sites (Tables 9.1 and 9.2).[3] As will be discussed below, this may have potential implications not only for optimal frequency of laser treatments, but also for determination of permanency of laser hair removal at a given site.

Table 9.1 Hair cycle based on anatomic location

Body site	Duration of anagen (months)	Duration of telogen (months)	% of hair in telogen
Scalp	48–72	3–4	10–15
Eyebrows	1–2	3–4	85–94
Moustache	2–5	1.5	34
Beard	12	2–3	15–20
Axillae	3–6	3–6	31–79
Arms	1–3	2–4	72–86
Pubic area	3–6	0.5	65–81
Thighs	1–2	2–3	64–83
Lower legs	4–6	3–6	62–88

Table 9.2 Example of treatment parameters

Skin type	Device	Setting parameters
I–III	LightSheer Diode 800 nm (Lumenis, Inc., Santa Clara, CA)	30 J/cm^2 12 mm spot size, 15 ms pulses with contact cooling
	GentleLase Alexandrite 755 nm (Candela, Corp., Wayland, MA)	20 J/cm^2 18 mm spot size, 3 ms pulses with cryogen cooling
IV–VI	GentleYAG 1,064 nm (Candela, Corp., Wayland, MA)	20 J/cm^2 18 mm spot size, 10 ms pulses with cryogen cooling
	CoolGlide Nd:YAG 1,064 nm (Cutera Inc., Brisbane, CA)	30 J/cm^2 10 mm spot, 20 ms pulses with contact cooling

The duration of anagen and telogen truncal hair cycles are not known. However, since the clinical response to treatment is much like that of the arms and thighs, it can be assumed that the cycles are similar to those seen in these two areas.

Precise timing of treatments is also not certain. It is assumed that early anagen may be more amenable to damage by laser beam.[4] As discussed above, the hair bulb is located superficially during this stage, allowing for adequate light penetration. Telogen hair is also superficial; however, the proximal hair shaft is depigmented and hence does not absorb laser energy well. On the other hand, fat is a better thermal insulator than collagen, so that damage to a hair bulb located in the subcutaneous tissue would be better confined to the hair follicle. Additionally, human hair cycles are not synchronized, which further complicates studies on the influence of hair cycle on laser hair removal. Consequently, results have been contradictory. Attempts to correlate effective hair removal with targeting anagen hairs have, in general, failed. Further research in this area is needed; in the meantime, most laser sessions for hair removal are currently carried out in 4- to 8-week intervals, with small, if any, regard as to the body site. There is, however, an apparent difference in response to laser treatment based on location. The upper lip, chin, scalp, and back are generally associated with weakest response, whereas the remainder of the face, chest, back legs, and axillae typically demonstrate higher clearance rates.

Most published studies with any laser hair removal systems do not distinguish response rates between different anatomic areas. One study of nonfacial skin, such as the trunk, did show a somewhat better clearance rate compared to facial sites when treated with a long-pulsed Nd:YAG laser.[5] Conversely, paradoxical hypertrichosis, a rare complication of laser hair removal, has also been reported on the trunk after alexandrite laser hair removal.

Conclusion

In general, the goals of truncal laser hair removal must be realistic. It is rare to see 100% total clearance of all treated hairs in this area. In general, male patients need to understand that the purpose of treatment is to thin the hair while decreasing the amount of hair in the treated sites. Younger treated males must also understand that they will continue to grow "new" hairs for decades. Thus periodic re-treatments will be required. Most males seeking truncal hair removal simply have excess hair without any underlying medical cause.

Women seeking truncal hair removal may have hypertrichosis. However, more commonly they seek truncal hair removal based on hirsutism, with underlying polycystic ovarian syndrome being a possible cause. As is the case, in general, thicker terminal hairs most readily respond. However, deep seated areolar hairs in women can be resistant to treatment. Treatment of underlying hormonal issues will only help the laser hair removal results.

Truncal hair removal is not an uncommon desire of both men and women. Today's technology can lead to dramatic results in realistic patients (Figs. 9.1–9.4).

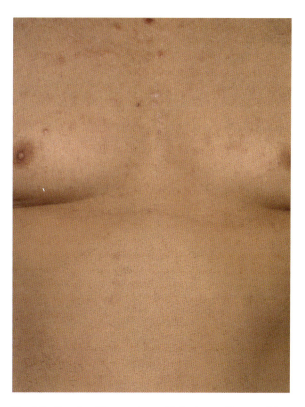

Fig. 9.1 Female with excess truncal hair. An excellent candidate for laser hair removal

Fig. 9.2 Male with excess truncal hair. An excellent candidate for laser hair removal

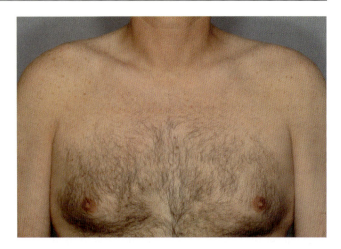

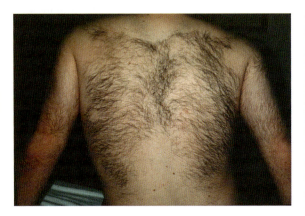

Fig. 9.3 Male with unwanted back hair before treatment

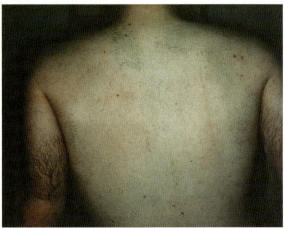

Fig. 9.4 Male with unwanted back hair after five laser hair removal treatments

References

1. Loo WJ, Lanigan SW. Laser treatment improves quality of life of hirsute females. *Clin Exp Dermatol*. 2002;27:439-441.
2. Headington JT. Transverse microscopic anatomy of the human scalp: a basis for a morphometric approach to disorders of the hair follicle. *Arch Dermatol*. 1984;120:449-456.
3. Olsen EA. Methods of hair removal. *J Am Acad Dermatol*. 1999;40:143-155.
4. Dierickx C, Alora MB, Dover JS. A clinical overview of hair removal using lasers and light sources. *Dermatol Clin*. 1999;17:357-366.
5. Alster TS, Bryan H, Williams CM. Long-pulsed Nd:YAG laser-assisted hair removal in pigmented skin: a clinical and histological evaluation. *Arch Dermatol*. 2001;137:885-889.

Chapter 10
Revision of Disfiguring Surgical Scars of the Back

Matthew J. Mahlberg, Julie K. Karen, and Vicki J. Levine

Introduction

Surgical procedures are performed on the back for a variety of reasons and universally result in some degree of scar formation. Optimally, these scars would result in a barely-perceptible, fine line that blends naturally with the color and texture of adjacent skin. Unfortunately, an optimal scar is rarely the end result, and a patient can be left with a scar that is deemed disfiguring. A disfiguring scar is one which has an appearance outside the accepted norm and which is deemed unsatisfactory by the patient and/or physician.

A variety of factors may contribute to the development of an unfavorable surgical scar on the back. Final scar cosmesis depends on many factors, including lesional dimensions and location, surgical technique, suturing materials, wound tension, and patient ethnicity. Suboptimal repair of the original surgical site is sometimes the culprit, although imperfect scars on the back plague even the most seasoned surgeons. Inadequate wound edge eversion may result in a depressed scar while insufficient undermining or improper design may lead to closure under excessive tension and consequent scar spread (Fig. 10.1). Infection, hematoma, dehiscence, and other postoperative complications can also contribute to suboptimal results. Of particular importance, the inherent anatomic features of the back contribute to an increased propensity to develop a widened (or spread) scar. For example, physical stress due to constant movement of the arms, torso, and even secondary to respiration is thought to result in shearing and opposing forces across a wound leading to scar spread.[1] Finally, the intrinsic aspects of wound healing can occur abnormally, resulting in keloidal or hypertrophic scar formation (Figs. 10.2 and 10.3). These lesions may be painful or pruritic or result in functional impairment (i.e., due to restricted range of motion). Both keloids and hypertrophic scars occur with greater frequency on the trunk and commonly result in significant cosmetic disfigurement (Fig. 10.4).

Because a wide variety of surgical procedures are performed on the back, disfiguring scars in this location are not uncommon. Biopsies or excisions of dysplastic nevi, cysts, and malignant lesions represent a large proportion of these procedures, especially in younger persons for whom the back may be a cosmetically sensitive area (Fig. 10.5). Thus, an appreciation of both prevention and correction of disfiguring scars on the back by the dermatologist is critical. Furthermore, patients should be counseled about the likelihood of scarring prior to any procedure being performed in this location.

Clinical Examination and Patient History

The approach to the correction of the disfiguring scar involves several components. First, assessment of the patient's concerns should be considered: are there functional limitations due to the scar or is the concern primarily cosmetic and does the patient hope to change the color, contour, size, or orientation with a corrective procedure? As with all cosmetic procedures, clarifying the patient's objectives is imperative in deeming the procedure a success. Secondly, the clinician's clinical history and examination can help to assess the factors contributing to the disfiguring scar. Exclusion of residual disease, infection, or neoplasia is necessary. Duration since the prior surgical procedure should be determined as surgical scars will continue to remodel

M. Alam and M. Pongprutthipan (eds.), *Body Rejuvenation*,
DOI 10.1007/978-1-4419-1093-6_10, © Springer Science+Business Media, LLC 2010

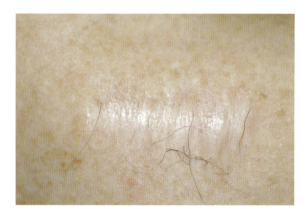

Fig. 10.1 Spread scar at site of prior excision

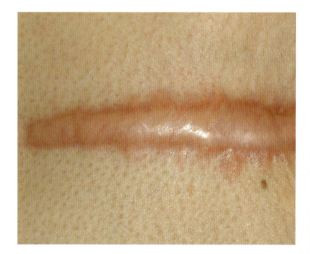

Fig. 10.2 Keloid scar at site of prior excision

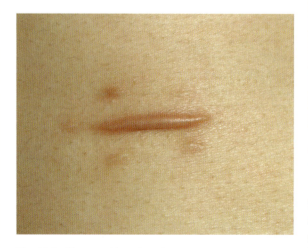

Fig. 10.3 Hypertrophic and erythematous scar

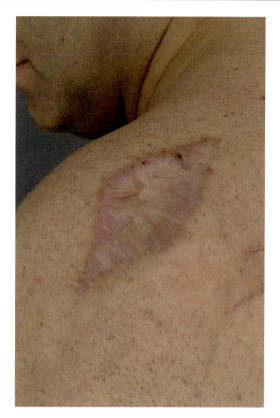

Fig. 10.4 Scar exhibiting features of spread and hypertrophy on upper back after excision of malignant melanoma

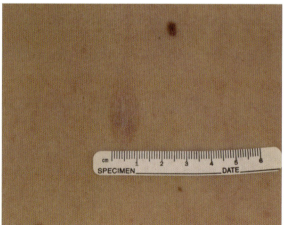

Fig. 10.5 Atrophic scar after deep shave biopsy of dysplastic nevus

for several months after surgery and premature correction may be unnecessary. Also, assessment of size, color, and orientation of the scar should be performed (Table 1). Measurement of a scar's length, width, height (or depth), and orientation provides important information that will further guide management. For example, scars <2 cm in length can often be improved through fusiform ellipse and reclosure alone. In cases where the scar is oriented away from relaxed skin tension lines (RSTL), reorientation may be necessary. Further, history guiding management includes color of the scar, patient's skin phototype, and whether or not the patient is prone to keloid or hypertrophic scar formation. Finally, pre-procedural photographs may be taken, and the patient should be given realistic expectations and counseled regarding the difficulties of scar revision on this part of the body.

Table 10.1 Scar Characteristics

1. Color
   - Red-violaceous
   - Hypopigmented
2. Contour
   - Depressed
   - Spread
   - Elevated
   - Hypertrophic
   - Keloid
3. Orientation
   - Along RSTL*
   - Not along RSTL*
4. Size
   - Length
   - Width

*RSTL: Relaxed Skin Tension Line

Treatment Methods

The history and physical examination as gathered above should provide some direction in choosing appropriate treatment options (Fig. 10.6).

Topical Treatments

Topical therapies, including silicone sheeting, massage, and other topical creams, are most appropriate for early intervention when scar formation is less than optimal. Creams containing such ingredients as Vitamin E, Vitamin A, and onion extract have long been availed with having the ability to limit scar formation, but studies have found minimal benefit and in some cases the studies have found that the ingredients have caused harm. Topical retinoic acid has been used with some success in treating keloids and hypertrophic scars. Topical silicone gels, ointments, and sheeting have demonstrated limited efficacy reducing the size, induration, erythema, and pruritus of pre-existing hypertrophic scars. Additionally, in high risk patients, silicone sheeting applied shortly after reepithelialization has been shown to reduce the formation of hypertrophic scar formation. Similarly, polyurethane occlusive dressings may help to improve the appearance of mature hypertrophic scars or prevent the formation

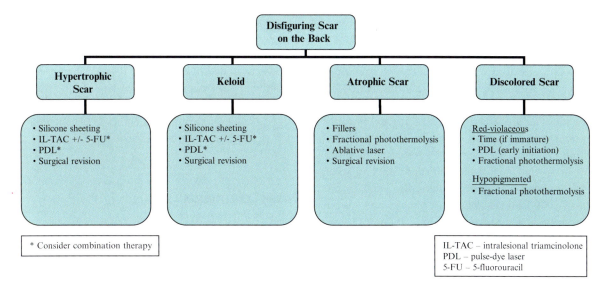

Fig. 10.6 Revision Technique Algorithm

of new ones. When utilized, both silicone sheeting and polyurethane dressings should be applied under occlusion, as a synergistic effect is likely.[2]

Imiquimod 5% cream, an imidazoquinoline, is a topical immunomodulator known to induce the synthesis of antifibrotic cytokines, IFN-alpha, and IFN-gamma. The success of imiquimod 5% cream in reducing earlobe keloid recurrences after excision is well documented and has raised interest in a possible role for this agent in the prevention of hypertrophic scars on the trunk. The authors of a recent, prospective, double-blinded, randomized, vehicle-controlled trial concluded that there was no benefit to the use of imiquimod 5% cream on healing surgical wounds with regard to the improvement of "normal" scar cosmesis.[3] However, a limited body of evidence suggests a possible role for imiquimod 5% cream in the prevention of presternal and breast hypertrophic scarring, although additional, larger studies with longer follow-up are needed.[4,5] There are currently no studies specifically looking at the use of imiquimod 5% cream in the treatment or prevention of disfiguring scars of the back.

Intralesional Injections

Minimally invasive treatment options such as intralesional injections and fillers can be used for keloids and hypertrophic scars or depressed scars, respectively. Intralesional triamcinolone injections in concentrations of 10–40 mg/mL administered approximately monthly over several months can have a profound effect on scar height although they do not affect the width. Higher concentrations can be used on the back than in other areas of the body, although as with other areas on the body, careful use is advised to minimize side effects of atrophy and hypopigmentation. Fitzpatrick reported the efficacy of intralesional 5-FU in the treatment and prevention of keloids and hypertrophic scars. In his experience in more than 1,000 patients, maximal benefit and minimal pain were achieved when a combination of 0.9 cc of 5-FU (concentration of 50 mg/cc) and 0.1 cc of triamcinolone (concentration of 10 mg/cc) was injected directly into the substance of the scar. In this report, injections were performed as frequently as thrice

weekly initially, with the frequency reduced as scars began to respond. Inflamed, indurated, erythematous, or otherwise symptomatic scars, as well as younger scars, were most likely to respond favorably. Side effects are generally limited to local pain or discomfort in all patients. Untoward effects commonly attributed to intralesional corticosteroids (i.e., atrophy, telangiectasia, hypopigmentation, and rebound) do not occur with 5-FU.[6] Treatment with the pulsed dye laser (see below) immediately prior to injection may improve response rates, particularly in more erythematous scars.[6] For atrophic scars, fillers such as silicone, bovine collagen, hyaluronic acid, calcium hydroxylapatite, and fat (lipografting) can be used.[7–9] However, due to their high cost, use of these filling agents has largely been limited to the management of atrophic scars in highly cosmetically sensitive regions such as the face.

Cryosurgery

Cryosurgery with liquid nitrogen has been successfully used to treat keloids and hypertrophic scars in areas including the back. Lesions that are most likely to respond include younger (<12 months), more vascular lesions. The therapeutic effects of cryosurgery are mediated by direct cellular and microvascular damage. Several, monthly treatments, consisting of two to three 30-s freeze-thaw cycles are typically required. Disadvantages include, but are not limited to, pain, atrophy, and hypopigmentation, rendering this modality of limited utility in dark-skinned patients. Irradiation has demonstrated disappointing results when used as monotherapy for the treatment of keloids and hypertrophic scars. However, when used as an adjunct to surgery, radiation therapy has achieved excellent scar cosmesis with low recurrence rates.[10]

Laser Treatments

Laser therapy has utility in cutaneous scar revision for hypertrophic scars, keloids, atrophic scars, and discolored scars although results are less impressive on the back. Limited long-term stability dampened initial enthusiasm about the use of the argon, Nd:YAG, and CO$_2$ lasers. More recently, promising results have been achieved with the pulsed dye laser (PDL) (585–595 nm) and fractional photothermolysis.

Pulsed dye lasers (PDL), specifically in the 585–595 nm range, are generally considered the laser therapy of choice for hypertrophic scars, keloids, and red-colored scars. Beneficial effects reported with PDL treatment include erythema reduction, textural improvement, and overall improved blending with surrounding skin. PDL therapy should be initiated with a spot size of 7 or 10 mm with fluences of 5–6.5 J/cm^2 or 4.5–5.5 J/cm^2, respectively. In patients with darker skin tones, additional fluence reduction may be necessary.[11] Variable pulse durations, ranging from 450 μs to 1.5 ms may be employed, depending on the degree of post-treatment purpura likely to be tolerated by the patient. Concomitant cryogen cooling should be applied during treatment. Unfortunately, multiple treatments (at 3–8 week intervals) are necessary, and complete resolution of scar erythema and/or thickness is not commonly achieved.

More recently, researchers have posited a role for PDL in the prevention of hypertrophic scar formation. Insofar as treatment with PDL may limit angiogenesis, upon which scar formation may depend, early intervention may prevent or minimize scarring. Two studies using three treatments with PDL, initiated at the time of suture removal, demonstrated efficacy in the prevention of unfavorable scars.[12,13] However, single treatment of PDL at suture removal is not efficacious, nor is there increased efficacy with concomitant use of intralesional corticosteroids.[14,15] In any case, in addition to its role in the treatment of disfiguring scars, PDL may play a role in preventing disfiguring scars and may be a useful adjuvant in surgical scar revision. Although there are reports documenting the efficacy of PDL as monotherapy, this modality is perhaps best utilized as one component of a multifaceted approach to suboptimal scars.[6]

The 308-nm excimer laser has some efficacies in the treatment of hypopigmented disorders, including vitiligo and mature striae. There may be a limited role for this laser in the treatment of hypopigmented scars on the back. However, since results are short-lived, ongoing treatments must be continued to maintain repigmentation.[16]

Fractional photothermolysis is increasingly considered a popular option for unfavorable scars in all loca-

tions. Since damage is restricted to noncontiguous microscopic arrays, obvious wounding is avoided, epidermal recovery is rapid, and bulk heating does not occur, minimizing the potential for scar exacerbation. With fractional photothermolysis, more subtle improvements should be expected, but there is less associated downtime and less risk of severe pigmentary alteration than with ablative lasers. Significant improvements in scar texture and blending can generally be achieved with a series of 3–5 treatments at approximately 3 week intervals. Newer devices achieve fractional photothermolysis utilizing ablative modalities. There are anecdotal reports of these devices effectively treating hypertrophic scars without the extended recovery time and other risks associated with conventional ablative resurfacing.

Several caveats should be considered in laser scar revision. Caution is advised when treating patients with darker skin tones (Fitzpatrick phototypes IV–VI). Melanin present in these patients' skin acts as a competing chromophore, thereby decreasing efficacy and increasing the risk of untoward effects. These patients should be counseled regarding the potential for dyspigmentation and close monitoring of this adverse effect is prudent. In all patients, if laser therapy is selected as a treatment option, patients should be instructed to refrain from tanning for several weeks prior to treatment. General techniques for laser therapy, such as using preprocedural anesthetics, are equally applicable to laser use on the back for scar revision.

Surgical Treatments

Surgical revision of disfiguring surgical scars is an option as on other parts of the body. However, because the back is inherently prone to disfiguring scars, aggressive surgical revisions should be approached with caution and should be avoided if possible. For very large procedures on the back, when complete and immediate removal is not mandatory, a staged resection may be considered, as this will permit skin stretch and thereby lessen wound tension. Fusiform or elliptical excisions of scars can be useful when the scar is small (preferably less than 2 cm) and when the scar is oriented along RSTL. Z-plasty repair may be useful for correction of scars that are not already oriented along RSTLs. However, the thickness of the dermis on the back may make the technique less favorable in that location as it makes transposition of the triangular flaps difficult. Techniques such as W-plasty and Geometric Broken Line Closure (GBLC) are also useful techniques elsewhere on the body for long scars along RSTLs, which help to create a less conspicuous scar line. However, the necessary removal of skin in these techniques increases the risk of scar tension and resultant spread in an area that is already under a great deal of tension. Thus, these techniques should be avoided on the back. As discussed above, surgical closure of primary wounds or revisions on the back require great care for optimal cosmetic outcome. Adequate undermining with placement of buried vertical mattress sutures minimizes wound tension and helps to create proper wound eversion. Use of a running subcuticular suture is an option to avoid "track marks," which may develop from cuticular sutures, and steristrips should be placed routinely after the removal of sutures to decrease cutaneous wound tension. Other adjuvant measures to be considered include PDL treatment at the time of suture removal as discussed above, and where cosmesis is to be achieved at any cost, temporary extremity immobilization with brace or sling can be considered.

Conclusion

In summary, a variety of treatment options are available for the revision of disfiguring surgical scars on the back though none is ideal. Important regional differences on the back alter choices and technique compared to other areas of the body. These difficulties, along with the risks inherent to surgical revision of scars anywhere on the body, should be discussed thoroughly with patients before embarking on a treatment course and realistic expectations should be established. In the future, development of newer techniques, including new types of lasers, the use of oral medications, and gene therapy techniques that suppress pro-fibrotic TGF-β, may bring improved novel approaches for scar revision.[17,18] For now, though, disfiguring scars on the back are a reality even in the setting of meticulous surgical technique and ideal post-operative care.

References

1. McGillis ST, Lucas AR. Scar revision. *Dermatol Clin.* 1998;16:165-180.
2. Zurada JM, Kriegel D, Davis IC. Topical treatments for hypertrophic scars. *J Am Acad Dermatol.* 2006;55:1024-1031.
3. Berman B, Frankel S, Villa AM, Ramirez CC, Poochareon V, Nouri K. Double-blind, randomized, placebo-controlled, prospective study evaluating the tolerability and effectiveness of imiquimod applied to postsurgical excisions on scar cosmesis. *Dermatol Surg.* 2005;31:1399-1403.
4. Prado A, Andrades P, Benitez S, Umana M. Scar management after breast surgery: preliminary results of a prospective, randomized, and double-blind clinical study with aldara cream 5% (imiquimod). *Plast Reconstr Surg.* 2005;115:966-972.
5. Malhotra AK, Gupta S, Khaitan BK, Sharma VK. Imiquimod 5% cream for the prevention of recurrence after excision of presternal keloids. *Dermatology.* 2007;215:63-65.
6. Fitzpatrick RE. Treatment of inflamed hypertrophjic scars using intralesional 5-FU. *Derm Surg.* 1999;25:224-232.
7. Barnett JG, Barnett CR. Treatment of acne scars with liquid silicone injections: 30-year perspective. *Dermatol Surg.* 2005;31:1542-1549.
8. Goldberg DJ, Amin S, Hussain M. Acne scar correction suing calcium hydroxylapatite in a carrier-based gel. *J Cosmet Laser Ther.* 2006;8:134-136
9. Coleman SR. Structural fat grafting: more than a permanent filler. *Plast Reconstr Surg.* 2006;118:108S-120S.
10. English RS, Shenefelt PD. Keloids and hypertrophic scars. *Dermatol Surg.* 1999;25:631-638.
11. Alster TS. Laser treatment of scars and striae. In: Alster TS, ed. *Manual of cutaneous laser techniques.* Philadelphia: Lippincott-Raven; 2000:89-107.
12. Conologue TD, Norwood C. Treatment of surgical scars with the cryogen-cooled 595 nm pulsed dye laser starting on the day of suture removal. *Dermatol Sug.* 2006;32:13-20.
13. Nouri K, Jimenez GP, Harrison-Balestra C, Elgart GW. 585-nm pulsed dye laser in the treatment of surgical scars starting on the suture removal day. *Dermatol Surg.* 2003;29:65-73.
14. Alam M, Pon K, Van Laborde S, Kaminer MS, Arndt KA, Dover JS. Clinical effect of a single pulsed dye laser treatment of fresh surgical scars: randomized controlled trial. *Dermatol Surg.* 2006;32:21-25.
15. Alster TS. Laser scar revision: comparison study of 585-nm pulsed dye laser with and without intralesional corticosteroids. *Dermatol Surg.* 2003;29:25-29.
16. Goldberg DJ, Sarradet D, Hussain M. 308-nm Excimer laser treatment of mature hypopigmented striae. *Dermatol Surg.* 2003;29:596-598.
17. Iannello S, Milazzo P, Bordonaro F, Belfiore F. Low-dose enalapril in the treatment of surgical cutaneous hypertrophic scar and keloid – two case reports and literature review. *Med Gen Med.* 2006;8:60.
18. Ono I, Yamashita T, Hida T, et al. Local administration of hepatocyte growth factor gene enhances the regeneration of dermis in acute incisional wounds. *J Surg Res.* 2004; 120:47-55.

Chapter 11
Breast Reduction Through Liposuction

Michael S. Kaminer

Introduction

Tumescent liposuction has revolutionized the surgeon's ability to remove unwanted fat in a minimally invasive, outpatient procedure. Requiring only local anesthetic, in some cases with the addition of oral or intramuscular analgesia, tumescent liposuction is a superb option for many women who are interested in breast reduction.[1-3]

Excessive breast tissue can be a physically impairing issue for women. Large, pendulous breasts can cause back pain, shoulder pain, and can lead to poor posture. For women with extremely large breast size, significant skin laxity, and/or downward oriented nipples (nipple ptosis), cold steel breast reduction is appropriate. For women with only 1–2 cup sizes over what they desire, in the absence of significant nipple ptosis or excess skin laxity, liposuction of the breasts may be an appropriate option. Liposuction can also be used for patients who have asymmetrical breasts and/or a modest amount of breast ptosis. It can also be useful in women who may be predisposed to poor wound healing.[4] Liposuction provides a quick, virtually scarless alternative to the traditional breast reduction procedure.

Clinical Examination and Patient History

The most appropriate female candidates are those with good skin tone, an anteriorly oriented nipple complex and lack of nipple ptosis, and relatively fatty breast tissue with the absence of a prominent glandular component. Younger women tend to have more glandular tissues than older women and are therefore less favorable candidates. The amount of fat that can be removed via liposuction is less than that achieved by excision, therefore patients who expect considerable reduction may not be good candidates. On average, breast size can be reduced by 1–2 cup sizes with liposuction alone. Although liposuction of the breast can give a certain amount of lift to the breast, it is not always predictable and should not be exaggerated when discussing results with the patient. However, for some women, the amount of correction of both nipple and breast ptosis can be significant. Ptosis of the breast is measured as the shortest distance between the infra-mammary crease and the lowest point of the breast profile (Fig. 11.1). There is a relative contraindication for patients who have a family history of breast cancer, and all women should have pre and 6–12 month postoperative mammograms performed.

Women with a history of polycystic ovary disease and breast cysts as well as significant swelling and pain with menstruation should be carefully screened prior to surgery. These women have a tendency to glandular, firm breast tissue that can be a challenge to remove with liposuction cannulas. Although in many cases these women can be effectively treated with liposuction, expectations as to final result should be carefully discussed and conservatively modified. Conversely, women who relate a history of significant breast size increase when they have gained weight can be superb candidates for breast reduction with liposuction.

Method of Device and Treatment Application

Perioperative antibiotics are begun 24 h prior to surgery (Cephalexin) and continued for a total of 7 days. Patients are also instructed to discontinue all medications and

M. Alam and M. Pongprutthipan (eds.), *Body Rejuvenation*,
DOI 10.1007/978-1-4419-1093-6_11, © Springer Science+Business Media, LLC 2010

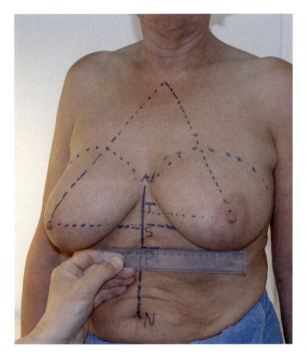

Fig. 11.1 Breast measurements. Breast ptosis is measured as the distance from the ruler (line P) to line S

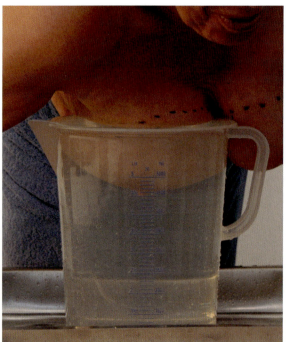

Fig. 11.3 The preoperative water displacement measurement technique for breast volume

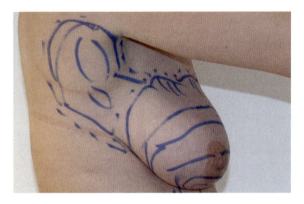

Fig. 11.2 Preoperative markings including the tail of the breast as well as lateral breast, axillary fat

vitamin supplements that can promote bleeding at least 10–14 days prior to the procedure.

After photographs have been taken, the patient's breast size may be measured via the water displacement method. A 4-liter beaker is filled to the brim, and with the patient standing, the breast is immersed in the beaker (Fig. 11.2). The water that is displaced is caught in an underlying bowl or pan, and that water volume is measured. This should be repeated twice on each breast to obtain precise measurements. Alternatively, a digital handheld scale can be used to measure breast weight. Preoperative markings should be made with the patient

in the upright position. It is important to draw the contours to include the inframammary crease as a landmark and to include the superolateral triangle of tissue near the axillae, if this area is to be treated in the cosmetic unit (Fig. 11.3).

It is imperative that sterile technique be used for all surgical aspects of the liposuction breast reduction procedure. The breast is anesthetized with 0.1% tumescent lidocaine anesthesia through small incisions placed inferolaterally, inferomedially, and in the anterior axillary line. These same incisions are used for the aspiration and heal nearly imperceptibly. Twenty gauge needles can be used to deliver the anesthesia, or the standard short sprinkler tip infusion cannula can be used. It is important to thoroughly anesthetize all levels of the breast tissue (superficial, mid, and deep). Typically, the volume of anesthesia required will be from 120 to 150% of the volume of the breast measured by the water displacement test. On average, this requires 750–1,250 cc per breast. After placement of the anesthesia is completed, it should be given 30–45 min to fully take effect.

Prior to suctioning, it is advantageous to position the patient on the operating table so that her back is approximately 30° above horizontal, with the side to be treated elevated on one to two rolled surgical towels.

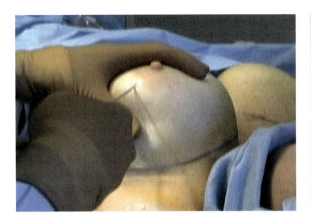

Fig. 11.4 Periareolar incision used for liposuction

In most cases, the ipsilateral arm is raised above the head to facilitate access to the cannula insertion sites. This positions the breast in the optimal neutral position and allows the surgeon to evaluate the progress of breast reduction more accurately.

Aspiration begins in the mid-layer of the breast with a mid-level aggressive cannula such as the 12 gauge Klein dual port spatula. It is important to use the smart (nondominant) hand to steady the breast tissue and allow for even planes of suctioning. After the mid layer is suctioned in all four quadrants, it is important to address both the superficial (cautiously) and deep levels. The central and superficial tissue often has a glandular component, and it may be difficult to remove sufficient fat from these areas. Using a 12 or 14 gauge Capistrano cannula can help to remove fat from these glandular areas. A stab incision on the upper outer perimeter of the areola can also be used to access the adipose, which is intertwined with the glandular tissue under the nipple (Fig. 11.4). Approximately, 25–50% of the volume of breast weight (based on the preop volume) should be removed. The better the skin quality and breast position preoperatively, the more aggressive the surgeon can be intraoperatively. After suctioning is complete, it is important to measure the amount of fat removed from one breast to be consistent with volume reduction in the other breast (Fig. 11.5).

Results and Postoperative Care

Postoperatively, absorbent padding and a chest-binding garment are worn for 24 h. The garment is then worn for 23 h a day for the first 3 or 4 days after surgery.

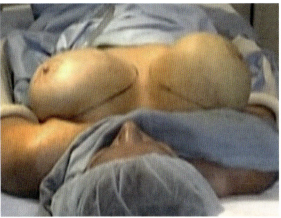

Fig. 11.5 Intraoperative assessment of liposuction after left breast has been treated

Thereafter, a supportive sports-type bra should be worn 23 h a day for 3 months. Most patients can resume normal activities within 5–7 days. Care should be taken when resuming upper body exercises, often requiring patients to use less weight and/or fewer repetitions.

Due to swelling, results are difficult to assess in the first 4–6 weeks. Patients will often reveal approximately 50% of their final breast reduction result at 6 weeks, and it can take as long as 4–6 months to see the full measure of improvement. The average patient will achieve a 1–2 cup size reduction at 6 months (Fig. 11.6). If a repeat procedure is to be considered to obtain additional breast size reduction, it is advisable to wait at least 6 months from the date of the original surgery.

Management of Adverse Events

Postoperative complications are uncommon. The most frequently seen events include pain, swelling, erythema, and edema. Occasionally, patients develop superficial blisters on the inferior surface of the breast 2–5 days after the procedure, presumably due to gravitational-related movement of fluid and swelling. These resolve without scarring and are treated with local wound care including the application of petrolatum based ointments.

Infection, bleeding, and necrosis as well as deep vein thrombosis of the legs are extremely rare events that, when present, require immediate and aggressive intervention. Contour irregularities of the breast are also

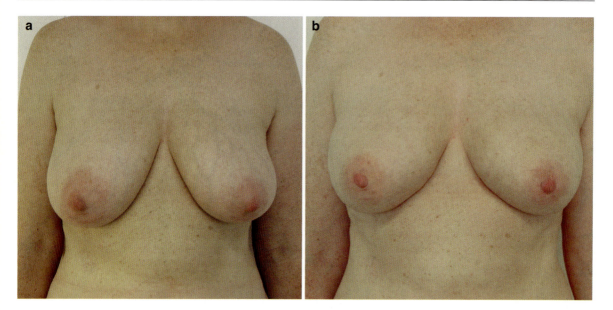

Fig. 11.6 (**a**) Before breast reduction with liposuction. (**b**) After breast reduction with liposuction

rarely encountered when proper technique is used and care is taken to avoid suctioning too much superficial breast tissue. Treatment of contour problems often requires a second liposuction procedure, which can present a challenge to the surgeon. Asymmetry of the breast following surgery can occur, and it is therefore important to have careful preoperative photographs and breast weight measurements to refer to in the postoperative period. Many women will have preexisting asymmetry, and the preoperative data can be incredibly useful when discussing results with patients. In almost all cases, it is advisable to point out to patients any preexisting asymmetry prior to the procedure. When asymmetry is surgically induced, a repeat procedure can be of significant benefit.

and shoulder pain is often significant.[5] Although nearly all women who desire a reduction in breast size can be treated, those with a predominance of fatty tissue (often associated with advanced age) are more suitable candidates.

Powered reciprocating liposuction cannulas, as well as some of the recently introduced laser-assisted technologies (SmartLipo, Cynosure, Inc. and ProLipo, Sciton, Inc.), may enhance results in the future. Although several noninvasive fat removal technologies are currently in the development phase, it remains to be seen whether these will be suitable and appropriate for breast reduction.

References

Conclusion

Minimally invasive breast reduction utilizing tumescent liposuction has become an accepted stand-alone treatment method. Previously performed only in conjunction with cold steel surgery, liposuction is now able to precisely and predictably reduce the size of the female breast by one to two bra cup sizes. In addition, natural shape and sensation are retained, and in some women, a modest amount of lifting and correction of breast ptosis can be achieved. Symptomatic improvement in neck, back,

1. Mellul SD, Dryden RM, Remigio DJ, Wulc AE. Breast reduction performed by liposuction. *Dermatol Surg.* 2006; 32(9):1124–1133.
2. Rohrich RJ, Gosman AA, Brown SA, Tonadapu P, Foster B. Current preferences for breast reduction techniques: a survey of board-certified plastic surgeons 2002. *Plast Reconstr Surg.* 2004;114(7):1724–1733.
3. Sadove R. New observations in liposuction-only breast reduction. *Aesthetic Plast Surg.* 2005;29(1):28–31.
4. Moskovitz MJ, Baxt SA, Jain AK, Hausman RE. Liposuction breast reduction: a prospective trial in African American women. *Plast Reconstr Surg.* 2007;119(2):718–726.
5. Moskovitz MJ, Muskin E, Baxt SA. Outcome study in liposuction breast reduction. *Plast Reconstr Surg.* 2004;114(1):55–60.

Chapter 12
Botulinum Toxin A for Upper Thoracic Posture and the Appearance of a "Breast Lift"

Kevin C. Smith

Introduction

The author (KCS) and others[1] have suggested that injection of BTX-A could, in selected patients, produce a pleasing change in upper thoracic posture and consequently in breast presentation such that the patient would obtain a "BOTOX® Breast Lift" (more properly termed a "BTX-A upper thoracic posture lift"). This could result if muscles responsible for a "head forward" posture were relaxed with BTX-A, so that opposing muscle groups responsible for erect upper thoracic posture could work with less opposition.

KCS has pointed out, in the New York Times[2] and elsewhere, that before any attempt is made to offer "BOTOX® Breast Lift" to patients, double-blind clinical trials should be done to determine whether the observed effect is the result of placebo or has a physiological basis. If there is a physiological basis for this observation, it will be necessary to optimize patient selection criteria and treatment protocols.

Clinical Examination

Recent contributions by Lang[3] and by Finkelstein and Katsis[4] have improved our understanding of the potential for the use of BTX-A to enhance upper thoracic posture, and in particular, they have provided evidence of improved results when a program of physiotherapy was added to the treatment with BOTOX®. When the patient has strengthened the interscapular muscles as a result of a program of prescribed exercises, improvement may be greater and may be maintained longer, with reduced long-term need for BOTOX® and a reduced rate of reversion to the "head forward" state of poor upper thoracic posture.

BTX-A has a long history of being used to improve posture in a variety of conditions.[5,6] The position of the shoulders is determined largely by the balance of forces between the pectoralis minor and pectoralis major muscles (Fig. 12.1), which tend to rotate the shoulders medially and depress them and the action of the opposing muscles of the back, for example, the rhomboids. The pectoralis minor muscles are accessory muscles that assist during strong exhalation. One author (KCS) has noted that three doses of 10 units of BOTOX® injected on each side into the pectoralis minor muscles in women who are slightly round shouldered can lead to a more erect posture with shoulders back – resulting in what they consider to be a more aesthetically pleasing presentation of the breasts (Fig. 12.2).

Patient Selection

KCS noted that the ideal candidate for this treatment is a slightly round-shouldered, physically fit, nonobese woman with a slightly "head forward" posture, between 35 and 50 years of age, with A or B cup-size breasts. These individuals could be described as having a mild degree of cervical hyperlordosis, forward head posture, and lumbar kyphosis. Older women, and those with larger breasts, tend to respond more slowly and to a lesser extent.

Treatment Application

The benefits of BOTOX® treatment usually develop over a period of 1–2 weeks, and persist for 3–4 months. The duration of effect is somewhat longer than might

M. Alam and M. Pongprutthipan (eds.), *Body Rejuvenation*,
DOI 10.1007/978-1-4419-1093-6_12, © Springer Science+Business Media, LLC 2010

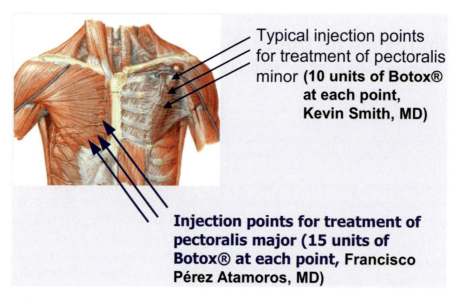

Fig. 12.1 BOTOX® injection sites reported by Drs. Smith and Atamoros

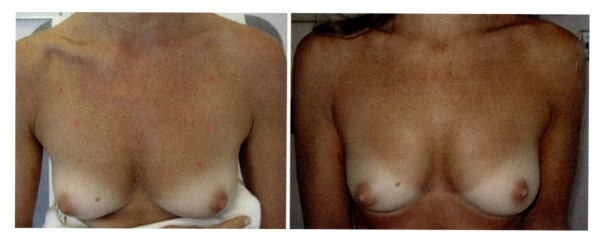

Fig. 12.2 Forty-eight-year-old woman before treatment of the pectoralis minor muscles with three 10 unit doses of BOTOX® on each side. There was improved posture with improved presentation of the breasts at 3 weeks follow-up, and the patient was very pleased

be expected considering the relatively low doses of BOTOX® in proportion to the size of the muscles. It may be that improvements in shoulder posture persist for a while once posture has been improved by BOTOX® altering the balance of forces between the pectoralis minor and/or major muscles and the opposing muscles in the back.

Some women have noted that not only are the breasts and nipples elevated by their more erect posture with shoulders back but that there is also a pleasing erection of the nipples, which develops about a week after BOTOX® treatment and persists for 3–4

weeks. The reasons for this are not known. Perhaps projection of the breasts as a result of improved shoulder posture leads to increased mechanical stimulation of the nipples under some circumstances.

Treatment Technique

BOTOX® is administered using a 30G 1 in. needle. One author (KCS) usually uses a reconstitution of 100 units of BOTOX® in 2.5 ml of normal saline with benzyl alcohol preservative. The pectoralis minor arises on the third, fourth, and fifth ribs and runs under the clavicle to insert on the coracoid process of the scapula. The pectoralis minor muscles are located by having the patient hold her arms up slightly above shoulder height, pressing the palms together when requested to do so, allowing the examiner palpate the pectoralis minor starting about 2.5 cm inferior to the lateral third of the clavicle. Injections points are generally about 2.5, 5, and 7.5 cm inferior to the lateral third of the clavicle. Injections are done at a depth of less than 2 cm. Apart from occasional muscle or fascia tenderness for several days, there have been no complications from this treatment. In particular, pneumothorax or bleeding have not been seen, but the possibility of such problems must be considered, even when working with a 30G 1 in. needle. The risk of entering the pleural space can be reduced by limiting needle insertion depth to less than 2 cm.

This proposed mechanism of action has been criticized by Dr. Otto Wegelin (personal communication, April 2004), who argues that:

1. The muscles (pectoralis minor and rhomboid minor) invoked to carry out the postural changes are far too small to do what is expected of them.
2. The muscles do not in fact rotate the shoulder but rather act primarily stabilize the scapula – an entirely different function.
3. The muscles are not antagonistic in action as are the frontalis and the orbicularis occuli but rather synergistic.
4. There is no way to determine how much, if any, of the Botox is actually acting on the pectoralis minor as the Botox can diffuse widely in a three dimensional plane unlike the forehead where there is the boney skull limiting diffusion.

Dr. Doris Hexsel (personal communication, July 2004) in a study of six women was not able to obtain satisfactory results, and in two cases noted that the nipples hung lower.

Dr. Francisco Pérez-Atamoros of Mexico City has obtained elevation of the breast on the side where the nipple is lower by injecting three doses of 15 units of BOTOX® into the parts of the pectoralis major muscle, which lies medial and inferior to the pectoralis minor muscles. In a series of almost 100 patients, Dr. Pérez Atamoros has obtained an elevation of the ptotic breast averaging 0.8 cm with the maximum elevation being 1.6 cm. Sixty-five of ninety-two patients rated the results good to very good, and 73 of 92 would repeat the procedure. Like Dr. Smith, Dr. Pérez Atamoros has noted that the best candidates are physically fit women in the age range 30–55 years, with small to moderate sized breasts. Five patients had pain lasting longer than a week. Dr. Pérez Atamoros has suggested that relaxation of the inferior portion of the pectoralis major muscle allows the superior portion to lift the ptotic breast. (Personal communications, Botox®, Fillers & More, Vancouver BC, August 2003; American Academy of Dermatology, Washington DC, February 2004, and April 2004). For a comparison of the injection sites used by Drs. Kevin Smith and Pérez Atamoros, see Fig. 12.1.

Issues that remain to be resolved include optimization of patient selection, Botox® dosing and the placement of Botox® doses, the issue of placebo effect vs. biomechanical effect, and elucidation of the mechanism of action if indeed there is a biomechanical effect from Botox® treatment of the pectoralis minor and/or pectoralis major muscles with Botox®.

Clinical Trial

A clinical trial could contain some of the following elements, depending on the resources available. The clinical trial would ideally be double-blind, placebo-controlled with respect to BOTOX®, and there might be an element of dose ranging, so that the patients would get either saline or 10 or 20 units of BOTOX® at each injection site. There would be three injection sites in each of the pectoralis minor muscles, and three in each of the horizontal components of the superior portions of the pectoralis major muscles (Fig. 12.3).

The patients could further be classified into two arms of the study: one receiving physiotherapy, which is intended to improve upper thoracic posture and a second group receiving no physiotherapy or sham physiotherapy. This could help to determine the role and relative contribution of physiotherapy to the overall improvement, if any. The physiotherapy program could be based on elements of O.N.E.U.P. (Optimizing Neurotoxin Efficacy Utilizing Physiotherapy) program, which includes a patient instruction booklet and an accompanying DVD with video clips illustrating the elements of the stretching and exercise program.[7]

Elements of that program intend to stretch the muscles involved in depression and internal rotation of the shoulders, to stretch the pectoralis major and minor muscles, and to strengthen the rhomboids. Exercises are also intended to strengthen the muscles responsible for erect upper thoracic posture and external rotation of the shoulders.

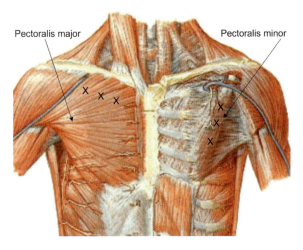

Fig. 12.3 Proposed sites for injections of BOTOX® 10 or 15 units in the pectoralis major and minor muscles

Standardized photography at baseline and at each follow-up visit could help to determine whether patient posture and breast presentation (in the case of female subjects) was improved by the interventions being studied. Patients could wear a thin "see through" white tank top for modesty during photography (Fig. 12.4). Standardized measurements on pre and posttreatment photos (using a vertical line from the tragus of the ear and comparing that with a marker on the anterior border of the acromion) could be used to determine whether or not there had been correction of "head forward posture", and to measure the degree of correction.

Special Considerations

- There is likely to be a strong placebo effect during the study; and so, patients can be put through a range of motions (perhaps on video) so that they will be caught "off guard". Then, standard frames at certain points could be extracted from the video and used for analysis.

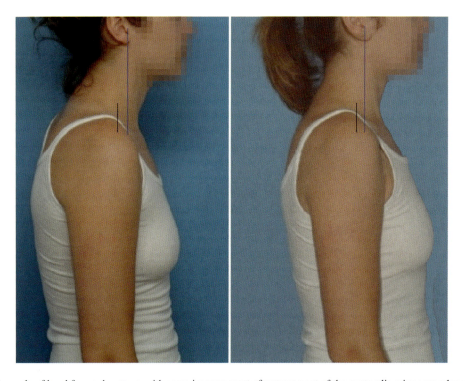

Fig. 12.4 Example of head forward posture, with some improvement after treatment of the pectoralis minor muscles with 30 units of BOTOX® on each side (Photo courtesy of Dr. S. Sapra)

- Because breast size and position may change at various points in the menstrual cycle, it will be optimal for treatments and assessments to be done as close as possible to the same point in the menstrual cycle at each visit.
- Changes in medications (particularly, those affecting breast size, including estrogens and medications affecting prolactin) will need to be carefully monitored at each visit.
- Patients should be weighed at each visit.

Subject and investigator global assessments, using a Likert scale, would also be taken at baseline and at each follow-up visit. Efficacy endpoints could also include the following measures (Fig. 12.5):

- Nipple to nipple Distance
- Nipple to Sternal Notch Distance
- Interscapular Distance could also be recorded, with the patient standing in a standard, relaxed posture

Functional magnetic image resonance (MRI) imaging before and after BTX-A treatment might provide useful insights. T-2 weighted MRI, with a repetition time of 1,500 ms, two echoes at 30 and 60 ms immediately after exercise can demonstrate areas of flaccid paralysis resulting from BOTOX® treatment.

It will be interesting to see if improved and more "positive" posture is reliably associated with improved mood, in a manner similar to improvements in mood associated with improved and more "positive" facial expressions, which are reported to result after interventions like treatment of negative facial expressions with BOTOX®.[8]

In this regard, assessments of depression (for example, Beck Depression Inventory, Hamilton Depression Rating Scale) might also be useful to determine if there was a relationship between objective improvements in upper thoracic posture and the patient's emotional state and self-image (for example, using the Rosenberg Self-Esteem Scale).

Because disorders of the soft tissues and structure of the cervical spine have been associated with cervical pain, thoracic pain, and headaches,[9] it will be important to collect information about those problems at baseline and at follow-up visits so that effects of BOTOX® and/or physiotherapy on those parameters will be detected and quantified.

Conclusion

There is increasing evidence that treatment with BOTOX®, or more likely a combined treatment with BOTOX® and a program of physiotherapy, may produce improvements in upper thoracic posture. These improvements in posture may result in a more aesthetically pleasing presentation of the female breast, creating the appearance of a "breast lift". Additional benefits, for both men and women, may include improved mood and/or reductions in some types of headache and other pain, which can be related to problems with upper thoracic posture. A properly designed and executed clinical trial is needed to determine whether or not, or to what extent, BOTOX® and physiotherapy are useful for the improvement of upper

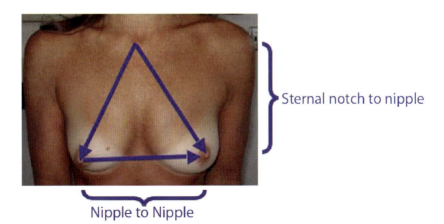

Fig. 12.5 Nipple to nipple and sternal notch to nipple measurements, with the patient standing in a standardized, relaxed posture. These distances are influenced by posture and by breast size, which can fluctuate with the menstrual cycle and with weight

thoracic posture and produce in women the appearance of a "BOTOX® Breast Lift." Such a trial could also help us to define optimal patient selection criteria and treatment protocols.

Disclosure: Dr. Smith is a consultant and investigator for Allergan.

References

1. Smith KC, Pérez-Atamoros F. Other dermatologic uses of botulinum toxin. In: Benedetto AV, ed. *Botulinum toxin in clinical dermatology*. London: Taylor and Francis; 2006: 219-236.
2. Cosmetic injections expand to points below the chin, New York Times, January 26, 2006 http://www.nytimes.com/2006/01/26/fashion/thursdaystyles/26sside.html?_r=1&oref=slogin Accessed 07.09.07.
3. Lang AM. Considerations for the use of botulinum toxin in pain management. *Lippincotts Case Manag*. 2006;11:279-282.
4. Finkelstein I, Katsis E. Botulinum toxin type A (BotoxR) improves chronic tension-type headache by altering biomechanics in the cervico-thoracic area: a case study. *Cephalalgia*. 2005;25:1189-1205.
5. Traba Lopez A, Esteban A. Botulinum toxin in motor disorders: practical considerations with emphasis on interventional neurophysiology. *Neurophysiol Clin*. 2001; 31(4):220-229.
6. Gallien P, Nicolas B, Petrilli S, et al. Role for botulinum toxin in back pain treatment in adults with cerebral palsy: report of a case. *Joint Bone Spine*. 2004;71(1):76-78.
7. Vad VB, Donatelli RA, Joshi M, Lang AM, Sims V. O.N.E.U.P. cervicothoracic & lumbar pain syndromes program. Beth Israel Medical Center, Office of Continuing Medical Education, 1st Avenue at 16th St., New York NY 10003. Accessed January 2008.
8. Alam M, Barrett KC, Hodapp RM, Arndt KA. The facial feed-back hypothesis applied to cosmetic procedures: change in emotions resulting from facial muscle activity and contour change induced by botulinum toxin injection. *J Am Acad Dermatol*. 2008;58:1061–1072.
9. Hurwitz EL, Aker PD, Adams AH, Meeker WC, Shekelle PG. Manipulation and mobilization of the cervical spine: a systematic review of the literature. *Spine*. 1996;21: 1746-1759.

Chapter 13
Treatment of Keratoses and Lentigines with Peels and PDT

John Strasswimmer

Introduction

The dorsum of the hands can portray an aged appearance due to sun damage. Contributing to the aged appearance are epidermal and dermal atrophy, prominent veins, solar lentigines, and actinic keratoses. Treatment of nonfacial solar lentigines and actinic keratosis is critical in providing a true age defying body rejuvenation. With actinic keratoses considered a precancerous disease state, treatment is not only cosmetically appealing but also medically pertinent. Treatment is often unrewarding using conventional approaches for facial lesions such as cryotherapy, topical fluorouracil, topical hydroquinone, and lasers due to discomfort, scarring, dyspigmentation, lack of efficacy, healing time, and cost.[1] Given how some treatments require a considerable amount of patience and patient compliance, practicality also becomes an issue. The lack of abundant sebaceous material, which confers suboptimal healing, in the hands does not allow for aggressive treatment. Ultimately, patients would like to achieve success with removing age defining lesions, such as solar lentigines and actinic keratoses with the same success and ease which clinicians have been performing on the face. Fortunately, two relatively old treatments for this situation, photodynamic therapy (PDT) and chemical peels, have been revisited with surprising success, offering good clearance and relative ease of application and most importantly excellent patient satisfaction.

Patient History and Clinical Examination

Just as in any procedure, patient identification and selection is paramount. When dealing with nonfacial areas, patient education must be thorough. Expectations not only of the clinician but also the patient must be delineated. Explanation to the patient of how the face is not the only indicator of age and how other sun exposed areas also incur damage is a must. With your treatment plan, the extent of sun damage must be portrayed to the patient. For example, an area such as the dorsum of the hands approaches the importance of facial lesions. Describing to patients the added benefit of removing potentially disfiguring skin cancers and the importance in removing them in general must also be emphasized. Examination should already be included with initial consultation for body rejuvenation. Clinically suspicious lesions for neoplasms should be treated before endeavoring on PDT or peels, as these are not conventional treatment options for both melanomatous and nonmelanoma skin cancers. With photodynamic therapy, concurrent photosensitive diseases such as lupus erythematosus, polymorphous light eruption, and xeroderma pigmentosa[2] might be a contraindication. Drug history is also critical. Known photosensitive drug eruptions (lupus such as toxic, etc.) may occur with its use. PDT is also considered pregnancy class C. Likewise, chemical peel patient selection is also important. Proper skin typing using a standardized scale such as the Fitzpatrick scale is essential for selecting not only the candidate but also concluding which peel would be most appropriate. Recent systemic retinoid therapy is also important. Previous peels, both facial and extrafacial, are part of obtaining patient history pertaining to scarring potential and previous successes and failures. As with any medical procedure, previous treatments the patient might have received must be known to help pinpoint the best options.

M. Alam and M. Pongprutthipan (eds.), *Body Rejuvenation*,
DOI 10.1007/978-1-4419-1093-6_13, © Springer Science+Business Media, LLC 2010

Method of Device and Treatment Application

For facial treatments, dosing and guidelines of performing PDT and peels are quite extensively found in the literature. However, very little data exist on nonfacial applications. The few reported studies are outlined in Table 1 for PDT and Table 2 for peels. Extrafacial PDT for photodamaged as not been widely reported, however, one report does show promise.[3] As with these treatments, like many others in dermatology, actual use differs greatly and ultimately rests on clinical confidence and personal experience. Finding the proper time for application of the photosensitizer for PDT also remains elusive. Peels will in general confer a better response with less risk of untoward effects in lighter skin types.

Photodynamic Therapy

PDT is useful in the treatment of photodamage and actinic keratoses (AK)[4]. Scaliness and redness of the hands may resolve after 1–3 treatments. For PDT, emphasis is placed on the patient receiving as little of ultraviolet radiation as possible leading up to their procedure. Initial consents should be completed along with any medical history. When utilizing this procedure for actinic keratosis (AK), we remove excess crust from the lesions to facilitate penetration; however, for rejuvenation, this is not needed. In the treatment of facial actinic keratoses, the topical 5-aminolevulinic acid (ALA) is allowed to preferently penetrate the parakeratotic skin found on AKs. This alone leads to most of the reported selectivity. In contrast, for a more broad rejuvenation, it is important to facilitate even penetration of the medication. The skin is first scrubbed with acetone to remove the lipid layer barrier. Second, a gentle (1–2 pass) microdermabrasion procedure might be done if the facility is available to allow penetration. Application of the sensitizing agent, topical 5-aminolevulinic acid (ALA), is completed first with varying time before treatment. We recommend 20% ALA with initially a 2 h incubation time. This is in contrast to the face, where even a 30 min incubation allows enough diffusion of the medication. On a cellular level, once the ALA has encountered a cell, it is metabolized to the photosensitizer protoporphyrin

IX (PPIX) within a few minutes. If a patient has not had significant response to this protocol, then the subsequent procedure may use an emollient applied after the ALA to maintain the ALA in solution and to facilitate penetration. The incubation time may also be expanded to overnight. We do not recommend this in the first treatment, as the reaction with light exposure can be quite robust.

The chemical is washed off with a soapy cleanser and water. This step removes the excess ALA from the surface, but there remains ALA within the skin for 48 h as discussed below. The choice light source then becomes another decision. Most decisions are obviously to use whatever equipment the clinician may already possess. The peak absorption curves occur at wavelengths in the 410 nm (blue) range (Fig. 13.1). However, additional minor absorption peaks can be found in the green, yellow, and red portions of the color spectra. Thus, light in these wave lengths can, in theory, activate. Blue light offers more extensive absorption (20-fold) and thus the most "potent" activation of PPIX. It also is not as deeply penetrating as the red light[3] If the goal is to target epidermal changes (keratoses, lentigos, epidermal atrophy), this is optimal. However, if the goal is to stimulate dermal remodeling then longer wavelengths are ideal. To this end, a continuous wave red light source might be ideal. The devices readily available and used to target other wavelengths are "pulsed" and thus are less likely to activate the PPIX.[3] Long

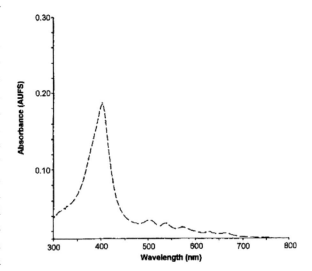

Fig. 13.1 Protoporphyrin IX absorption curve with visible light absorption

pulsed pulse dye laser (585–595 nm), with the non-purpuric setting, can be used.[5] In addition, intense pulse light (IPL) may be used and is frequently one of the choices since it is present in many cosmetic offices, it alone is able to treat lentigenes, and various filters can be used to treat. Because of the extremely short pulse time, there might not be enough oxygen available to produce a true "photodynamic" response, but might rather produce a "photothermal" effect to good benefit. The standard treatment is to use the laser or IPL as if one were treating with out the ALA. Immediately following, the patient must practice total avoidance of visible (not just UV) light, because the ALA remains in the skin and can be metabolized to PPIX for up to 48 h. Inadvertent light exposure, such as a 20 min drive home after the procedure, may be enough to produce a brisk phototoxic reaction manifested by excess erythema, swelling, and pain. Instruct patient that a reaction similar to a light sunburn, burn and peel can be expected after 72 h. Follow visits should be around 72 h for reassurance and again at 2–4 weeks for re-evaluation and possible reapplication. For the weeks following the procedure, such as for peels, UV protection helps to prevent dyspigmentation.

Chemical Peeling

Chemical peeling on the hands and arms is more of a challenge because of the uneven nature of the skin thickness and the dramatic hyperkeratosis seen on some portions of the hand. Depending on patient medical history, pertinent prophylactic antimicrobial therapy should be instituted, especially for impetigo and herpetic infections. Prior to peeling, one needs to decide whether superficial peeling (Jessner's solution, glycolic acid, low percentage of trichloroacetic acid (TCA) that targets epidermis is the goal or if deeper medium depth (35% TCA pretreated by Jessner's solution) is to be performed. While a superficial chemical peel is optimal for patients with mild photodamage and color abnormalities, a medium depth chemical peel is effective for patients with lots of pigment alterations, especially brown and tan pigmentations and seborrheic keratoses. However, the medium depth chemical peel will require longer healing times than the superficial chemical peel and PDT treatment.

We usually opt for the medium depth because the goal is to get a permanent improvement. Patients are pretreated with topical retinoids at least 14 days before the procedure to help with even penetration and this is particularly important for the thicker areas of skin such as the hands[6]. The retinoid is stopped 5 days prior to treatment. Acetone scrub is done to degrease the area. This is followed by one even application of Jessner's solution. Subsequently, 25–35% TCA is applied in an even pattern in perpendicular directions to maximize even coverage. The chemical should be layered cautiously and before starting a new application, waiting for frost to appear. TCA and Jessner's solution are "self neutralizing" and the frost is the endpoint. The procedure should not be painful. An even frost demonstrates a successful application. Spot treating difficult lesions such as hyperkeratotic actinic keratosis with increased number of applications may be necessary. If a patient has not responded to this protocol, it may be repeated in 1–2 months with additional "spot" touching of 50% TCA after the application of the 35% TCA. We do not recommend higher concentration because of the risk of scarring. Likewise, we do not recommend "deep" chemical peels (such as phenol containing peels) in nonfacial locations due to the risk of scarring.

Postoperative care for chemical peels is usually simple and straightforward. There is a wide array of options for patient comfort post procedure ranging from simple cool compresses with cold water to emollients to more sophisticated topical treatments including hyaluronic acid and other anti-inflammatories. Restarting previous topical therapy is also advised including retinoids and any topical bleaching agents. Follow up is again simple. A 24–48 h check would reassure patient and would be a good indicator of success of application. Following that, a recheck at 4 weeks would be prudent as this would be an opportune time for an additional peel if necessary.

When adverse effects do arise, and they will, proper anticipation and treatment options must be recognized by the clinician. The main side effects of both procedures include erythema (overabundant and nonexistent), edema, and crusting. There are many variables that can be changed with PDT to decrease these side effects, including decreasing incubation time and using less irritating light sources such as long pulse laser. If they do occur, topical mid potency corticosteroids often will suffice. Adjunct topical anti-inflammatories can also be used. Posttreatment hyperpigmentation that can occur with both treatment modalities can be remedied with use of bleaching agents. Most often times, reassurance is warranted and review of preoperative education will alleviate most concerns. Post treatment hypopigmentation is rare with peeling and rarer with PDT, but can be permanent.

Conclusion

The future of these treatment modalities is promising. As popularity increases especially in the field of photodynamic therapy, this will become more and more popular. Advances in sensitizers, incubation times, and tailoring light sources to each patient to ensure a great cosmetic result with minimal side effects will occur as more and more clinicians become familiar with this technology. As literature prevails pointing out the possible preventative nature of PDT for nonmelanomatous skin cancers, medical and cosmetic indications will meld and make this much more of a viable option, even in noncosmetic based offices. Peels have been stalwart and remain effective for numerous applications. Using less destructive peels with combinations products (retinoids and other peels) may make these procedures

extremely safe and still yield significant results. Overall, PDT and chemical peels are viable, safe, and relatively simple treatments to help eliminate solar lentigines and actinic keratoses on photodamaged hands. This is an important component of total body rejuvenation.

Acknowledgments Dr Strasswimmer gratefully acknowledges the assistance of John Mini DO and Danika Przekop DO, resident physicians from the Palm Beach Centre for Graduate Medical Education.

References

1. Todd MM, et al. A Comparison of three Lasers and liquid nitrogen in the treatment of solar lentigines: a randomized controlled comparative trial. *Arch Derm.* 2000;136:841-846.
2. Leonard AL, Hanke CW. *Cosmetic Dermatology Procedure Manual.* New York: Physicians' Continuing Education Corp; 2007:168.
3. Strasswimmer J, Grande DJ. Do pulsed laser activate PDT? *Lasers Surg Med.* 2006;38:22–25.
4. Gold MH, Nestor MS. Current treatments of actinic keratoses. *J Drugs Dermatol.* 2006;5(Suppl):17–24.
5. Alexiades-Armenakas MR, Geronemus RG. Laser-mediated photodynamic therapy of actinic keratoses. *Arch Derm.* 2003; 139:1313–1320.
6. Nemeth HO, Taylor JR AJ. Tretinoin accelerates healing after trichloroacetic acid chemical peel. *Arch Derm.* 1991;127(5): 678–682.

Chapter 14
Off-Face Laser Treatment of Keratoses and Lentigines

Paul M. Friedman and Brenda Chrastil-LaTowsky

Introduction

Laser procedures for the skin continue to become more and more popular: 590,000 procedures were performed in 2004, up by 300% since 2003, according to the American Society for Aesthetic Plastic Surgery. Many dermatologists have been asked by patients, friends, and relatives: "What can I do about these brown and red spots on my neck and chest?"

Traditionally, treatment modalities of keratoses and lentigines have been focused on facial lesions. With greater treatment success, coupled with modern dress, patients now demand treatment options for lesions off the face. Laser treatment of these lesions will be discussed in this chapter, including the Q-switched (QS) Nd:YAG laser (532 nm), QS ruby laser (694 nm), fractional photothermolysis (1,550 nm erbium laser), and pulsed dye laser-mediated photodynamic therapy (PDT). Intense pulse light therapy, which is noncoherent light, will not be discussed in this chapter, but has also been used to treat lentigines. Of note, traditional ablative resurfacing is not used on nonfacial skin in our practice because of the risk of scarring, although fractional CO_2 treatment will likely play a role in the future.

Clinical Examination and Patient History

The most important aspect of the pretreatment history and physical exam is the establishment of the patient's expectations as well as communicating the importance of realistic expectations. The patient must be educated that usually more than one treatment will be required. More than one modality should be offered, based on the patient's concerns, physical findings, and other pertinent factors. Baseline and posttreatment photographs of previous patients treated with different treatment options are helpful, as are photographs of immediate posttreatment findings, such as erythema and edema. A detailed description of the treatment, expected downtime, and posttreatment protocol are important parts of the treatment process.

Method of Device and Treatment Application

532 nm Q-Switched Nd: YAG and 694 nm QS Ruby Lasers

The QS ruby and 532 nm QS Nd:YAG lasers have been found to be effective in the removal of lentigines on the dorsal hands, forearms, chest, and back (Figs. 14.1–14.3). When compared, the QS ruby laser produced slightly better treatment results, but caused more discomfort during treatment. However, the 532 nm QS Nd:YAG laser produced more posttreatment discomfort.[1] The 532 nm QS Nd:YAG has been found to produce superior results when a head-to-head comparison was performed with cryotherapy. Patients also preferred laser therapy over cryotherapy.[2]

Please see Table 14.1 for suggested settings in the treatment of lentigines and seborrheic keratoses with the 532 nm QS Nd:YAG based on skin type.

Treatment technique is similar to on-face treatment. It should be emphasized that using subtherapeutic fluences in patients with darker skin types may cause posttreatment hyperpigmentation, lasting weeks to months. Aggressive fluences may cause skin

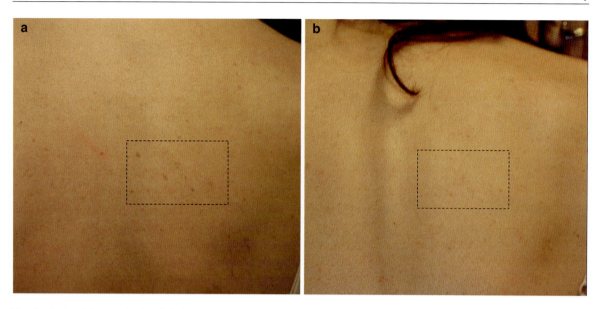

Fig. 14.1 Lentigines and seborrheic keratoses treated with 532 nm QS Nd:YAG and QS ruby. (**a**) Patient's back at baseline. (**b**) Three months after treatment. The patient had one treatment with the QS Nd:YAG (fluence of 3 J/cm², spot size of 3 mm). Two weeks later, the patient was treated with the QS ruby laser (fluence of 3.5 J/cm² and spot size of 5 mm)

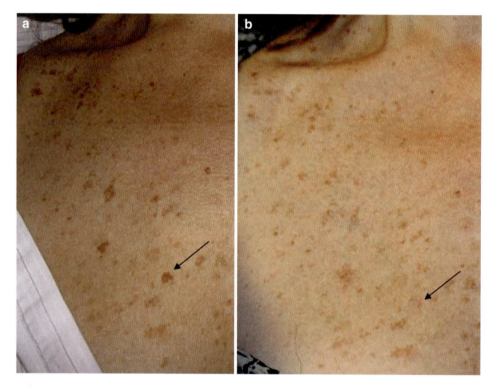

Fig. 14.2 Lentigines and seborrheic keratoses treated with 532 nm QS Nd:YAG. (**a**) Patient's chest at baseline. (**b**) Ten months after a single treatment with the 532 nm QS Nd:YAG (fluence of 3.2 J/cm², spot size 3 mm)

sloughing and postinflammatory hypo- or hyperpigmentation. The clinical endpoint of whitening should be sought during treatment and used to adjust laser settings (Fig. 14.4). Wound healing is

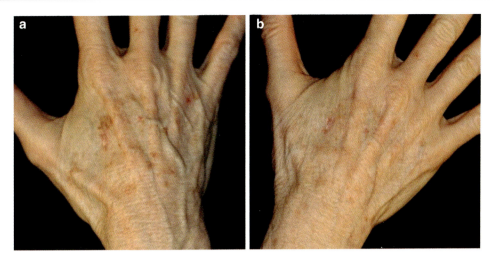

Fig. 14.3 Treatment of lentigines of the dorsal hand with the ruby laser. (**a**) Patient's hand at baseline. (**b**) Patient's hand 9 months after a single treatment with the ruby laser

Table 14.1 Suggested treatment settings of lentigines and macular seborrheic keratoses with the QS Nd:YAG (532 nm). Standard Treatment of Lentigines and Macular Seborrheic Keratoses with the QS Nd:YAG (532 nm)

Fitzpatrick Skin Type	Spot Size (mm)	Fluence (J/cm^2)
I–III	3	3.0
IV–V	3	1.4–1.6

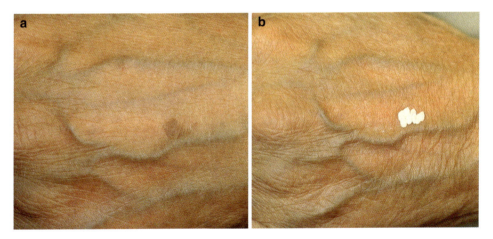

Fig. 14.4 Treatment of a macular seborrheic keratosis in a patient with Fitzpatrick skin type IV. (**a**) Patient at baseline. (**b**) Patient immediately after treatment. Note the clinically-apparent white endpoint of the treated lesion

fastest when the lowest therapeutic fluences are used. One to three treatment sessions every 3–4 weeks are generally recommended, but adjusted to patient's clinical response. Post-op care instructions are generally consistent with that of the treatment of facial lentigines (Table 14.2).

Table 14.2 An example of posttreatment instructions given to patients after Q-switched Ruby & Nd:YAG laser therapy. *Courtesy of Dr. Roy G. Geronemus*

DermSurgery ◈ Laser Center

POST-OPERATIVE INSTRUCTIONS

Q-SWITCH YAG / RUBY LASER TREATMENT

WHAT SHOULD I EXPECT AFTER MY Q-SWITCHED RUBY LASER AND Q-SWITCHED YAG LASER TREATMENT?

The treated area will turn white in color immediately following your treatment and some swelling may occur. A small blister may form in some of the exposed areas in 24 to 48 hours after the treatment. You may experience some swelling and redness of the area surrounding the treatment site and it is possible that some scaling or crusting may occur following the procedure.

Please note: The lesion might temporarily return to its original color shortly after the procedure.

CARE FOLLOWING TATTOO TREATMENT

On the day following treatment, begin <u>gently</u> cleansing the area two times a day with mild soap and water followed by <u>Aquaphor or bacitracin ointment</u>. **If the area has increased redness and itching, discontinue the ointment and call the office**. The object of cleaning the wound is to keep the treated lesions moist, which aids in the healing process.

CARE FOLLOWING TREATMENT OF <u>PIGMENTED LESIONS</u>

On the day of treatment, apply <u>Aquaphor or bacitracin ointment</u> to the treated area two times a day and continue applying twice daily until the treatment site(s) are healed. **If the area has increased redness and itching, discontinue the ointment and call the office**.

MAY I BE EXPOSED TO THE SUN FOLLOWING THE PROCEDURE?

Direct exposure of sunlight must be avoided following ruby and YAG laser therapy. If there is no crusting or blistering, a sunscreen of SPF-15 or higher should be applied to the treated area for two months following the treatment to avoid sun damage. Sunscreen is available at our Center.

HOW LONG MUST I WAIT BEFORE I AM ALLOWED TO USE MAKE-UP OVER THE TREATED AREA?

Make-up should not be used over the treated area until it has completely healed.

WHEN SHOULD I RETURN TO HAVE MY TREATED AREA RE-EVALUATED?

Please make a follow-up appointment within 3 - 6 weeks following the treatment. Should you have any questions or concerns before your follow-up visit, please feel free to call the office at (713) 791-9966 and ask to speak with a nurse.

F:\ORIGINAL FORMS\COSMETIC\YAG POST INST.doc REV. 06.25.07

1,550 nm Erbium-Doped Fractional Photothermolysis (Fraxel™)

Fractional photothermolysis can safely be used off the face and is routinely used in our practice for photorejuvenation of the neck, chest, dorsal hands, and extremities (Figs. 14.5–14.7).[3] We have also had outstanding results using this device to treat disseminated superficial actinic porokeratosis (DSAP).[4] In a series of 4 patients, we found that two patients using the Fraxel SR 750 achieved a 50–75% improvement of DSAP lesions and skin texture after 3–6 treatments (Fig. 14.8). Two patients treated with more aggressive treatment settings using the Fraxel SR 1500 device achieved greater than 75% improvement after 5–6 treatments every 4 weeks[4] (Figs. 14.9–14.11). Additionally, preliminary results

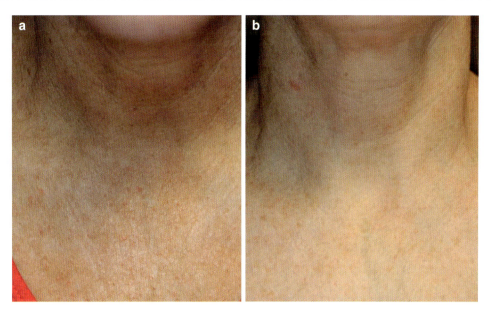

Fig. 14.5 Lentigines and photodamage treated with fractional photothermolysis. (**a**) The patient's chest at baseline. Note lentigines, keratoses and poikiloderma. (**b**) The patient after only one treatment. Treatment settings: energy of 11 mJ, 15 mm spot, 6–8 passes 1,500–2,000 microscopic treatment zones/cm^2 (MTZs/cm^2). Zimmer cooling system was set at level 3

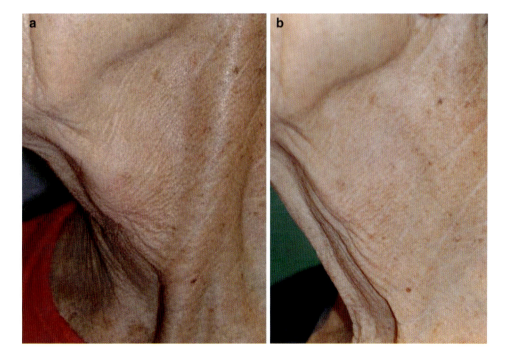

Fig. 14.6 Dyschromia treated with fractional photothermolysis. (**a**) The patient's neck at baseline. (**b**) The patient after three treatments with fractional photothermolysis. Note marked improvement of the dyschromia, as well as skin texture. Treatment settings were: energy setting of 40 mJ, 15 mm spot size, 8 passes. Total kJ ranged from 4.02–4.88. Zimmer cooling system settings ranged from 3 to 5

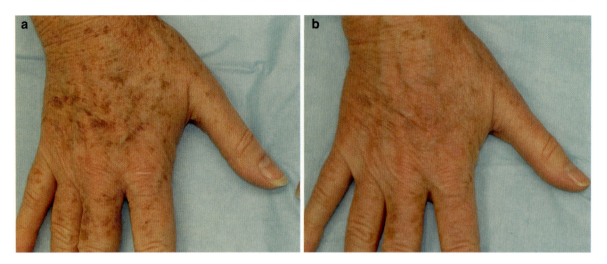

Fig. 14.7 Fractional photothermolysis for the treatment of lentigines of the hand. (**a**) Patient's dorsal hand at baseline. (**b**) Dorsal hands three months after 5 treatments of fractional photothermolysis. Treatments were spaced at 2–3 week intervals. Treatments settings were: energy of 8–9 mJ and density of 2,500 microscopic treatment zones/cm². *Photographs courtesy of Dr. Ming Jih. Permission for publication given by Dermatologic Surgery*[3]

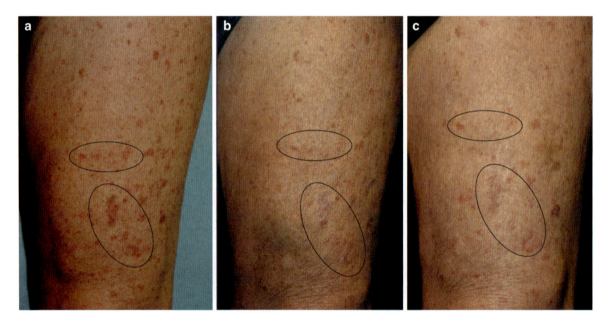

Fig. 14.8 DSAP treated with fractional photothermolysis. (**a**) The patient's thigh at baseline. (**b**) Thigh one month after three treatments with fractional photolysis (Fraxel SR 750). Ecchymosis is unrelated to treatment. (**c**) Thigh one month after 6 treatments. Energy settings ranged from 8 to 12 mJ and a final treatment density of 2,000–2,500 MTZs/cm²

of an ongoing study at our facility have shown that fractional photothermolysis may effectively treat actinic keratoses.

Energy parameters should be appropriate for the indication being treated (Table 14.3). Usually, energy parameters range from 10 to 40 mJ when treating off-face for improvement of pigmentation and texture. High energies (50–70 mJ) should be used with caution and in limited areas only when the maximum penetration and remodeling are required, such as

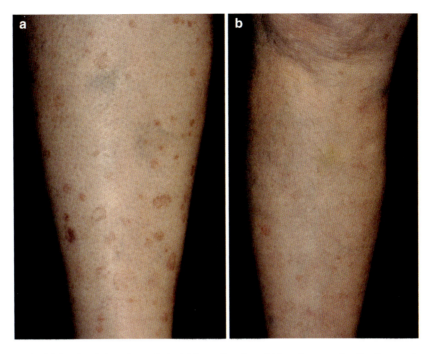

Fig. 14.9 DSAP treated with fractional photothermolysis. (**a**) Leg at baseline. (**b**) Leg three months after three treatments with fractional photothermolysis (second model, Fraxel SR 1500). Energy ranged from 35–50 mJ and treatment level was 10

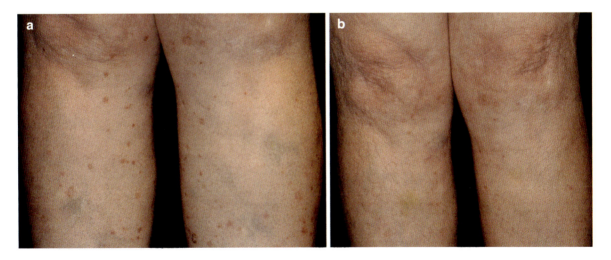

Fig. 14.10 DSAP treated with fractional photothermolysis. The same patient as in Fig. 14.7: (**a**) legs at baseline. (**b**) Three months after three treatments. Patient reported complete resolution of pruritus associated with the DSAP and was completely satisfied with treatment

hyperkeratotic lesions. Wound healing is prolonged off-face and treatment levels (TL) should be conservative (i.e., TL 6-TL 9).

Treatment technique is similar to facial fractional resurfacing. The laser handpiece should be held per-pendicularly to the skin surface. Treatment density is maximized when treating keratoses, including actinic keratoses, in our practice. Thicker, hyperk-eratotic lesions should receive 2–4 extra passes. The treated skin edges should be feathered, especially on

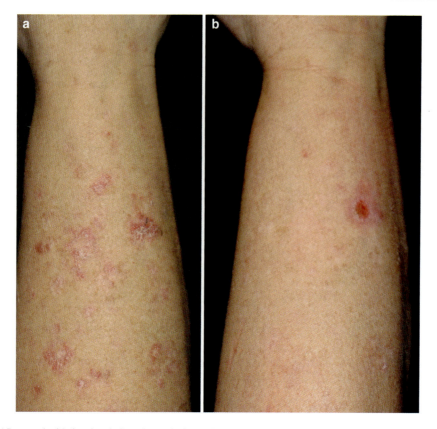

Fig. 14.11 DSAP treated with fractional photothermolysis. (**a**) Patient's forearm at baseline. (**b**) Two months after four treatments with fractional photothermolysis (Fraxel SR 1500). Note biopsy site (biopsy showed actinic keratoses). Energy ranged from 35–50 mJ and treatment level was 10. Patient reported >90% improvement. Physician improvement graded as >75% improved

Table 14.3 Examples of recommended treatment parameters using Fraxel™ off the face

Off Face Indication	Energy	Treatment Level Fitzpatrick Skin Type I–III	Treatment Level Fitzpatrick Skin Type IV–V
Resurfacing and Lentigines	10–40 mJ	7–11	4–7
Acne and Surgical Scars	20–50 mJ	7–11	4–7

Note that for off-face applications, a more conservative treatment level, or density, is used than for face treatments.

darker skin types, to avoid potential (transient) postinflammatory hyperpigmentation. This is done by performing fewer passes further out from the central treatment area.

Posttreatment care is similar to that of facial treatment (Table 14.4). The patient should wear loose-fitting clothing for more comfort posttreatment.

In our experience, there have been no severe adverse events, such as blistering or scarring. Posttreatment erythema and edema may be prolonged compared to facial treatments and ranges from 5–21 days posttreatment.

Laser-Mediated Photodynamic Therapy with Pulsed Dye Laser (PDL) (595 nm)

Laser-mediated PDT may be used for keratoses, lentigines, and photorejuvenation. Previous studies utilizing the pulsed-dye laser as a light source have found that extremity lesions cleared in 83.1% at 10-day posttreatment evaluation and 70.9% at 4-month follow-up, which is less clearance than that of the face.[5] These results are consistent with those experienced in our practice. Figure 14.12 demonstrates a patient's scalp one month after a single treatment.

Table 14.4 An example of posttreatment instructions given to patients after fractional photothermolysis treatment. *Courtesy of Dr. Roy G. Geronemus*

DermSurgery ◇ Laser Center

POST-TREATMENT INSTRUCTIONS

FRAXEL LASER TREATMENT

WHAT WILL I LOOK LIKE AFTER MY LASER TREATMENT?

The treated area will be sunburn pink and there will be some swelling. The pinkish tone may last for 5-7 days. This is a sign that your skin is healing properly. Make-up may be applied immediately following the treatment to cover the redness. Swelling should be minimal to moderate and will resolve within 3-5 days.

A bronze appearance may occur around 3 days post treatment and may last up to 2 weeks. Flaking of the skin, similar to that of a sunburn, also may occur anytime following treatment. This natural exfoliation is a sign of the reorganization of the skin cells as new cells replace the old.

MAY I WEAR MAKE-UP FOLLOWING THE PROCEDURE?

Make-up may be worn immediately following the procedure. Particular care must be taken to avoid irritation of the skin while removing the make-up. You should avoid abrasive or irritating make-up removers.

MAY I BE EXPOSED TO THE SUN FOLLOWING THE PROCEDURE?

Direct exposure of sunlight should be avoided following treatment. A sunscreen of SPF-45 or higher should be applied to the treated area for two months following the treatment to avoid sun damage.

WHAT SHOULD I DO IF THE TREATED AREA BEGINS TO CRUST OR BLISTER?

The skin should then be treated gently with twice daily applications of Polysporin or Aquaphor ointment. **If the area has increased redness and itching, discontinue the ointment and call the office.** It is not necessary to wear a bandage. However, if a bandage is preferred, a telfa (non-adhesive) bandage should be used. It can be cut to size and secured with paper tape. The area may get wet while bathing, but swimming should be avoided for one (1) week following treatment.

AFTER THE PROCEDURE—

- Use hydrating gel mask or ice packs to treated area every hour for 15-20 minutes as needed for swelling.
- Apply Bionect gel twice a day for 3-5 days.
- After treatment to the face, sleep with head elevated at a 45° angle (2 pillows.)
- Take an anti-inflammatory (Motrin/Ibuprofen) every six hours as needed for swelling
- Take an antihistamine (Zyrtec/Claritin) as directed when needed for swelling– use with caution, as may cause drowsiness.
- Moisturize the treated area twice daily. May moisturize more frequently for dryness when needed.
- Apply sunscreen every morning (after moisturizer.)

WHEN SHOULD I RETURN TO HAVE MY TREATED AREA RE-EVALUATED?

Treatments are spaced 4 – 6 weeks apart, depending on the nature of your skin condition. Should you have any questions or concerns prior to your next visit, please feel free to call our office at (713) 791-9966.

C:\Documents and Settings\Linda\Desktop\FRAXEL POST INST new doc rev. 10.11.07

Pre-op treatment of pulsed-dye laser-mediated PDT is similar to treatment of the face (Table 14.5).

In our practice, the following parameters are used for the pulse dye laser after 20% ALA application: 10 mm spot size, fluence range of 7.5–9 J/cm^2, and 10 msec pulse width. A dynamic cooling (tetrafluoroethane) spray is used for pre-treatment and posttreatment cooling. The spray is fired twice: 30 msec prior to each laser pulse followed by a 30 msec post-laser pulse delay.

See Table 14.5 for the laser-mediated PDT protocol used in our office. Treatment technique is the same as that of facial treatment.

Posttreatment care is similar to treatment of the face and is listed in Table 14.5.

One of the challenges in using PDT off the face is ensuring sun avoidance post-therapy. Any type of ambient light may augment the treatment; however, excess exposure may cause complications such as increased edema, erythema, and blistering. The

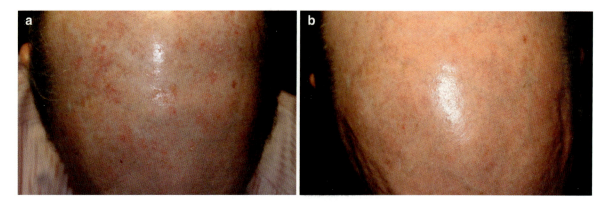

Fig. 14.12 Actinic keratoses of the scalp treated with laser-mediated PDT. (**a**) Patient's scalp at baseline. (**b**) Patient's scalp one month after a single treatment of laser-mediated PDT using the PDL. Please see text for suggested treatment settings

Table 14.5 Pre-treatment protocol, treatment technique, posttreatment protocol used for laser-mediated PDT using the 595-nm pulsed-dye laser

Pretreatment	Confirm diagnosis: lentigines versus AKs
	Acetone applied to treatment area
	Microdermabrasion of treatment area
Treatment technique	20% ALA application with three-hour incubation
	20% ALA re-applied 60 min after first application
	Topical anesthetic applied 45–60 min before laser treatment
	595-nm pulsed dye laser, 1–2 passes to treatment area (see text for laser parameters)
Posttreatment technique	Treatment area cleansed with soap and water
	Apply physical sunscreen such as titanium dioxide or zinc oxide
	Vigilon hydrogel dressing applied to treatment area for 30–60 min
	Patient instructed on strict sun avoidance for two days
	Patient instructed to expect desquamation and erythema for 2–3 days.
	Biafine emollient is applied to treatment area twice a day for 5–7 days
	Aquaphor ointment is applied to rough, dry or scaly areas as needed
	Follow-up in 4–6 weeks for evaluation

patient should be counseled that driving gloves and long sleeves are necessary, even indoors and during driving time.

Conclusion

Clinicians should tailor their treatment approach based on clinical setting and maximum benefits for the patients. PDT parameters: ALA incubation time and delivery, light source settings, number of treatments, and treatment intervals will be continually refined to deliver maximum efficacy. Future treatment of lentigines and keratoses will also focus on fractional CO_2 devices.

References

1. Tse Y, Levine VJ, McClain SA et al. The removal of cutaneous pigmented lesions with the Q-switched ruby laser and the Q-switched neodymium: yttrium-aluminum-garnet laser. A comparative study. *J Dermatol Surg Oncol* 1994; 20(12):795–800
2. Todd MM, Rallis TM, Gerwels JW et al. A comparison of 3 lasers and liquid nitrogen in the treatment of solar lentigines: a randomized, controlled, comparative trial. *Arch Dermatol* 2000; 136(7):841–846
3. Jih MH, Goldberg LH, Kimyai-Asadi A. Fractional photothermolysis for photoaging of hands. *Dermatol Surg* 2008; 34(1):73–78
4. Chrastil B, Glaich AS, Goldberg LH et al. Fractional photothermolysis: a novel treatment for disseminated superficial actinic porokeratosis. *Arch Dermatol* 2007; 143(11):1450–1452
5. Alexiades-Armenakas MR, Geronemus RG. Laser-mediated photodynamic therapy of Actinic Keratoses. *Arch Dermatol* 2003; 139:1313–1320

Chapter 15
Treatment of Hand Veins with Sclerotherapy

Neil S. Sadick

Introduction

Sclerotherapy is not a new science, but has evolved into a more exact and effective way to shrink aesthetically undesirable veins, including those of the dorsum of the hand. The technique for treating hand veins by sclerotherapy is similar to the technique for treating leg veins.[1]

In sclerotherapy, a sterile "sclerosing" solution is injected into the target vessels that induce inflammation of the intima layers and destroys the endothelial cells, causing the vessels to collapse and dissolve. Sotradecol (sodium tetradecyl sulfate (STS), ESI Lederle Generics, Philadelphia, PA) (0.25%) is the only FDA-cleared sclerosing solution available and is administered by traditional injection technique.

A newer option is foam sclerotherapy. Since commercial preparations of the foam are not available, STS (0.2%) foam, fluid or viscous, must be made in the physician's office by either the Tessari or double-syringe technique. A 3-way stopcock, sclerosing solution, 3-mL disposable plastic syringe, and 30-gauge needle are needed. First, a syringe containing liquid is connected to a similar air-containing syringe via the 3-way stopcock. Then, for fluid foam, the liquid and air are pumped back and forth 20 times and for viscous foam, five times with additional pressure and seven times without additional pressure.[2,3] Local anesthesia is given before injection and ultrasound is used to visualize the target vein. When the foam sclerosing solution is injected into the vein, the foam forces blood from the vein, oxygen bubbles dissolve, and the vein deflates.

Foam sclerotherapy is currently safe, effective, rapid, sterile, and reproducible. Compared with traditional sclerotherapy, foam sclerotherapy is associated with fewer adverse effects, fewer required treatments, and superior overall benefit. The sclerosing solution and blood have greater contact with each other as the air presses the blood cells against the wall of the vein. Other advantages are that the foam, rather than mixing with the blood, actually replaces the blood and is in contact with the vein for a longer period.[3]

Clinical trials to evaluate the long-term efficacy and safety of foam sclerotherapy are in progress in Europe and the US. In the meantime, the following consensus statements for foam sclerotherapy have been published[2]:

- Sclerosing foam is an appropriate treatment for varicose veins
- Foam sclerotherapy is a powerful procedure when performed by an experienced surgeon
- Sclerosing foam is more powerful than liquid sclerosing solution
- Most recommendations for conventional sclerotherapy are applicable to foam sclerotherapy

Traditional and foam sclerotherapy are the gold standards for treating hand veins. Ambulatory phlebectomy, endovascular laser treatment, and radiofrequency closure are less commonly used.[3] Sclerotherapy causes less trauma than surgical procedures. It is also safe, effective, economical, and less dependent on technique than other procedures. On the downside, sclerotherapy may cause bruising, require several sessions to achieve maximum clinical benefit, and may result in extravasation of the sclerosing solution into the perivascular tissue, leading to localized cutaneous ulcers. (Even the most experienced physician may accidentally inject a small amount of sclerosing solution into the perivascular tissue[4]).The advantages and disadvantages of sclerotherapy vs. endovenous laser hand vein ablation (EVLH) are shown in Table 15.1.

M. Alam and M. Pongprutthipan (eds.), *Body Rejuvenation*,
DOI 10.1007/978-1-4419-1093-6_15, © Springer Science+Business Media, LLC 2010

Table 15.1 Comparison of hand vein sclerotherapy and endovenous laser hand vein ablation (EVLH)

	Advantages	Disadvantages
Sclerotherapy	Nonsurgical	May require multiple treatments
	Cost effective	Risk of extravasation
		Increased bruising
EVLH	Usually single treatment	High cost
	Requires minor surgical intervention	Requires knowledge of tumescent anesthesia
	Use of laser fiber	Risk of laser skin burns

Clinical Examination and Patient History

Potential candidates for sclerotherapy have protuberant veins. Patients can be told that the procedure is simply the injection of a solution that irritates the lining of the vein which causes the vein to become inflamed, collapse, and be absorbed by the body. Patients should withdraw from antiplatelet medicines, NSAIDS, and aspirin before treatment. Stopping the of antiplatelet and antithrombotic medication is not recommended except in consultation with and in approval of the prescribing physician. There is an evidence that perioperative discontinuation of such agents is rarely associated with serious adverse events increasing pulmonary embolus, stroke, and valvular dysfunction. If a patient is taking daily aspirin for routine health maintenance without the instruction of a physician, this may be discontinued as early as 2 weeks before the procedure and resumed 2–3 days after the procedure. Physicians should review the histories for anticoagulant, disulfram, antabuse, and other sclerosant interactive medications; coagulation disorders; bruising easily; and hand rejuvenation procedures. Pregnancy, hypercoagulable disorder, recurrent thrombophlebitis, connective tissue disease, disabling arthritis, severe asthma and allergies, soft-tissue infection, severe neurologic or circulatory disease, and chronic hand problems (pain, weakness, edema, carpal tunnel syndrome) are contraindications for sclerotherapy.[1]

Hand veins range from 1 to 6 mm in diameter and are identified by their ropey, protuberant appearance. Unlike leg veins, which protrude due to valvular incompetence, hand veins protrude as we age due to muscle atrophy, bone demineralization, and loss of

volume of adipose tissue and dermal collagen. A loss of elasticity occurs in both the skin and superficial blood vessels. Sun exposure, in turn, produces wrinkles, dyschromia, and protuberant, tortuous varicosities of the superficial hand veins. Patients consider these veins cosmetically unacceptable and seek treatment to remove them.[1]

Method of Device and Treatment Application

The size and diameter of hand veins do not determine the treatment modality. Rather, the choice is determined by the physician's experience and preferences and by the patients' desires. For hand veins, sclerotherapy requires multiple sessions while intravenous laser procedures require only a single session. The appropriate concentrations of foam sclerosing solution for vessels of various diameters are shown in Table 15.2.

The technique for treating hand veins is a simple injection. Injecting one hand at a time permits the patient to have the use of the other hand while the treated hand recovers. It is possible, however, to treat multiple vessels in one session. Posttreatment compression for a few days enhances the results and prevents hyperpigmentation.[5] Excessive compression of the skin covering the treated vein should be avoided, as it may produce tissue anoxia and subsequent localized cutaneous ulceration.[4] Hand sclerotherapy is technique dependent and should be performed only by physicians with training and experience. Other than the face, hands are the most commonly noticed anatomical area of the body and should be protected from photodamage with regular use of sunblocks or antioxidant creams. Clinical examples are shown in Figs. 15.1–15.4.

Table 15.2 Suggested concentration of foamed sclerosant for management of dorsal arch hand veins with sclerotherapy based upon vein diameter

Vein diameter (mm)	STS (%)
1–2	0.1–0.2
2–4	0.2–0.25
4–6	0.25–0.5
6–8	0.5–1.0

STS sodium tetradecyl sulfate

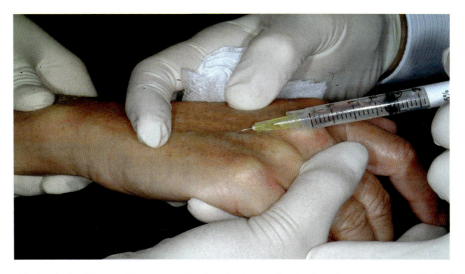

Fig. 15.1   The right hand of a 64-year-old woman as her dorsal veins receive the first of two treatments with the foam sclerosing solution. Photographs courtesy of Neil S. Sadick, MD

Fig. 15.2   Gauze secured by elastic adhesive bandage covering the dorsal vein areas after injection of the foam sclerosing solution. Both hands were injected in a single treatment session. Photographs courtesy of Neil S. Sadick, MD

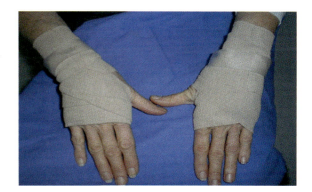

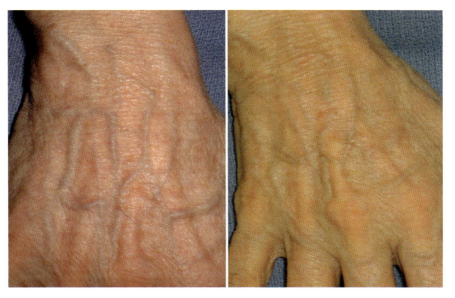

Fig. 15.3   The right hand before the first treatment (*left*) and 3 months after the final of two treatments (*right*) with the foam sclerosing solution. Photographs courtesy of Neil S. Sadick, MD

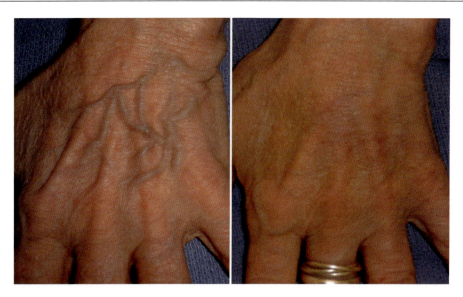

Fig. 15.4 The left hand before the first treatment (*left*) and 3 months after the final of two treatments (*right*) with the foam sclerosing solution. Photographs courtesy of Neil S. Sadick, MD

To prepare the foam sclerotherapy solution, the following are needed:

- Syringe (3 mL)×2
- Bacteriostatic water, 30-mL vial
- STS (3%), 2-mL vial
- Fluid Dispensing Connector or adaptor
- Drape (nonsterile)
- Gloves (nonsterile)
- Gauze (nonsterile, 4×4 cm)
- Alcohol prep pads
- Elastic adhesive bandage (5-cm wide, 1 roll)

The sclerosing solution (STS, 0.25%) is prepared by diluting 2 mL STS (3%) with 22 mL bacteriostatic water. Remove 8 mL from a 30-mL vial of bacteriostatic water and transfer the entire contents of a 2-mL vial of STS (3%) to the remaining 22 mL of bacteriostatic water. Fill one syringe with fresh sclerosing solution and draw 1 mL of air into the other syringe. Connect the two syringes to a Fluid Dispensing Connector (B. Braun Medical Inc., Bethlehem, PA) and depress the plungers to push the sclerosing solution and air back and forth until the mixture becomes a foam. Then, attach a 30 G ½″ hypodermic fine-inject needle to the syringe with the foam sclerosing solution.

The tray (Fig. 15.5) should include the drape, gloves, gauze, alcohol prep pads, syringe of foam sclerosing

solution, and postprocedure wound care materials (elastic adhesive bandage and gauze) for cleaning purposes and if needed, for compression on injection sites that bleed.

Posttreatment care focuses on appropriate compression of the treated veins. The treated hand is cleaned with either hydrogen peroxide or alcohol and gauze. If bleeding persists at the injection sites, gauze is rolled or folded and placed on the bleeding site. Gauze is then secured by elastic adhesive bandage wrapped with appropriate compression (according to the patient, not too tight or too loose) distally from the wrist, then proximally toward the fingers around the dorsal and palmar areas of the hand. The compression bandage should be worn for 24 h after treatment.

Adverse effects with sclerotherapy are minimal; hyperpigmentation and ulceration are extremely rare. For Posttreatment care, our patients receive 1–3 treatments with healing ointment (Aquaphor, Beiersdorf AG, Hamburg, Germany) at 4 to 6-week intervals. We treat bruising with vitamin K cream and use arnica to accelerate wound healing. Hydroquinone cream can be used for whitening skin and retinoid creams for repairing photodamage.

Other therapies can be used in combination with sclerotherapy. Dermal fillers such as Radiesse (Bioform Medical, Inc., San Mateo, CA) or Sculptra (Dermik

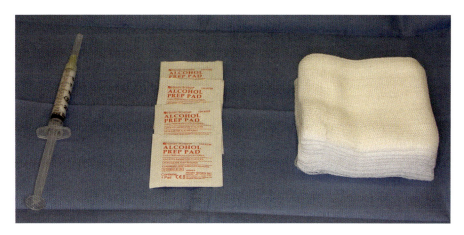

Fig. 15.5 Tray setup. Photographs courtesy of Neil S. Sadick, MD

Laboratories, Inc., Berwyn, PA) correct volume loss in the hands, thus improving the appearance of the elevated veins. Fractional laser procedures or plasma portrait technology can correct skin wrinkling or discoloration, and radiofrequency can improve laxity. Sclerotherapy will eventually give way to endovenous laser therapy for vein removal because fewer treatments are required and bruising occurs less frequently with the laser procedure.

Conclusion

Full-body rejuvenation is the future of aesthetic medicine. Many technologies are available to improve the face and more people are looking for ways to improve the look of their aging hands as well. Combination approaches that include radiofrequency, fractional laser treatment, injectable dermal fillers, and endovenous laser treatment can improve the hands as well as the face.

Training in sclerotherapy for hand veins is available through the American College of Phlebology at http://www.phlebology.org/.

References

1. Duffy DM, Garcia C, Clark RE. The role of sclerotherapy in abnormal varicose hand veins. *Plast Reconstr Surg*. 1999;104: 1474-1479.
2. Breu FX, Guggenbichler S. European consensus meeting on foam sclerotherapy, April, 4–6, 2003, Tegernsee, Germany. *Dermatol Surg*. 2004;30:709-717.
3. Sadick NS. Advances in the treatment of varicose veins: ambulatory phlebectomy, foam sclerotherapy, endovascular laser, and radiofrequency closure. *Dermatol Clin*. 2005;23: 443–455.
4. Goldman MP, Sadick NS, Weiss RA. Cutaneous necrosis, telangiectatic matting, and hyperpigmentation following sclerotherapy. Etiology, prevention, and treatment. *Dermatol Surg*. 1995;21:19-29.
5. Weiss RA, Sadick NS, Goldman MP, Weiss MA. Post-sclerotherapy compression: controlled comparative study of duration of compression and its effects on clinical outcome. *Dermatol Surg*. 1999;25:105-108.

Chapter 16
Treatment of Hand Atrophy with Fat Transplantation

Samuel M. Lam

Introduction

The aging process is multifaceted, encompassing the manifestation of wrinkles, gravity, and volume loss. The last – soft-tissue, bone, and fat loss – is a relatively new concept of how aging occurs, and it has become the cornerstone to my rejuvenation practice. I truly believe that volume loss, especially around the eyes, is the principal expression of aging and merits the most attention. Fat grafting, which is the subject of this chapter, is the main method by which I restore lost volume to the face as well as to the hands. When a person is clothed, the two exposed parts of the body that give away aging are the face and the hands. Therefore, I believe that hand rejuvenation can be secondary only to the face in terms of importance in overall face/body rejuvenation.

Clinical Examination

When approaching hand rejuvenation, there are obviously two major components to aging: aging of the skin as exhibited by rhytids, dyschromias, and poor texture/tone and the focus of this chapter, volume loss with concomitant exposure of deeper structures such as the veins and bones. Fat grafting to the hands is targeted to manage volume loss. However, I have seen some textural improvements to the skin along with reduction in surface dyschromias over a period of a year or more. The current thinking as to why this may occur focuses on possible stem-cell changes to the skin overlying the transplanted fat. This dermatologic improvement does not consistently occur and should not be proffered as a guarantee of any kind. If the patient

is seeking hand rejuvenation that is office-based, I offer them either hyaluronic-acid-based products or calcium hydroxylapatite injections to improve the lost volume, albeit temporary as compared to the relative permanence of fat injections to the hand. Office-based alternatives to hand volume replacement lie beyond the scope of this chapter.

Treatment Application

Anesthesia Considerations

I perform all fat grafting under either intravenous sedation or full general anesthesia in my own private surgical suite. Therefore, the techniques that I will elaborate upon have that inherent bias disclosed. After the patient is properly sedated, a 50/50 mixture of 1% lidocaine with 1:100,000 epinephrine and sterile saline, 10 cc of each, is injected with a spinal needle into the fat pad intended for harvesting. Generally, I would place one 20 cc mixture into the lower abdomen, although I prefer placing a 20 cc mixture into each thigh planned for harvesting.

The hand is then anesthetized with a ring block consisting of straight 1% lidocaine with 1:100,000 epinephrine across the dorsum of the wrist, with a second ring placed just distal to that first block, again along the dorsum of the wrist. A total of usually 2–3 cc per hand is all that is necessary to achieve adequate anesthesia to the entire dorsum of the hand with this double-ring block technique to the dorsal half of the wrist. Finally, additional local anesthesia of 1% lidocaine with 1:100,000 epinephrine is infiltrated into the sites where skin entry will be undertaken with the 18-gauge

M. Alam and M. Pongprutthipan (eds.), *Body Rejuvenation*,
DOI 10.1007/978-1-4419-1093-6_16, © Springer Science+Business Media, LLC 2010

Triport Harvester

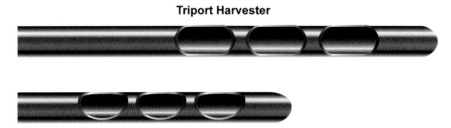

Fig. 16.1 Triport cannula (Tulip, Inc.)

needle (through which the cannula will be introduced). More specifically, each quadrant of the dorsum along with access points for each proximal phalanx is infiltrated with a small aliquot of local anesthetic. Direct local anesthesia into the entire dorsal hand is unnecessary and will cause unwanted ecchymosis and tissue distortion.

Fat Harvesting

Fat is harvested from the areas where a patient is most recalcitrant to lose fat, e.g., lower abdomen for men and either lower abdomen or thighs for women. Fat harvesting is undertaken with a harvesting cannula (I prefer the Triport model (Fig. 16.1) manufactured by Tulip Inc., San Diego, CA)[1] attached to a 10-cc Luer-Lok syringe. A 16-Gauge Nokor needle is used to make the stab incision through the skin as an entry point, inferior aspect of the umbilicus to access the lower abdomen and along the inguinal line for the thighs. I have also found that a Johnny Lock device (Tulip Inc.) (Fig. 16.2) can help maintain 2–3 cc of negative suction pressure on the syringe without manually having to hold that pressure with one's fingers, which greatly alleviates strain injury. With the aforementioned 2–3 cc of negative pressure on the syringe, the fat is harvested and then prepared for processing, to be described.

A few technical points should be emphasized for the novice surgeon undertaking fat harvesting. It is important to retract the harvesting cannula almost all the way back to the skin entry point before readjusting the cannula tip to the next adjacent site for harvesting. Simply twisting the cannula tip over to the adjacent fat

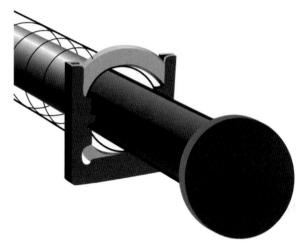

Fig. 16.2 Johnny Lock (Tulip, Inc.)

bed will promote overharvesting of one area since the cannula tip in effect has not moved over to the adjacent site, which can in turn create contour problems in the donor area. When harvesting the inner thigh, the surgeon should keep the leg to be harvested straight and not bent to minimize the occurrence of a contour problem. Furthermore, the cannula should pierce through an initial fascial layer so that the cannula cannot be seen abrading the skin or causing tenting changes to the overlying skin, which would indicate too superficial a harvest and the potential for contour problems in the donor area.

The total amount of fat to be transplanted per hand varies between 20 cc for a conservative injection and 30 cc for a more aggressive transplant and 25 cc on average. For a normal harvest that is not too bloody, expect about 50% of the 10 cc syringe to contain usable fat. Accordingly, to attain 25 cc per hand or 50 cc total of viable fat, one will most likely need 10 syringes. I typically place between 35 and 55 cc of fat into the

---

[1] I have no financial affiliation with any medical device or any medical companies.

face for facial rejuvenation, so you can see that the hands require quite a bit of fat to achieve a durable and appreciable change. Whereas I do not overfill the face, I tend to overfill the hands by about 20% since they are highly mobile and are prone to a little bit of absorption. Also, a hand that is slightly overfilled and maintains the fat will not in most cases be noticeable to an observer. Conversely, a face that is even slightly overfilled can be deforming.

Fat Processing

To attain a purified column of fat, free of lidocaine, blood and lysed fat cells, centrifuge the syringe outfitted with specialized caps and plugs at 3,000 rpm for 3 min duration then pour off the supranatant consisting of oily lysed free fatty acids and then drain off the infranatant consisting of blood and lidocaine. Place a 4 × 4 gauze into the open back side of the syringe to wick away any remaining oily supranatant for 5–10 min before loading the fat into 1 cc syringes in preparation for injection.

Fat Injections

Fat injection into the hand is one of the technically easiest procedures to perform when undertaking fat grafting. If one is just starting out with fat transfer, comfort level can be attained by starting with some hand fat transfers. Unlike the face where fat grafting into a prescribed area cannot be readily adjusted after injection, the fat immediately just transplanted into the hand can be easily spread out and smoothed with gentle digital manipulation.

Fat transfer to the hand is directed at two principal areas for correction: the dorsum of the hand and the sides of the proximal phalanges, with the former area being the most important aesthetic area to rejuvenate. As mentioned, all entry sites are created with an 18-gauge stab incision. Starting with the fingers, the injection cannula (I prefer the Tulip 1.2 mm cannula as my workhorse injection cannula) is used to inject approximately 0.5 cc into each side of the proximal phalanx. The easiest port of entry is at the base of the proximal phalanx in the interphalangeal space, which can be used to access the sides of two adjacent fingers. For the dorsum of the hand, I like to divide the dorsum into

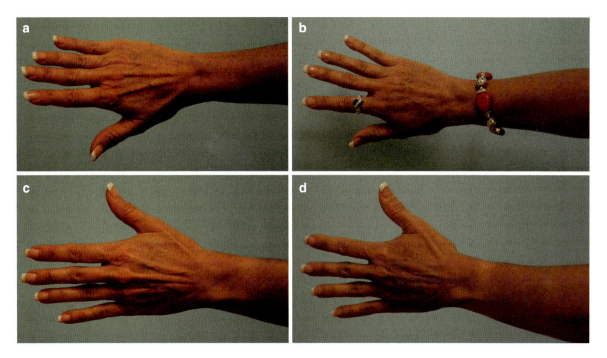

Fig. 16.3 Hand fat transfer using 20 cc per hand across the dorsum and proximal phalanges and shown before (**a,c**) and a year after surgery (**b, d**)

four quadrants and place between 4 and 5 cc per quadrant. Then, feather between 1 and 3 cc of fat into the dorsum of the hand by coming back through the points that were used to access the proximal phalanges and spread the fat in a wide arc to make sure that the grafted fat that was originally performed per quadrant appears smooth and free of any abrupt transitions. Again, any fat that appears lumpy after transplantation can be easily remedied by gentle digital manipulation immediately after injection.

Postoperative Management

There is really no postoperative management except application of ice to minimize edema and soreness for the first 48–72 h following surgery. There is no need for compressive dressings of any kind. Although no strict restrictions in hand movement are required, a general limitation in excessive manual labor should be entertained for the first 7–14 days. The hand will in general look a bit puffy for the first 4–6 weeks, but as the hands are an area that is not often studied in detail, the distortion oftentimes escapes detection. Hand rejuvenation with fat grafting can provide a wonderful and durable aesthetic enhancement with minimal morbidity (Fig. 16.3).

Reference

1. Lam SM, Glasgold MJ, Glasgold RA. *Complementary Fat Grafting*. Philadelphia, PA: Lippincott, Williams, & Wilkins; 2007.

Part V
Arms (and Legs)

Chapter 17
Reduction of Arm Fat by Liposuction

Hayes B. Gladstone

Introduction

While liposuction of the abdomen, flanks, and hips remains the most popular areas for contouring, the upper arm is a significant esthetic concern for most women. A properly contoured arm enhances the fit of blouses and dresses. Tapered upper arms are viewed as a sign of youth and vigor. Despite vigorous activity and weight training, fatty deposits and lax skin may remain in the posterior triceps aspect of the arm extending to the axilla. This upper arm deformity progresses with age into what is known as "butcher" arms.

The surgical rejuvenation of the upper arm remains a persistent challenge despite the many techniques that have been proposed for its improvement.[1] With the advent of tumescent liposuction of the arm, removal of excess fat can be accomplished easily with minimal scarring and fewer complications.[2,3] The problem of newly created or preexisting skin ptosis remains in those patients with poor elasticity of the skin. For excess skin, a limited excision brachioplasty can be performed.

Indications

Tumescent liposuction of the medial and posterior arm is indicated for the recontouring of the arm in patients with excess fat and good skin elasticity.

Clinical Examination and Patient History

Upper arm changes can be divided into four general categories with different treatment options for each. These groups include group 1: minimal to moderate subcutaneous fat with minimal skin laxity, group 2: generalized accumulation of subcutaneous fat with moderate skin laxity, group 3: generalized obesity and extensive skin laxity, and group 4: minimal subcutaneous fat and extensive skin laxity.[1] In all patients, it is essential to evaluate the skin tone with the pinch test to ensure that the skin will shrink adequately to give a cosmetically acceptable result. Patients with minimal to moderate subcutaneous fat with minimal skin laxity have a circumferential increase in fat volume but adequate skin turgor and elasticity. These individuals can benefit greatly from tumescent liposuction of the posterior arm without the need for brachioplasty. Patients described in groups 2 through 4 will require increasingly more aggressive surgical interventions, with more noticeable scarring, to address the ptosis of the skin.

Contraindications

Absolute contraindications include active infection, blood clotting disorders, and pregnancy. Relative contraindications include a history of keloids, hypertrophic scarring, or any condition with healing abnormalities. Relative contraindications include significant weight loss resulting in very loose skin. A full brachioplasty would be indicated.[4,5]

Treatment Application

Procedural Protocol

Tray Setup

There should be up to three trays. The first is for the tumescent anesthesia. A 20-gauge spinal needle is

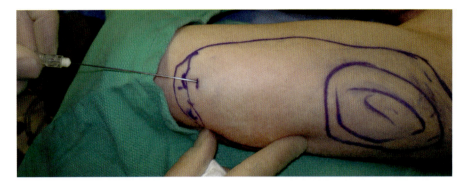

Fig. 17.1 Infiltrating the tumescent anesthesia

attached to a Klein pump. The second tray contains the cannulas for this procedure, 16- and 14-gauge micro-cannulas should be used. These are used with suction. Though some practitioners use ultrasound liposuction, this increases the risk of burns, particularly in this anatomic region. A third tray with an excision tray is needed if a limited excision brachioplasty is being considered.

Relevant Anatomical Structures

The main venous drainage of the arm is provided by the basilic vein on the medial arm and the cephalic vein overlying the biceps brachii muscle. The posterior cutaneous and inferior lateral cutaneous nerves of the arm, which are derived from the radial nerve, providing sensation to the posterior and lateral arm. Sensation of the superior posterior arm is provided by the superior lateral cutaneous nerve, which is derived from the axillary nerve. The ulnar nerve, which has no branches above the elbow, is most superficial at the medial epicondyle. Unlike the cutaneous nerves of the posterior arm derived from the radial nerve, the ulnar nerve is deep to the fascia enveloping the muscles of the arm.

Anesthesia

One percent lidocaine with 1:100,000 epinephrine is used to anesthetize the puncture sites and 0.1% lidocaine with 1:1,000,000 epinephrine is infiltrated using a Klein pump. Depending on the size of the arm, 200–400 cc's are infiltrated (Fig. 17.1). Because this procedure is minimally invasive, sedation is not required.

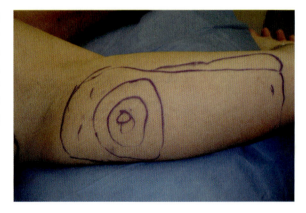

Fig. 17.2 Marking the upper arm

Technique

Following informed consent and photos from the anterior, oblique, and posterior perspectives, the skin is marked. The patient should be sitting with the arm abducted. The distal extent of the liposuction is approximately 1 cm proximal to the epicondyle groove. At the lowest point of the posterior upper arm, the skin is pinched between the finger and thumb. This maneuver will determine the medial and lateral boundaries of the liposuction. The proximal border of the liposuction is in the preaxillary groove just distal to the axilla proper. A line should connect these boundaries creating a rectangular area where the liposuction will be performed. The sidewall of the chest extending posteriorly to the back is often included in the liposuction since it further defines this region (Figs. 17.2 and 17.3). As for most patients, there will be at least some ptotic proximal skin which would benefit from the additional tightening provided by a limited excision axillary brachioplasty.[6]

This excision is defined by a simple ellipse hidden within the axilla. Its anterior and posterior apices are defined by those respective borders of the axilla. The width of the ellipse is determined by the amount of posterior arm skin that can be grasped between finger and thumb. A typical ellipse is between 2 and 4 cm in width.

While external ultrasound can be used, it is not usually necessary since the fat is not very fibrous in the posterior arm. Following tumescent anesthesia, a nick incision with an 11 blade is made just proximal to the elbow. Using a microcannula, for instance, an 18-, 16-, or 14-guage Capistrano, or a 16-, or 14-guage Klein, long sweeping strokes are used in order to prevent an uneven result (Fig. 17.4). Similar to other anatomic areas, a layer of fat should be left to avoid dimpling. While the patient may want dramatic results, over liposuctioning will result in an unnatural appearance and disharmony with the forearm. A liposuction entry point should also be made at the edge of axilla so that liposuctioning can also be performed from a proximal to distal manner. This will result in a smoother result. If a brachioplasty is being performed, then the liposuction can enter through this excision.

The excision is performed down to the subcutaneous plane avoiding deeper vessels and nerves in this area. Some sweat glands may also be removed, and the patient should be educated before the procedure that there may be less perspiration in this area following the surgery – most patients welcome this added benefit. Undermining is performed in order to reduce tension on the wound (Fig. 17.5). It is then closed with 3–0 vicryl buried sutures and 4–0 nylon running epidermal sutures (Fig. 17.6). Occasionally dog ears may form, and should be removed which may extend the incision on to the posterior arm. A postoperative dressing is applied which should have a Coban wrap (Fig. 17.7a–d).

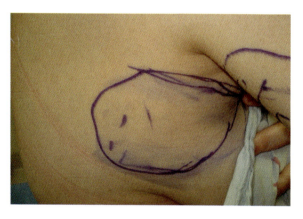

Fig. 17.3 Marking the chest wall and posterior extension

Postoperative Instructions

Patients should keep the arms wrapped for the first 24 h. Unlike tumescent liposuction of other areas where there may be significant drainage, it is minimal in this location. At the first dressing change, the wounds should be cleaned with dilute hydrogen peroxide and polysporin and nonstick Telfa bandages should be applied. A coverlet band aid can cover the Telfa. Bandages are changed on a daily basis. A compression arm garment should be worn for up to 2 weeks which will decrease swelling and bruising and may aid in uniform skin contraction. When the limited excision

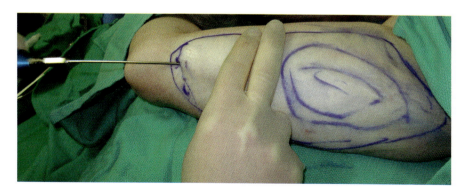

Fig. 17.4 Using a 14G microcannula and liposuctioning in broad, crisscrossing strokes

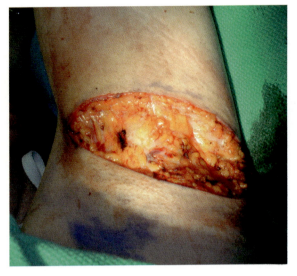

Fig. 17.5 Following the limited axillary brachioplasty incision

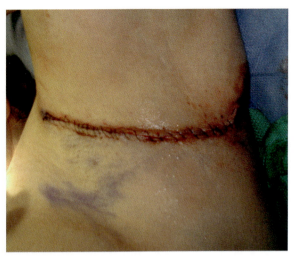

Fig. 17.6 Brachioplasty incision closed with 3-0 vicryl and 4-0 nylon. No drain is needed since this is a superficial excision

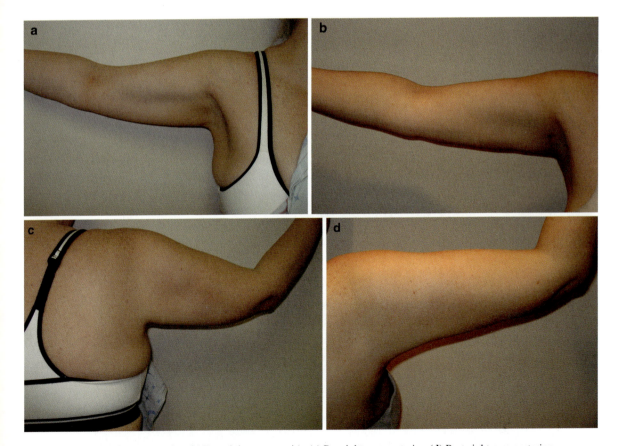

Fig. 17.7 (**a**) Pre-right arm anterior. (**b**) Post-right arm anterior. (**c**) Pre-right arm posterior. (**d**) Post-right arm posterior

brachioplasty is performed, it is imperative that the patient does not extend her upper arms beyond ninety degrees, or lift objects for 4–6 weeks.

Complications

Minor complications include ecchymosis and swelling. Other complications include hematoma, infection, keloid or hypertrophic scarring, nerve damage, and asymmetry. There can also be dimpling if a thin layer of fat is not maintained as well as striae if the liposuction is too superficial. Dehiscence of the incision is a risk for the limited excision brachioplasty if the upper arm is extended.

Pearls

1. Tumescent anesthesia is the key to this procedure and allows it to be performed under local anesthesia in an office setting.
2. When performing liposuction, use 12 inch cannulas so that there are long smooth strokes. As with any other anatomic region, multiple entry points will result in a smoother outcome.
3. At the distal aspect of the upper arm near the elbow, avoid suctioning medially since this may increase the risk of ulnar nerve injury.
4. If liposuction is indicated, then in most of these patients, there will also be sufficient skin laxity at the proximal upper arm to perform a limited excision brachioplasty. This excision will produce much tauter skin and contour when compared with liposuction alone or a skin tightening device.

5. The depth of the brachioplasty incision only needs to go to the subcutaneous level. This will prevent any type of potential nerve damage or lymphedema.
6. Because the brachioplasty ellipse is within the axilla, the patient may have the added benefit of decreased axillary hidrosis.

Conclusion

The upper arm is often an overlooked cosmetic unit. Yet, it plays an important role in fashion and what society considers being active and fit. Upper arm rejuvenation with tumescent liposuction and limited excision brachioplasty is a minimally invasive method for producing more esthetically appealing arms. Recovery time is relatively short and serious complications are rare. This procedure should be in every dermatologic surgeon's cosmetic procedure armentarium.

References

1. Teimourian B, Malekzadeh S. Rejuvenation of the upper arm. *Plast Reconstr Surg*. 1998;102(2):545-551.
2. Lillis PJ. Liposuction of the arms. *Dermatol Clin*. 1999;17(4): 783-797.
3. Lillis PJ. Liposuction of the arms, calves and ankles. *Dermatol Surg*. 1997;23(12):1161-1168.
4. Appelt EA, Janis JE, Rohrich RJ. An algorithmic approach to upper arm contouring. *Plast Reconstr Surg*. 2006;118(1): 237-246.
5. Hurwitz DJ, Holland SW. The L brachioplasty: an innovative approach to correct excess tissue of the upper arm, axilla, and lateral chest. *Plast Reconstr Surg*. 2006;117:403-411.
6. Trussler AP, Rohrich RJ. Limited incision medial brachio-plasty: technical refinements in upper arm contouring. *Plast Reconstr Surg*. 2008;121:305-307.

Chapter 18
Reduction of Excess Arm Skin via Surgical Excision

John Y.S. Kim, Robert D. Galiano, and Donald W. Buck

Introduction

With natural aging or with significant weight loss, the skin and soft tissue of the upper arm undergo changes in their fat-skin composition and elastic properties. The relative laxity of supportive tissue and the relative excess of skin vis-à-vis underlying subcutaneous fat will lead to varying degrees of upper extremity *ptosis*. Not only is the appearance of this excess skin cosmetically problematic, but can also be functionally impairing with redundant soft tissue hampering adduction of the arm and occasionally leading to dermatitis within the folds.

In cases of milder upper arm excess and milder ptosis, where the skin has retained elasticity, liposuction alone may be an option. However, when the skin excess and laxity are more pronounced, direct surgical excision – brachioplasty – is necessary. Since brachioplasty was first described in 1954 by Correa–Iturraspe and Fernandez, the essential promise and pitfall of brachioplasty have remained the same: to restore normal contour by excision of excess skin while concomitantly minimizing visible scars.

There has certainly been a recent surge of interest in brachioplasty with the heightened interest in both aesthetic and bariatric surgery. According to recent statistics from the American Society of Plastic Surgeons (ASPS), there were 14,886 brachioplasty procedures performed in 2006 alone – an increase of over 4,300% since 2000.[1] Moreover, as bariatric surgery continues to improve technologically and command a greater presence in the modern healthcare milieu, subsequent postbariatric surgery for the body contouring, including the upper arms, is projected to increase significantly.

Clinical Examination and Patient History

Patients seeking brachioplasty should be approached in a similar fashion as those seeking any cosmetic surgical intervention. A thorough history should be obtained, with a focus on existing comorbidities, such as cardiopulmonary disease, diabetes, or other chronic illnesses, which could place them at risk for adverse events. Sound clinical judgment should be used when determining a patient's candidacy for exposure to surgical and general anesthetic risk. It is also important to obtain a detailed past surgical history, documenting any prior upper extremity procedures that might alter the anatomic position of integral upper arm and axillary structures. Prior surgery of the arms or axilla could affect the viability of brachioplasty flaps and also – in the case of axillary node dissection – enhance the risk of lymphedema. It is imperative over the course of the consultation to establish the patient's motivation for seeking out surgical assistance and to counsel them regarding their overall expectations and the expected surgical outcome.

Finally, after a thorough history has been obtained, it is important to conduct a detailed physical examination, including documentation of cardiopulmonary exam findings. In addition to the overall appearance of the skin and soft tissue of the upper extremity, it is imperative to conduct a full neurovascular examination. Preoperative assessment of upper extremity motor and sensory function is crucial and becomes important in the postoperative period if motor or sensory deficits are encountered. The proper physical exam should be conducted with the patient standing or seated in an upright position, with both arms abducted at 90° from the trunk. In this position, excess skin is easily visualized and can be better characterized via palpation and the "pinch test."

Several surgeons have attempted to establish grading systems of upper extremity skin ptosis as a way to determine the appropriate surgical technique for upper extremity rejuvenation.[2,3] In general, it is best to approach the upper arm with regard to two major factors: the degree of subcutaneous fat deposition and overall amount of skin excess. Patients who suffer from excess fat deposition, but lack skin excess, probably benefit most from upper extremity suction lipectomy. Patients who have excess skin, regardless of fat deposition, will require brachioplasty for best results. If patients have both excess fat deposition and excess skin, suction lipectomy and brachioplasty can be judiciously performed in tandem.

Some cosmetic surgeons prefer to use suction lipectomy on all patients undergoing brachioplasty, regardless of fat deposition characteristics. It is their belief that suction lipectomy reduces upper arm volume without damaging important lymphatics, nerves, or vessels, and allows better tissue mobilization.

Treatment Application

On the day of surgery, it is imperative to mark the patient preoperatively. Again, have the patient standing, or seated in the upright position, with both arms abducted 90° from the trunk. With your hands, palpate the intermuscular groove on the inferomedial aspect of the upper arm, between the biceps and triceps muscles. With a skin marker, trace along the intermuscular septum from the axilla to the medial epicondyle of the humerus. This line will act as a reference, and represents the positioning of the future scar. Next, using the pinch test centered about your reference line, you can easily trace out the borders of your upper and lower incision lines, creating an ellipse of "excess" skin that can be excised. A conservative approach is generally preferred, as it is easy to remove extra skin margins in the operating room if warranted.

With regard to the axillary skin excess, several techniques have been described and are available to the surgeon, including the use of a wedge, L, or T pattern incision.[5,6] Axillary and trunk skin excess is discussed in a separate chapter, thus only upper arm skin excess is presented here. It is important to keep in mind that massive weight loss patients may require reduction of both upper arm and axillary skin for optimal results.

At the proximal aspect of the upper arm, within the axillary fold, it is best to tailor the incision by first generating an axillary reference line. The axillary reference line is highlighted by drawing a short line within the axillary fold, at the proximal aspect of the upper arm, which is perpendicular to the upper arm reference line. Along the axillary reference line, you can again use the pinch test to set your incisional borders and determine an acceptable amount of skin excess to excise. Some surgeons have advocated the use of a z-plasty within the axillary fold, instead of a wedge pattern, to reduce the overall tension within the fold after excess skin has been excised (See Fig. 18.1).

After generating skin markings, finish the preoperative assessment by reexamining both arm markings together to assess for symmetry and accuracy. If discrepancies are apparent, repeat the marking process to insure accuracy, remembering the tenet: look twice, cut once. The above marking technique, without z-plasty, will generate a closure pattern and scar in the shape of a T.

The patient should be placed under general anesthesia for the procedure. They should be placed in the supine position on the operating room table, with both arms abducted to 90°. The upper extremities should be prepped circumferentially with sterile prep solution, remembering to apply also a wide prep to the axilla. Routine sterile draping should also be used.

Of note, if suction lipectomy of the upper arms is also being performed, it is generally performed first, prior to skin excision. Depending on the degree of elasticity of the skin and overall surgical plan, the liposuction can be performed just prior to the excision or staged as a separate earlier procedure.

Once the patient is prepped and draped, incise the skin along your preestablished incision borders. It is imperative to remain superficial with your incisions, as only the excess skin should be removed. Incision into and dissection of deeper tissue planes places important neurovascular structures at risk, especially those structures with a superficial course, including the medial antebrachial cutaneous nerve and the medial brachial cutaneous nerves which perforate the intermuscular septum to supply the skin and soft tissue of the medial upper arm. In addition, deep dissection could lead to lymphatic disruption and the development of a lymphocele or seroma (Fig. 18.2).[4] Particular attention should be paid to the axillary incisions, so as to avoid injury to both major vascular and lymphatic networks.

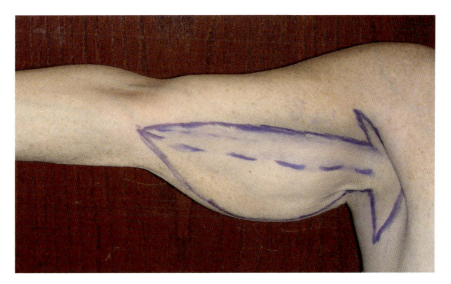

Fig. 18.1 Preoperative skin markings. This image shows the proper preoperative markings for the brachioplasty procedure. The reference line is indicated by the dotted line. The upper and lower incision lines were created by using the pinch test about the reference line. The elliptical incision marking within the axilla were also created using the pinch test. Orienting the axillary incisions perpendicular to the upper arm incision will help to pull the skin taught into the axilla, enhancing the upper arm "lift"

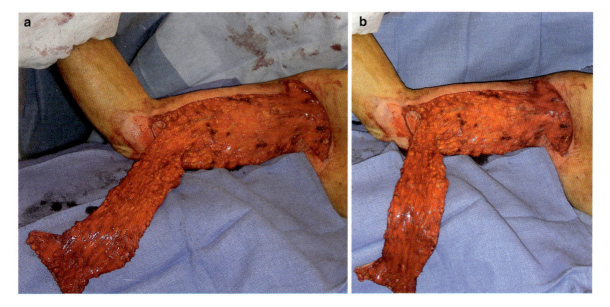

Fig. 18.2 Intraoperative skin excision. This image details the dissection plane for proper excess skin excision. Carrying your dissection plane too deep within the subcutaneous tissue can injure the lymphatics and lead to an increased risk of seroma formation

Once the skin is incised and the superficial layer is dissected free from the field, it is time to turn your attention to wound closure and skin approximation. Adequate hemostasis is crucial to limit the risk of hematoma formation. The remaining wound should be closed in layers. The deepest layer is closed using a 3–0 absorbable suture (Fig. 18.3). This deep layer serves two major functions: minimizing deadspace and reducing tension on the epidermal layer. If a large deadspace exists, a small Jackson-Pratt (JP) drain can be placed to reduce the risk of postoperative hematoma/seroma. After adequate deep dermal closure, a 4–0 absorbable suture can be used to approximate the epidermis via a subcuticular stitch. Alternatively, a 4–0 nonabsorbable

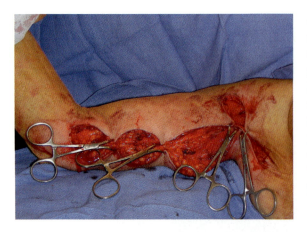

Fig. 18.3 Intraoperative skin closure. This image depicts the brachioplasty defect just prior to skin closure. Penetrating towel clips can be used to help align the skin edges and reduce the tension while sutures are being placed

suture can be used to close the epidermis in a running fashion. Steri-strips can be applied to add an extra element of support. The incision should be dressed with sterile gauze and the entire upper extremity wrapped with ACE bandages. The compressive dressing should be kept in place for 5–7 days. JP drainage should be carefully monitored. To reduce seroma formation, the drain should not be removed until there is less than 30 mL of drainage over 24 h.

Outcomes and Complications

The most common complications resulting from brachioplasty are similar to other procedures involving excess skin excision. In a recent review within the literature, the reported incidence of complications after brachioplasty was approximately 25%.[4] The majority of these complications were minor, requiring reoperation in only 5% of cases. The most common complications encountered were seroma formation and hypertrophic scarring (10%), followed by cellulitis and wound dehiscence (7.5%). Although complications can occur commonly, when encountered they can generally be treated conservatively with good results.

The most difficult aspect to address following brachioplasty is overall scar cosmesis. It is important that patients undergoing brachioplasty understand that they will have a visible scar postoperatively. Unfortunately, despite numerous technique modifications, unsightly and/or hypertrophic scars have not been eliminated altogether. Patients should be instructed on appropriate postoperative care, including the reduction of suture line stress and tension, as well as how to recognize infection/dehiscence. They should be seen in clinic for follow-up examination on regular intervals to insure proper wound healing. If hypertrophic scarring develops, steroid injections and pressure dressings have been used with variable results. In severe cases, where possible, scar revision may be necessary.

Conclusion

The number of patients seeking surgical assistance with upper extremity rejuvenation is rising exponentially (over 4,300% increase since 2000). This number will only continue to climb as the baby boomers age and the number of bariatric procedures increases. Brachioplasty remains the gold-standard treatment of upper extremity skin excess, and can be performed in conjunction with liposuction when indicated. There are a number of standard incisions, technical modifications, and evolving strategies regarding differential liposuction which will continue to enhance outcomes and scar cosmesis after the brachioplasty procedure. With proper patient selection and counseling and a thorough understanding of upper extremity anatomy, brachioplasty can be performed safely with excellent cosmetic results and overall patient satisfaction.

References

1. 2000/2005/2006 National plastic surgery statistics. American Society of Plastic Surgeons. http://www.plasticsurgery.org. Accessed 1.30.2008.
2. Cannistra C, Valero R, Benelli C, Marmuse JP. Brachioplasty after massive weight loss: a simple algorithm for surgical plan. *Aesth Plast Surg*. 2007;31:6-9.
3. Khatib HA. Classification of brachial ptosis: strategy for treatment. *Plast Reconstr Surg*. 2007;119:1337-1342.
4. Knoetgen J, Moran SL. Long-term outcomes and complications associated with brachioplasty: a retrospective review and cadaveric study. *Plast Reconstr Surg*. 2006;117(7):2219-2223.
5. Pascal JF, Le Louarn C. Brachioplasty. *Aesth Plast Surg*. 2005;29:423-429.
6. Strauch B, Greenspun D, Levine J, Baum T. A technique of brachioplasty. *Plast Reconstr Surg*. 2004;113(3):1044-1048.

Chapter 19
Skin Tightening of the Arms and Legs with Radiofrequency and Broadband Light

Matthew J. Mahlberg, Julie K. Karen, and Elizabeth K. Hale

Introduction

With increasing age, skin that was once full and firm begins to sag, developing laxity and redundancy. Traditionally, a surgical procedure was required for treatment of this laxity as in rhytidectomy, browlift, or brachioplasty. More recently, technological advances have shifted the treatments toward nonsurgical alternatives in place of plastic surgery. Further refinement toward nonablative tissue remodeling has proven popular because of its efficacy and markedly reduced downtime and complication rate. The major emphasis in the field of nonablative tissue remodeling has been on facial rejuvenation; however, these techniques can be applied to other areas of the body as well. Of particular interest has been the development of the nonsurgical techniques for areas of loose skin on the posterior upper arms and around the knees, sites of concern particularly for many women. These areas of tissue redundancy are troublesome as they can be difficult to otherwise treat and are not necessarily a reflection of body weight or thinness. Certain devices, particularly radiofrequency (RF) and broadband light sources, have demonstrated utility for tightening and nonsurgical contouring of mild to moderate skin laxity in these regions.

RF and broadband light sources are well-established, nonablative modalities for the treatment of unwanted structural changes and can be particularly useful for body contouring and the treatment of mild to moderate laxity on the arms and legs. These noninvasive devices produce directed delivery of energy to deep dermal tissue, inducing collagen contraction and dermal remodeling eventuating in neocollagenesis. However, these techniques differ substantially with respect to their specific mechanisms.

In contrast to most dermatologic lasers that are coherent light sources and target-specific chromophores, RF energy is produced by an electrical current. RF energy produces a thermal effect when its high-frequency electrical current flows through target skin and encounters tissue of high impedance in the deep dermis and subcutaneous fat.[1] These properties allow RF to circumvent energy scatter and absorption by epidermal pigment and therefore, generate significant thermal energy within deeper tissue layers. This three-dimensional volumetric heating of the deep dermis leads to collagen denaturation, remodeling, and tissue contraction.[2] Ultimately, these effects lead to improvement in skin laxity without alteration of the superficial portions of skin.

RF devices have one of two different electrode configurations–monopolar or bipolar. Monopolar devices have two electrodes, one that emits the RF energy and a second dispersive electrode that serves as a grounding pad. Monopolar devices are characterized by high power density and relatively deep penetration (Fig. 19.1). In contrast, bipolar devices have two identical electrodes set at a short, fixed distance. Electrical current flow is restricted to this small distance, resulting in a more controlled current distribution, but significantly less depth of power penetration.[3] Examples of currently available RF devices are found in Table 19.1.

Intense pulsed light (IPL), a form of broadband light, is frequently used for photorejuvenation. Traditionally, IPL uses a flashlamp combined with optical filters selective for wavelengths between 500–900 nm to target melanin and hemoglobin. This form of IPL is well established as a nonablative method to reduce telangiectasias and pigmentary alteration and improve superficial skin texture.[4] Histologic examination of

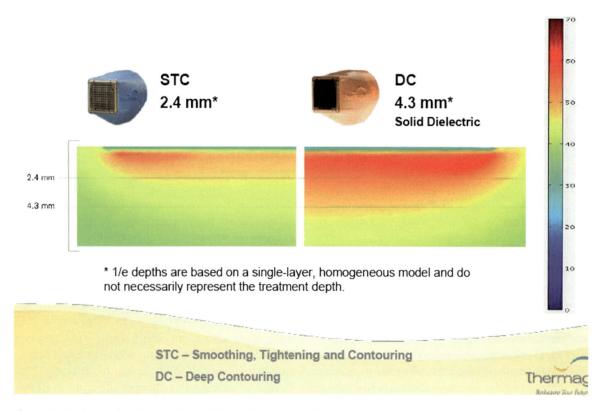

Fig. 19.1 Heating profile of the STC tip and DC tip (Thermage, Inc.)

Table 19.1 Devices utilizing radiofrequency for tissue tightening

Device name	Manufacturer	Type
ThermaCool NXT™ and TC™	Thermage	Monopolar RF
Polaris™	Syneron	Bipolar RF with diode (900 nm)
ReFirme™	Syneron	Bipolar RF with diode (900 nm)
Aluma™	Lumenis	Bipolar RF with vacuum
Accent/Accent XL™	Alma Lasers	Unipolar and bipolar RF

Table 19.2 Devices utilizing broadband infrared light for tissue tightening

Device name	Manufacturer	Wavelengths targeted
Starlux IR® and DeppIR®	Palomar	850–1,350 nm
Titan™	Cutera	1,100–1,800 nm
SkinTyte™	Sciton	800–1,400 nm

skin after treatment with these devices exhibits new upper papillary dermal collagen formation.[5] More recently, though, IPL devices utilizing broadband infrared light (wavelengths: 800–1,800 nm) have been introduced. These longer wavelength devices target water as a chromophore and achieve penetration to the deep dermis, thereby eliciting collagen denaturation with subsequent remodeling.[6] The epidermis is protected through contact cooling allowing for deep heating without epidermal damage. Examples of broadband infrared light devices are found in Table 19.2.

Combination treatment options utilizing radiofrequency with a variety of light sources have been designed with the hope of augmenting the actions of both treatments while minimizing adverse effects. Examples of such devices are outlined in Table 19.3. Termed electro-optical synergy, the optical energy provided by the light source preheats dermal structures, creating a temperature differential between targeted structures and adjacent tissue. The temperature changes allow for more targeted RF energy application, reduced impedance, and ultimately lowered optical energy levels.[1] In addition to improving skin texture and laxity, other aspects of skin rejuvenation are improved such as rhytides, pigmentation, and vascularity.

Table 19.3 Combination radiofrequency and light devices for tissue tightening

Device	Manufacturer	Components
Aurora SR™	Syneron	RF + IR (400–980 nm; 580–980 nm; 680–980 nm)
Polaris WR™	Syneron	RF + Diode $_{(900\,nm)}$
ReFirme™	Syneron	RF + IR (700–2,000 nm)
VelaSmooth™	Syneron	RF + IR (700–2,000 nm) + Vacuum

Clinical Examination

These nonsurgical skin tightening modalities can provide skin tightening and improvement of skin redundancy with minimal complications, no downtime, and no surgical incision. Still, appropriate patient selection and counseling is essential to ensure procedural success and patient satisfaction. The best candidates for the procedure are those with mild to moderate skin laxity and minimal excess fat in the treatment area. Common areas for treatment include the posterior upper arms and the anterior thighs, just proximal to the knees. Patients with more severe laxity, excess fat, or those who want more dramatic improvement should be counseled to consider an alternative surgical procedure. Prior to performing the procedure, all patients should be counseled to ensure realistic expectations. Pre- and postprocedural photographs and measurements may be taken with standardized lighting and positioning to illustrate treatment outcome which may be subtle to the patient's eye. Finally, as with any medical procedure, a thorough medical history should be performed to ascertain the patient's general health and exclude patients with specific contraindications. Special consideration should be given to patients with tattoos over the areas to be treated given the potential for bulk heating.

Treatment Application

Patients are usually offered some combination of an oral or intramuscular analgesic and/or a mild anxiolytic before the procedure. A topical anesthetic may be used to ease patient anxiety, but because these devices generally produce deep dermal heat, anesthetic applied to the surface does little to reduce discomfort.

To minimize the risk of burn injury while using these tissue tightening devices, all residue on the skin surface should be removed with a gentle cleanser. This includes wiping the skin clean of any topical anesthetic. Infiltration of local anesthesia should be avoided as this may unpredictably alter tissue resistance and potentially increase the risk of thermal injury.

The skin must always have a generous layer of coupling fluid (before radiofrequency) or cooling gel (before broadband light sources) to further minimize the risk of burn injury. Grid markings may be applied before the procedure is initiated to facilitate tracking which areas have already been treated. These grid patterns are often included with the device. Alternatively, a white gel pen can be used to mark the skin before the procedure. Care must be taken to avoid any type of marking which may contain metal, as there is a theoretical risk of inadvertent burn if the device comes into contact with metal residues. It is helpful to mark the areas to be treated while the patient is standing, so that the dependent areas are more prominent. This is especially useful for the loose skin which is common around the knees. When the patient assumes a recumbent position, a return pad needs to be affixed to the patient if a monopolar radiofrequency device is being utilized.

When treating nonfacial skin, treatment parameters should be adjusted to reflect anatomic differences such as increased skin thickness and the absence of underlying vital structures. Particular attention should be paid to sensitive areas including the inner arm and inner thighs. In general, higher energy levels are used to treat the arms and legs relative to the face. For certain devices (i.e., Thermage™), a designated tip with a larger surface area is used to treat the arms and legs.

Patient feedback is very important with these tissue tightening devices, as the patient should be able to feel warmth. Initial treatment parameters were associated with significant, sometimes intolerable pain. Newer parameters, however, rely on multiple passes at lower fluences and are generally well-tolerated. There is significantly less pain associated with treatment with certain vacuum-assisted bipolar RF devices (i.e., Aluma™, VelaSmooth™). Prior to treatment with more painful devices, the patient is provided with a 4-point feedback scale (0-nothing, 1-warm, 2-hot, 3-very hot, 4-intolerable). The patient is instructed to anticipate accumulating warmth, which should be uncomfortable but still tolerable (a 2 or 3 on the feedback scale).

After the initial treatment, a patient may appreciate some initial improvement of the treated areas due to immediate collagen contraction. Generally, the treated collagen remodels over a course of several months. The patient is seen back 3–4 months after the procedure, and the patient and treating physician can decide together whether or not a second procedure is indicated. Postprocedural care after both RF and IPL is minimal. Patients may experience a warm sensation in the skin for several hours after the procedure. In addition, there may be mild edema and/or erythema that can last for 1–2 days. Water or cooling gels can be applied to the skin for patient comfort. Follow up in cases without complications should be in 4–6 weeks and then spaced several months apart to monitor for continued tightening from a single treatment which may continue up to 6 months after the procedure in studies on facial and neck skin.[7,8] (Figs. 19.2 and 19.3). Durability of effect on the arms and legs has not yet been reported.

Adverse events are uncommon in RF and IPL when used for tissue tightening. Both modalities may produce prolonged erythema or edema which may be treated with a tapering course of corticosteroids. Superficial burns are very uncommon and usually only occur from electrical arcing due to uneven contact between electrode and skin. They should be treated with local wound care. In one report, infrared-based IPL caused scarring due to bulk heating and consequent third-degree burns.[9] Overall, though, both therapies are well tolerated, and the incidence of complications is extremely rare.

Conclusion

Although radiofrequency and broadband light sources are effective in skin tightening, they are only able to make an impact in cases of mild to moderate skin laxity

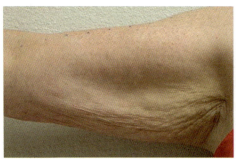
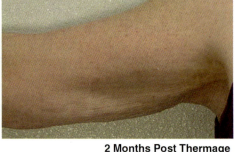

Before Thermage   **2 Months Post Thermage**

All before and after photos are un-retouched.
Results vary depending on age and skin condition   **Treatment by Martin Safko, M.D.**

Fig. 19.2 (**a**) Before and (**b**) 2 months after Thermage procedure to treat the arm

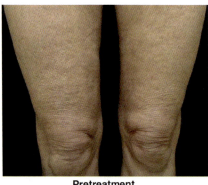

Pretreatment   **12 Months Post Treatment**

All before and after photos are un-retouched.
Results vary depending on age and skin condition   Suzanne Kilmer, M.D.

Fig. 19.3 (**a**) Before and (**b**) 12 months after Thermage procedure to treat thighs

and the results may be suboptimal when compared to more invasive options. Ideally, a device could even more precisely and dramatically contour and tighten with results approximating a surgical approach. Newer technologies and techniques are being investigated to assist in this goal. These include more precise methods of delivering energy such as an RF device with fine needle electrodes[10] and an infrared light device that allows for variable depth heating.[11] An alternative treatment option, transcutaneous ultrasound, has shown promise in tissue tightening of the forehead, cheek, and neck in a preliminary study.[12] While these newer technologies are developed, more detailed and longer-term studies of current devices should help to better define the role of radiofrequency and broadband light sources in the nonsurgical treatment of skin laxity of the arms and legs.

References

1. Alster TS, Lupton JR. Nonablative cutaneous remodeling using radiofrequency devices. *Clin Dermatol.* 2007;25: 487-491.
2. Zelickson BD, Kist D, Bernstein E, et al. Histologic and ultrastructural evaluation of the effects of radiofrequency based nonablative dermal remodeling device: a pilot study. *Arch Dermatol.* 2004;140:204-209.
3. Gold MH, Goldman MP, Rao J, Carcamo AS, Ehrlich M. Treatment of wrinkles and elastosis using vacuum-assisted bipolar radiofrequency heating of the dermis. *Dermatol Surg.* 2007;33:300-309.
4. Narurkar VA. Lasers, light sources, and radiofrequency devices for skin rejuvenation. *Semm Cutan Med Surg.* 2006;25:145-150.
5. Goldberg DJ. New collagen formation after dermal remodeling with intense pulsed light sources. *J Cutan Laser Ther.* 2000;2:59-61.
6. Gold MH. Tissue tightening: a hot topic utilizing deep dermal heating. *J Drugs Dermatol.* 2007;12:1238-1242.
7. Alster TS, Tanzi E. Improvement of neck and cheek laxity with a nonablative radiofrequency device: a lifting experience. *Dermatol Surg.* 2004;30:503-507.
8. Fitzpatrck R, Geronemus R, Goldberg D, Kaminer M, Kilmer S, Ruiz-Esparza J. Multicenter study of noninvasive radiofrequency for periorbital tissue tightening. *Lasers Surg Med.* 2003;33:232-242.
9. Narukar V. Full thickness permanent scars from bulk heating using an infrared light source. *Lasers Surg Med.* 2006;S18:S96.
10. Laubach HJ, Manstein D. Histologic evaluation of minimally invasive radiofrequency exposure. *Lasers Surg Med.* 2006;S18:S28.
11. Ross EV, Thomas BC, Clinton TS, Paithankar DY. Variable depth laser skin heating and tightening. *Lasers Surg Med.* 2006;S18:S96.
12. Alam M, White L, Majzoub R, Martin N, Yoo S. Safety and efficacy of transcutaneous ultrasound for forehead, cheek, and neck tissue tightening. *Laser Surg Med.* 2007;S19:S56.

Chapter 20
Sclerotherapy of Leg Veins

Mary Martini and Katherine K. Brown

Introduction

Sclerotherapy is the injection of a chemical irritant into small and large venous varicosities to create complete destruction of the vessel wall via irreversible endothelial damage and localized thrombosis. The aim is improved hemodynamics, elimination of symptoms, and achievement of an improved aesthetic result.[4] Sclerotherapy is a first-line treatment for small intracutaneous varicosities, and is ideally suited for vessels measuring 0.3mm-0.5 mm.

Clinical Exam and Patient Selection

Achieving good outcomes with sclerotherapy begins with appropriate patient selection and a thorough medical history. The presence and extent of symptoms of venous insufficiency, should be addressed during initial patient assessment. Absolute and relative contraindications to fluid and foam sclerotherapy are reviewed here. The most commonly encountered side effects include pain and edema at injection site, hyperpigmentation, and matting. Despite these, in experienced hands, sclerotherapy remains the most effective technique to treat small venous varicose vessels of the lower extremities.

Physical evaluation should include both standing and supine inspection and palpation. Keys for an effective clinical evaluation include adequate even lighting and use of a handheld Doppler auscultation device to detect points of reflux. Incompetent varicose veins will be distinguished on Doppler by retrograde flow. Large vessel disease of reticular veins, perforators, or deep incompetent veins exist must be addressed before treating superficial telangiectasias with sclerotherapy. For small vessels, check for rapid capillary filling, which suggests high flow rate and possible resistance to sclerotherapy. One primary goal of the exam is to create a topography of all known areas of superficial reflux. After marking the venous map, photographs should be included in the medical record to assist with accurate operative planning and to serve as a comparison tool illustrating posttreatment results.

In selecting appropriate candidates, it is helpful to understand patient goals and expectations for the procedure. Are they considering treatment for cosmetic reasons or do they expect relief of symptoms? Do they understand the expected, as well as rare, sequelae and risks? Are they willing to utilize short- and long-term compression to maximize outcome? During the preoperative evaluation, one should discuss postoperative care and downtime. Downtime depends on the scope of treatment, but one can expect 2 or 3 weeks of restrictions on lifting and intense exercise. Expected side effect is pain with injection and edema. Minor risks include hyperpigmentation, local thrombosis, and matting. Rare and serious adverse events are anaphylaxis, nerve damage, thrombophlebitis, skin necrosis, and complications of thromboembolism, including deep venous thrombosis, pulmonary emboli, and visual disturbances.

M. Alam and M. Pongprutthipan (eds.), *Body Rejuvenation*,
DOI 10.1007/978-1-4419-1093-6_20, © Springer Science+Business Media, LLC 2010

Table 20.1 Preoperative interview- pertinent findings

HPI elements	Medical history elements
Age	Hypertension
Weight, height, BMI	Diabetes mellitus
Duration/progression of varicosities	Cardiovascular disease
Associated symptoms	Vasculitis
Exacerbating factors	Thromboembolic disease
Prior treatment	Coagulopathy
Venous trauma or disease	Malignancy
Obstetric history	Allergies/anaphylaxis
Family history of vascular/ venous disease	Tobacco, alcohol, illicit drug use
Lifestyle factors (active vs. sedentary, occupational sitting/standing)	Use of medications (hormones, anticoagulants, NSAIDS)

Table 20.2 Contraindications to sclerotherapy

Absolute	Allergy to sclerosant
	Acute DVT
	Local infection
	Severe systemic infection
	Immobility
	Peripheral arterial disease (stage 3 or 4)
	Hyperthyroidism
	Pregnancy 1st trimester or late 3rd trimester
Relative	Leg edema/ulcer
	Peripheral arterial disease (stage 2)
	Hypercoagulability
	Thrombophilia with history of DVT
	Bronchial asthma
	Extensive comorbidity
	Diabetic polyneuropathy

Treatment Application

Sclerosants

The four most commonly used liquid sclerosants are compared in Table 20.3 to highlight the advantages and disadvantages of each. The detergent class of sclerosants act by disrupting the vein cell membrane and include polidocanol and sodium tetradecyl sulfate (STS). STS has FDA approval for the treatment of varicosities of the lower extremity, while polidocanol is widely used outside the US, but is not currently an FDA approved sclerosant. Hypertonic saline is a hyperosmolar agent used off-label for sclerotherapy. It has a good safety profile and may be the ideal choice for a patient at risk for allergy to other agents; however, it is

very painful and has inconsistent results, especially on larger vessels. Chromated glycerin is in the irritant class of sclerosants. This practitioner finds it useful on only the very smallest (<0.2 mm) veins. Individual practitioners vary in their preference of sclerosant, but in general, the detergents are the most widely used because of their efficacy and versatility.

Treatment Algorithm for Large and Small Vessels

Regional variation in response and efficacy is common; therefore, it is helpful to divide the lower extremity into treatment regions that correspond to venous beds. In the authors' experience, we find the posterior thigh responds well, the medial and lateral thighs are prone to matting, and the ankles are often treatment resistant and prone to ulceration. As a general rule, large vessel sclerotherapy, which would address saphenofemoral and saphenopopliteal junctions, perforators and large (>3 mm) reticular veins, should be completed before proceeding to small vessel sclerotherapy to treat small (<3 mm) reticular veins and surface spider veins (Fig. 20.1).

A treatment algorithm based predominantly on vessel size is summarized in Table 20.4. When measuring veins, one should avoid stretching the skin, which may falsely widen visible vessels. Helpful supplies include a clear plastic ruler, a magnifying eyepiece, and both a 25 gauge and a 30 gauge needle for comparison, which measure 0.3 and 0.5 mm diameter, respectively (Table 20.5).

The dose of detergent sclerosants should be adjusted to fit the clinical scenario. Lower concentrations should be considered in a patient who bruises easily, who is older than 60, and for thin-walled vessels. For a vessel less than 0.3 mm, increasing concentration threefold rarely improves result but may increase pigmentation. For a vessel 0.5–0.9 mm, the practitioner may be able to increase sclerosant twofold with beneficial results. For a vessel greater than 2 mm, the sclerosant concentration often must be increased to overcome high volume blood flow within the vessel.

To inject large varicose veins, it is important to place the leg in a horizontal position, occasionally elevating it 5–30°, to obtain adequate emptying.[2] This technique helps maximize sclerosant contact with the

Table 20.3 Comparison of common sclerosants

Solution	Concentration	Max dose	Advantages	Disadvantages	Complications
Sodium tetradecyl sulfate	0.1–3%	10 cc per session	FDA approved for sclerotherapy. Most potent agent, useful for large veins at high strengths and small veins at low strengths	Mild discomfort on injection. No more effective than saline for small veins. May cause significant hyperpigmentation	PE, anaphylaxis, DVT; deaths reported at therapeutic volumes and concentrations; CTN at 1% and greater
Polidocanol	0.5–5%	20 cc of 3% (max 2 mg/kg)	May be used to treat wide range of vessel sizes. Nearly painless to inject; no CTN at 3% intradermally, no deaths reported at therapeutic doses or concentrations	Not FDA approved. Transient urticaria and pruritus	PE, anaphylaxis; death from pulmonary failure after overdose (600 mg)
Hypertonic saline	23.40%	20 cc per session	No reported allergies. Pigmentation is mild	Injections moderately painful; muscle cramps; ineffective for large veins. Use for sclerotherapy is off-label	PE; no reports of deaths; CTN at >10%
Chromated glycerin	1.11%	10 cc of pure solution per session	No CTN at full-strength. Most effective on the very smallest vessels (e.g., 0.2 mm or less)	Not FDA approved. Painful to inject. Not effective for large veins	Necrosis and allergic reactions very rare. Hematuria

CTN contact tissue necrosis, *DVT* deep vein thrombosis, *PE* pulmonary embolism. Adapted from Duffy DM. Sclerotherapy. In: Alam M, Nguyen T, eds. *Treatment of Leg Veins*[1], 87–88

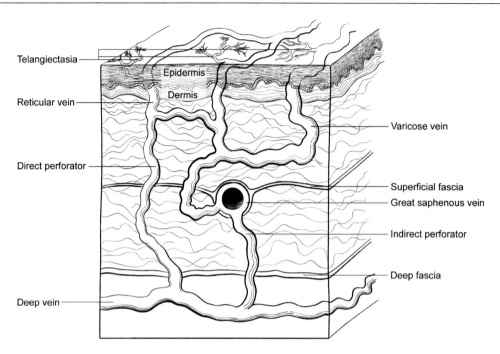

Fig. 20.1 Cross-sectional anatomy of superficial venous system depicting relationship between large and small vessels, including small reticular veins and surface telangiectasias. Adapted from Bogle MA, Sadick NS, Laser Surgery. In: Alam M, Nguyen T, eds. Treatment of Leg Veins.[1] (Illustration by Alice Y. Chen)

Table 20.4 Treatment algorithm based on vessel size

Vessel size	Color	Sclerosant concentration	Number of treatments	Treatment interval (weeks)
0.1–0.2 mm	Red	P = 0.5% HS = 23.4% S = 0.2–0.3% CG = 1.11%	2–4	4–6
0.3 mm	Red	P = 0.5% HS = 23.4% S = 0.2–0.3%	2–6	4–6
0.5 mm	Red/magenta	P = 0.5–0.75% HS = 23.4% S = 0.2–0.3%	1–4	1–2
0.6–0.9 mm	Magenta/ blue–green	P = 0.5–0.75% HS = 23.4% S = 0.2%–0.3%	1–2	1–2
1–1.6 mm	Blue–green	P = 0.75%–1.5% S = 0.3–0.5%	1–2	1–2
1.6–2.5 mm	Blue–green	P = 1–3% S = 0.5–1.5%	1–2	1–2
2.5+ mm	Blue–green	P = 1.5–3% S = 0.5–1.5%	1–2	1–2

S Sodium tetradecyl sulfate, *CG* Chromated glycerin, *P* polidocanol, *HS* hypertonic saline. Adapted from Duffy DM. Sclerotherapy. In: Alam M, Nguyen T, eds. Treatment of Leg Veins.

vein wall and minimizes dilution of the sclerosant. With the non-dominant hand, countertraction is applied to the injection site. For spider veins, a small needle ½″ 30 gauge needle is ideal; for larger veins, a 25-gauge short bevel is appropriate. The vein is punctured with the needle placed at 30°. The practitioner then checks for intravascular placement before slowly and steadily injecting the sclerosant. If placement is correct, there should be very little resistance during injection and immediate blanching of the target vessel is seen (Fig. 20.2). Immediately after removal of the needle, compression is applied along sclerosed vein. The patient should briefly walk afterwards to dilute sclerosant, while monitoring for signs of an allergic reaction or vasovagal response.[5]

Duplex ultrasound-guided sclerotherapy is a visualization technique to gain more control, improve efficacy, and minimize complications. If used successfully, the physician is able to confirm the intraluminal localization of the needle tip and visualize the infusion of sclerosant. There are different views regarding whether this technique adds significant information; however, it may be most helpful when the target vessel is not visible from the skin surface or when sclerosing near the saphenofemoral junction to confirm placement of the needle at a safe distance from the junction.

Table 20.5 Sclerotherapy supplies

Rubbing alcohol
Needle (25′ and 30′)
Syringes 1 cc and 3 cc
Disposable basin
Sclerosant
Cotton balls
Compression bandages/hose
Gauze
Paper tape
Three-way stopcock
Plastic ruler
Camera
Magnifying eyepiece
Surgical marking pen

Foam Sclerotherapy

To target larger varicosities and recurrent varicose veins resistant to fluid sclerotherapy, foam sclerotherapy is another option. It involves the injection of detergent sclerosants (polidocanol, STS) that have been converted into finer foam preparations. Foam sclerosants, due to the increased amount of displaced blood, allow for more intimal contact over a greater distance and for a longer duration. Due to increased potency, smaller volumes and lower concentrations can be used and puncture sites are minimized. However, foam sclerosants can be difficult to use, there are no standardized preparations available, and the FDA has not examined or approved the use of foam for sclerotherapy.

To prepare the foam sclerosant, the Tessari technique is commonly used and involves filling one syringe with air and another with sclerosant in a 4:1 air to sclerosant ratio. To mix, one passes the materials back and forth vigorously through a 3-way stopcock until viscous foam is produced (Fig. 20.3). A maximum of 6–8 ml per session should be injected using this technique, and far less if treating the lesser saphenous vein.[5] Delaying compression by a few minutes prevents premature displacement of the foam and maximizes contact with the vessel lumen. Elevation of the extremity during the injection of large veins will help to slow absorption into the deep venous system. The addition of Duplex ultrasound guidance for saphenous veins, recurrent varicose veins, and perforating veins has been recommended by some authors.

Concerns about the safety profile of foam preparations remain. There is a slightly higher risk of transient visual disturbances than with traditional fluid sclerotherapy, particularly in patients with a history of

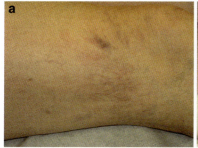 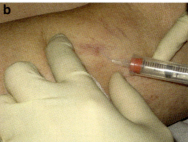 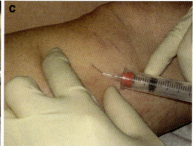

Fig. 20.2 (**a**) Visualization of the target vein. (**b**) Application of two-point couterpressure assists needle placement into vein at 30°. (**c**) Steady injection produces immediate blanching of target vessel

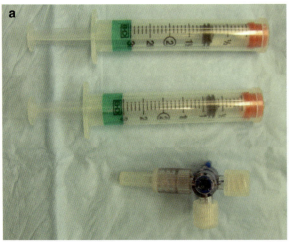

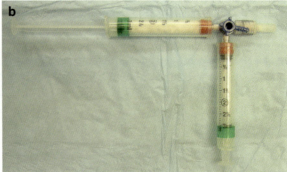

Fig. 20.3 The Tessari method to produce foam requires two syringes and a three-way stopcock to facilitate rapid mixing of air and detergent sclerosant

migraine headaches.[5] Another consideration is the presence of a patent foramen ovale, which is present in 10% of individuals. This predisposes to the possibility that a foam embolus may pass through the opening and cause transient visual changes or more serious embolic events. A recent large meta-analysis reported the median rate of serious adverse events in foam sclerotherapy, including pulmonary embolism and deep venous thrombosis was less than 1%; the median rate of visual disturbances was 1.4% and headache 4.2%.[3]

pression stockings routinely used for vessels >2 mm in diameter and in those with symptomatic reflux. Light compression hosiery (Class 0, 10–20 mm/hg) is a good adjunct when treating small fragile vessels <2 mm and can be used to enhance long term treatment results for patients whose occupation requires prolonged standing or sitting. There are no firm guidelines on the desired duration of compression. Some authors suggest that duration of 2–8 weeks may be required, but utilization is often limited by patient compliance.[2]

Compression

Immediate compression applied after treatment and sustained compression in the days to weeks following sclerotherapy are critical to maximizing efficacy.[5] The immediate technique diminishes the return of blood thereby minimizing displacement of sclerosant. Compression decreases the size of intraluminal thrombus at site of injection, which will lessen time required for full-thickness mural destruction, thereby reducing the risk of recanalization.

Immediate posttreatment compression is achieved with application of cotton balls and tape or elastic bandages at injection site. A few hours following the treatment session, patients are instructed to replace bandages with compression hose. Class 1 (20–30 mm/hg) com-

Postoperative Care

Postoperative instructions should include directions for short showers during sustained compression period and warning signs of circulatory compromise, such as numbness, tingling, and swelling in the case of over-compression. If travel occurs in the immediate postoperative period, frequent ambulation every 1–2 h and support hose is recommended. Further recommendations are to ensure adequate hydration, avoidance of alcohol, and consideration of aspirin supplementation if large vessels have been treated. Patients are encouraged to take short daily walks with appropriate support hose; however, intense exercise, hot baths, or saunas should be avoided for the first week posttreatment.

Management of Adverse Events

Most adverse reactions from sclerotherapy are mild and may resolve with treatment. Hyperpigmentation occurs in 0.3–10% of cases and is seen more commonly with higher sclerosant concentration and with rapid vessel destruction in larger vessels. It regresses slowly and fading can be accelerated with laser treatment. When involution of the treated vessel is followed by distal proliferation of fine vascularity, this is known as matting. This unpredictable and undesirable result may resolve spontaneously, respond to repeat sclerotherapy, or be diminished by various laser treatments.

Posttreatment local thrombosis is a common adverse outcome, heralded by the development of a tender palpable cord. Because spontaneous resolution is prolonged, thrombectomy may be attempted as early as 2 weeks after sclerotherapy for symptomatic thrombi. This involves incision with a No. 11 scalpel blade and evacuation of clot under local anesthesia. Skin necrosis leading to ulceration in its most severe form is a rare complication that occurs most often when a paravascular injection of high concentration sclerosant has occurred. If extravasation is suspected at the time of the procedure, diluting the area with injection of warm saline may minimize tissue damage.

Conclusion

Sclerotherapy remains the most effective technique to treat small venous varicose vessels of the lower extremities. In skilled hands, it is relatively safe and well-tolerated. Laser treatment of leg telangiectasias often produces the less desirable result of increased pigmentation.

References

1. Alam M, Nguyen TH. *Treatment of Leg Veins*. Philadelphia, PA: Elsevier Saunders; 2006.
2. Green D. Sclerotherapy for the permanent eradication of varicose veins: theoretical and practical considerations. *J Am Acad Dermatol*. 1998;38:461-475.
3. Jia X, Mowatt G, Burr JM, et al. Systematic review of foam sclerotherapy for varicose veins. *Br J Surg*. 2007;94:925-936.
4. Kahle B, Leng K. Efficacy of sclerotherapy in varicose veins – a prospective, blinded, placebo-controlled study. *Dermatol Surg*. 2004;30:723-728.
5. Rabe E, Pannier-Fischer F, Gerlach H, et al. Guidelines for sclerotherapy of varicose veins. *J Dermatol Surg*. 2004; 30:687-693.

Chapter 21
Ambulatory Phlebectomy

Marisa Pongprutthipan, Girish Munavalli, and Simon Yoo

Introduction

Ambulatory phlebectomy (AP) is a common, minor, office-based procedure using a specially designed hook inserted through a minute stab incision to avulse and completely remove superficial varicose veins. AP is generally well tolerated and results in a high degree of patient satisfaction. Advantages of AP include short surgical time, ability to be performed under local tumescent anesthesia, low recurrence rate compared to sclerotherapy, minimally obtrusive scars and dyschromia compared to other methods, and immediate postoperative ambulation, which helps prevent vascular complications.[1–4]

Indications

- Superficial varicose venous tributaries of the great saphenous vein (GSV) or small saphenous vein (SSV), perforator veins, and reticular varicose veins when distended, visible, and palpable on the surface of the skin (Fig. 21.1 and 21.2(a))
- Preferred for varicosities greater than 4 mm in diameter and flesh-colored (which are thicker wall and more resistant to treatment with sclerotherapy)
- Large tortuous distal veins (which are difficult to treat with endovascular procedures)

Contraindications

- Infection in the treatment area
- Severe arterial occlusive disease
- Bleeding tendency or coagulopathy
- Allergy to local anesthetics
- Severe peripheral edema or severe lymphedema
- Seriously ill patients (i.e., cardiovascularly compromised, etc.)
- Very elderly patients

Relative Contraindications

- Recent deep vein thrombosis
- Hypercoagulable states
- Pregnancy
- Untreated or poorly managed diabetes mellitus

Clinical Examination and Patient History

Before stripping any vessels or performing extensive phlebectomies, a preoperative evaluation must be completed. The deep venous system should be interrogated, and any source of venous hypertension needs to be identified by using duplex ultrasound.[1]

M. Alam and M. Pongprutthipan (eds.), *Body Rejuvenation*,
DOI 10.1007/978-1-4419-1093-6_21, © Springer Science+Business Media, LLC 2010

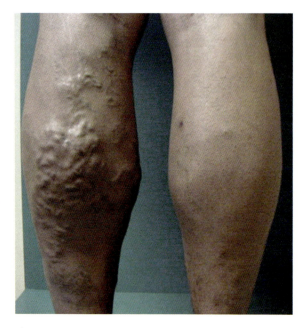

Fig. 21.1 Varicose veins. The bulging veins on the calf of an African-American female in her 40 s. AP would be preferred to sclerotherapy due to the size of the vessels and high probability of postsclerotherapy hyperpigmentation

If reflux is demonstrated at the saphenofemoral or saphenopopliteal junctions, procedures such as endovascular radiofrequency, endovascular laser, or ligation and short stripping should be performed.[3,5] This will decrease venous pressure, prevent recurrence, reduce the size of the superficial veins, and ease the phlebectomy procedure. AP can be done concurrently or several weeks after endovenous ablation.

Treatment Application

Procedural Protocol

Tray Setup

1. Indelible skin marking pen
2. Iodine prep solution
3. Disposable face mask, sterile gloves
4. Local anesthetic, syringes, needles
5. Ambulatory phlebectomy hooks: Mueller, Oesch, Ramaelet, Varady (Table 21.1)
6. Sterile 4×4 gauze pads

7. Instruments for creating incisions: 18-gauge Nokor needle, no. 11 scalpel blades or 15-degree ophthalmologic Beaver blades.
8. Mosquito clamps (6–12)
9. Postoperative washing solution (i.e., 0.9% normal saline solution or hydrogen peroxide)
10. Absorbent dressing (i.e., Telfa, sanitary pads, etc.)
11. Inelastic compression wrap (i.e., cotton roll gauze)
12. Elastic graduated compression stockings (ABD pads, Webril, Kerlix, Ace Wrap, Coban, Comprilan)
13. If needed, suturing material (needle holder, suture material, suture scissors and Adson forceps)

To avoid any possible injury to superficial neurovascular structures, use caution when treating deeper superficial veins along the common femoral artery, superficial femoral artery, popliteal artery, anterior and posterior tibial artery, and superficial nerve supplies of the lower limb below the knees (the superficial peroneal nerve and saphenous nerve) (Fig. 21.2(b)). If inadvertently hooked, patients will experience sharp burning pain radiating proximally or distally. Special attention should be paid to difficult anatomical zones such as the ankles, feet, and knees where injuries to the superficial cutaneous nerves are common. Injury to the sensory cutaneous nerves may cause paresthesia and dysesthesia. In most cases, this is only temporary and resolves within 2–3 weeks. However, there are case reports of foot drop that may or may not resolve over time, depending on the extent of nerve damage.

Technique (Fig. 21.3)

1. *Venous Marking*: Accurate and comprehensive venous marking on the skin with an indelible marker should be done while the patient is standing (Fig. 21.4). Marking should be done in a consistent, standardized way, so as to highlight straight and tortuous segments. The choice of marking pen is important, as even the most tough markings can easily wear off during the procedure as the area is exposed to surgical prep washes and interoperative blood and oozing. Marking is a critical aspect of the procedure, allowing the surgeon to quickly locate the desired venous segments. The standing position increases venous hydrostatic pressure, making them easily visible. Mapping may be done via visual inspection and palpation. An intense point light

Table 21.1 Ambulatory phlebectomy hooks

	Mueller's hooks	Oesch's hooks	Ramelet's hooks	Varady's hooks
No. of size	4	3	2	4 hooks and 2 phlebodissectors
Left-handed availability	Yes	Yes	Yes	May be used by both

Photographs provided by Venosan North America, Inc.

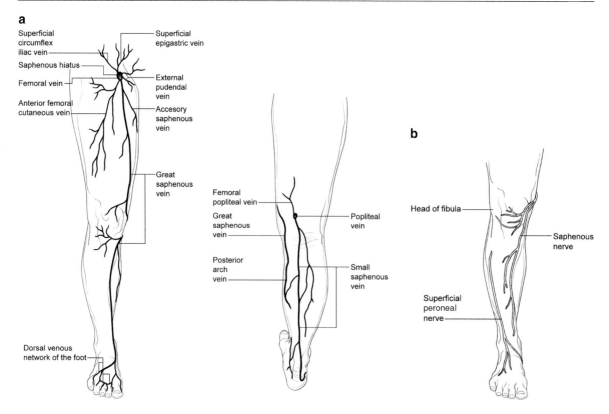

Fig. 21.2 Relevant anatomical structures: (**a**) veins and (**b**) nerves (Illustration by Alice Y. Chen)

source can be used to transilluminate the skin, making it much easier to visualize less superficial segments of the vein.

2. *Anesthesia*: Tumescent anesthesia is a safe and easy technique for use with AP. The technique involves infiltration of the subcutaneous fat compartment by using an irrigation pump with a 0.05–0.1% preparation of lidocaine with epinephrine[1,6] (Table 21.2). Advantages of tumescent anesthesia include elimination of multiple needle sticks, rapid-onset of anesthesia, and an extensive anesthetic field. Additionally, the temporary turgor and hydrodissection of surrounding adventitia can facilitate vein identification and extraction, reduce blood loss, diminish bruising, shorten postoperative recovery, and allow for greater postoperative comfort.[7]

3. *Incisions*: When the patient is in the supine position, the vein may shift from the initial markings. Confirm the vein location with transepidermal illumination or Doppler ultrasound mapping. This will allow better vein visualization, fewer incisions, and less operative time. Depending on vein size, incision lengths vary from 0.5 to 4 mm, or as long as the diameter of the hook curvature. Place incisions just lateral to the targeted vein, and parallel to the long axis of the extremity following tension lines. This allows approximation of the wound edge with the force of a circumferentially placed compression dressing. Incisions are made by a needle for small varicose veins or a scalpel for larger ones. Horizontal stab incisions, following the relaxed skin tension lines, are preferred around the knees and ankles. Incision through marking ink should be avoided to prevent tattooing the skin. Avoid stretching or traumatizing the wound edge. The interval between incisions varies from 3 to 5 cm depending on the patient's veins. Verify the location of subsequent incisions by simply pulling the vein gently to observe depression of the skin along the venous course.

4. *Hooking and Extraction*: Vessels are grasped by either using a hook or using fine hemostats to elevate the vein. Hooks should be inserted very gently to grasp veins 2–3 mm in depth to avoid unnecessary trauma to the wound margins and avoid injury to the deep structures. Ultrasound may be used to guide hooking especially for deeper or subtle veins.

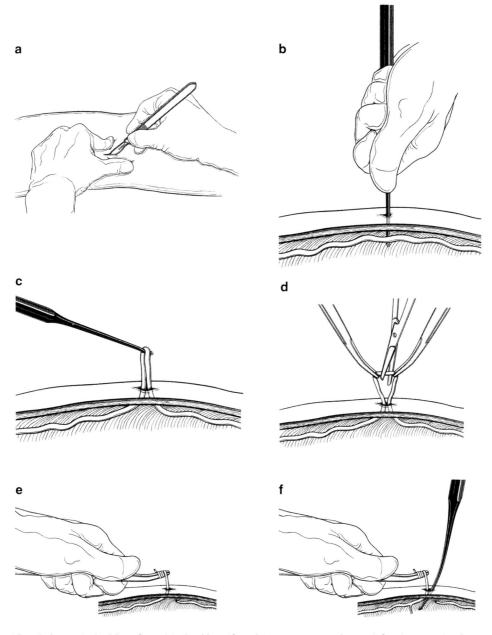

Fig. 21.3 AP techniques: (**a**) incision, (**b**) and (**c**) hooking, (**d**) and (**e**) venous extraction, and (**f**) vein separation from surrounding tissue using the spatula component of Varady's hook (Illustration by Alice Y. Chen)

The authors typically use blunt dissection with the blunt end of the Varady hook to release the vein from the surrounding dermis prior to inserting the hooked end of the instrument. Due to the availability of a variety of hooks, it is recommended that the surgeon try each to determine which fits his style best. Different hooks have different advantages; for example, the Ramelet hook is more pointed and smaller in size, thus easier in tight spaces. Once the vein or its adventitia are hooked, the vein should come out easily through the stab incision. If the effort is met with resistance or requires a lot of traction, it is possible that another structure has been hooked; remove the hook and reattempt.

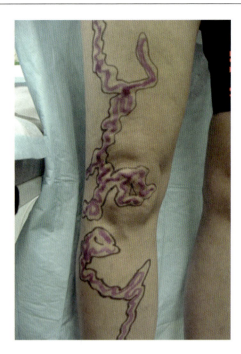

Fig. 21.4 AP markings. A water-resistant, indelible marker is used to clearly mark the varicose veins while the patient is standing

Table 21.2 Tumescent anesthesia preparation (0.05% lidocaine)

In 1 L of 0.9% normal saline solution:
Lidocaine 500 mg (50 ml of 1% lidocaine solution)
Epinephrine 1 mg (1 ml of 1:1,000 solution)
Sodium bicarbonate 12.5 mg (12.5 ml of an 8.4% NaHCO$_3$ solution)

Separation of the vein from the surrounding adventitia may be necessary by using iris scissors or the spatula component of a phlebectomy hook such as the Varady. Veins are exteriorized by the phlebectomy hook. The exteriorized vein is then clamped proximally and distally and cut in between. A gentle rolling motion of the clamp in the same or opposite direction pulls and frees the vein from its surrounding tissue (Fig. 21.5). Dissection of the vein from its adventitia should be done at the skin level to avoid injury to the unseen structures. Lack of subcutaneous tissue in the anterior of the knee and dorsum of the foot may cause difficulty when extracting the vein. Do not forcibly pull the vein. Instead, either locate and ligate the perforator, or make a larger incision. Perforators may be identified by their perpendicular course and by evaluating patient discomfort when retracted.[2] Hemostasis is achieved by

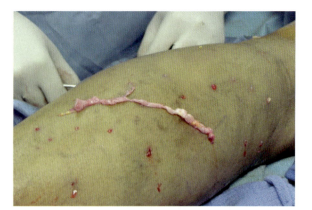

Fig. 21.5 Avulsed vein segment

applying gentle pressure over the incision site and by placing the patient in Trendelenburg position to reduce the venous hydrostatic pressure. Venous ligation is not necessary, as stretching of the vein causes rapid hemostasis most likely due to an increase in exposed endothelial sites for platelet aggregation.[8] If the vein is difficult to compress, ligation may be performed in areas such as the inner thigh.

Special attention should be paid to difficult anatomical zones such as:

- Below the knee: The saphenous nerve is particularly prone to injury. If this nerve is injured, the patient may experience shooting pain radiating into the foot.
- Pretibial area: This area contains many lymphatic vessels. Accidental trauma to lymphatic vessels will cause lymphatic pseudocysts and swelling may follow.[6]
- Popliteal fossa: The skin is very soft and easily torn. Be very gentle when handling the wound edge, especially with the elderly.
- Ankle and foot: Superficial sensory cutaneous nerves and vascular structures may be easily injured on the ankle and foot. Multiple attempts or traumatized manipulation in the wound may produce swelling, hematomas, and nerve damage. If a sensory cutaneous nerve is avulsed, paresthesia and dysesthesia may follow. In most cases, this is temporary.

5. *Incision Closure*: Cleanse the area postoperatively (i.e., with 0.9% normal saline solution or hydrogen peroxide), and apply antibiotic ointment to the puncture sites. Spontaneous wound healing facilitated by sterile adhesive tape to approximate wound

edges is preferred by most surgeons. This spontaneous healing allows blood and anesthetic fluid to drain. Sutures may be required if the surgical incision is longer than 3 mm, or if the incision is near the foot and ankle, which is subject to potential bleeding and wound dehiscence. In some cases, steristrips can be used to facilitate epidermal skin approximation, while allowing for mild drainage to continue.

6. *Dressing Compression Bandage*: After applying absorbent sterile dressings to the incision site, a compression bandage is applied to prevent bleeding and hematoma. Careful precautions must be observed to avoid ischemic nerve damage and blistering.

   - Apply extra padding over the lateral fibular head to avoid foot drop from a pressure-induced injury to the deep and superficial peroneal nerves.
   - Wrap the leg circumferentially from foot to groin, first with inelastic compression dressing and then with an elastic compression dressing. This dressing helps to promote hemostasis, to reduce swelling of the foot and leg, and to promote wound healing.
   - Take heed of patient's complaints, such as pain, numbness, and tightness, to guide assessments and complication prevention. These complaints can herald nerve compression.
   - Observe the patient for at least 15 min after the three-layer compression bandage is in place.
   - Encourage ambulation of all patients while still in the office to help mold the pressure wrap, generate normal function of the calf muscle pump, and minimize potential thromboembolic complications.

Postoperative Instructions

Patients should return to the office 2 days after the procedure for dressing removal and follow-up. Consideration of a duplex ultrasound to exclude the presence of deep venous thrombosis may be performed. Some ecchymosis or some minor leakage of blood and anesthetic fluid from the open wound is expected near the treated areas. After the compression bandage is removed, class II (20–30 mmHg) graduated compression stockings are indicated during daytime hours for 2 weeks.

Alternative Treatment Methods

Sclerotherapy is the alternative treatment for truncal varicosities or perforators especially in thin-walled venules. It may be performed 4–6 weeks after AP to clear up residual, smaller caliber vessels. Endovascular laser and endovascular radiofrequency may be combined with AP for maximal removal of GSV branches from the saphenofemoral junction, or deeper GSV and SSV.

Complications

Proper patient evaluation selection and operator experience are the most important elements to prevent complications. The most common postoperative event is hematoma or ecchymosis (Table 21.3), which resolve within 2–3 weeks. The majority of neurologic complications is temporary and usually resolves within a few months.

Pearls

- Use of tumescent anesthesia is key to an easy, successful procedure.
- Prevent recurrence by evaluating for venous reflux.

Table 21.3 Complications of Ambulatory Phlebectomy[6,8]

Frequent complications
- Transient hyper- or hypopigmentation
- Vesicles or blisters from pressure dressing
- Hematoma and ecchymosis

Uncommon complications
- Skin: allergic contact dermatitis, infection, scar, tattoo from marking pen, skin dimpling, skin necrosis, indurations, swelling
- Vascular: postoperative bleeding, matted telangiectasias, superficial thrombophlebitis
- Lymphatic: persistent edema, seroma (Fig. 21.6)
- Neurologic: postoperative pain, transitory sensory defect or dysesthesia (temporary/permanent), neuroma

Rare complications
- Keloid and hypertrophic scar
- Lymphatic pseudocyst
- Infection
- Talc granuloma
- Deep vein thrombosis
- Pulmonary embolism
- Foot drop

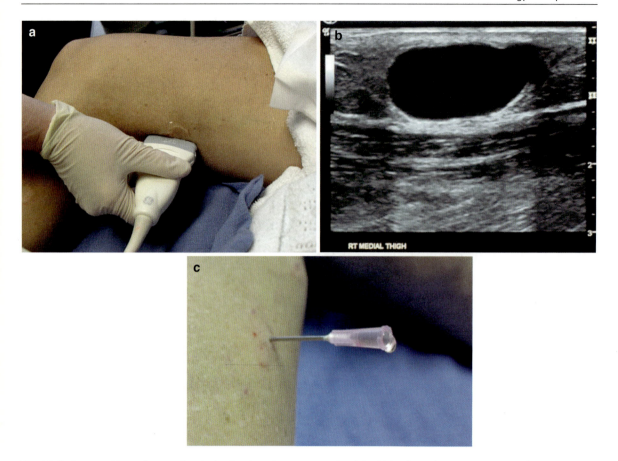

Fig. 21.6 Seroma: (**a**) an ultrasound probe is placed on the seroma on the right thigh of a patient 1-week post-op from AP, (**b**) the duplex ultrasound image shows the seroma fluid collection under the skin, and (**c**) an 18-G needle is being used to drain the seroma. The clear fluid being drained from the seroma can be seen at the hub of the needle.

- Minimize the size and number of incisions and decrease operative time by mapping veins with transepidermal illumination (venoscope) or Doppler ultrasound.[9]
- Avoid complications such as swelling, hematoma, and nerve damage by exercising caution when the procedure is performed around the knee, ankle, or foot.
- Correct GSV and axial vein reflux by combining AP with saphenofemoral ligation or endovenous ablation prior to AP. This will reduce the vein size and make it easier to remove.

- Manage patient expectations by educating patients about recurrence and possible complications.

Conclusion

Ambulatory phlebectomy is a simple, minor surgical procedure for complete removal of large superficial varicose veins. By combining AP with endovenous ablation or PIN stripping, complete removal of all varicose veins can be accomplished in-office. With proper and careful operation, AP is safe, effective, and achieves successful cosmetic results.

References

1. Almeida JI, Raines JK. Ambulatory phlebectomy in the office. *Perspect Vasc Surg Endovasc Ther*. 2008;20(4): 348-355.
2. Ricci S. Ambulatory phlebectomy. Principles and evolution of the method. *Dermatol Surg*. 1998;24:459-464.
3. Sadick NS. Advances in the treatment of varicose veins: ambulatory phlebectomy, foam sclerotherapy, endovascular laser, and radiofrequency closure. *Dermatol Clin*. 2005;23(3):443–455.
4. Ramelet AA. Phlebectomy. Technique, indications and complications. *Int Angiol*. 2002;21:46-51.
5. Weiss RA, Dover JS. Leg vein management: sclerotherapy, ambulatory phlebectomy, and laser surgery. *Semin Cutan Med Surg*. 2002;21:76-103.
6. Olivencia JA. Pitfalls in ambulatory phlebectomy. *Dermatol Surg*. 1999;25:722-725.
7. Cohn MS, Seiger E, Goldman S. Ambulatory phlebectomy using the tumescent technique for local anesthesia. *Dermatol Surg*. 1995;21:315-318.
8. Olivencia JA. Complications of ambulatory phlebectomy. Review of 1,000 consecutive cases. *Dermatol Surg*. 1997;23: 51-54.
9. Weiss RA, Goldman MP. Transillumination mapping prior to ambulatory phlebectomy. *Dermatol Surg*. 1998;24(4): 447–450.

Chapter 22
Endovenous Laser and Radiofrequency Treatment of Leg Veins

Marisa Pongprutthipan and Jeffrey T.S. Hsu

Introduction

Superficial varicosity is a common medical condition that is symptomatic in 20–30% of the US population. Classic symptoms of venous insufficiency are ankle edema, leg fatigue, aching, discomfort, and muscle cramps. Some patients develop associated complications, including stasis dermatitis, lipodermatosclerosis, skin atrophy, superficial thrombophlebitis, and venous ulcers. The treatment of varicose veins reduces symptoms and complications of chronic venous insufficiency and improves quality of life. Superficial varicose veins are often due to failure of the valves in the saphenous vein and at the saphenofemoral junction (SFJ), causing venous reflux. Until recently, traditional ligation and stripping has been the standard of care in the treatment of truncal varicosities. But there are some disadvantages, including a 20% recurrence rate in 5 years, requirement of 2–6 weeks of downtime, associated risks of general anesthesia, scars, and possible neurovascular and lymphatic vessel damage. As an alternative, there are currently available endovenous treatment options for superficial varicose veins: ultrasound guided foam sclerotherapy, endovenous radiofrequency, and endovenous laser treatment. These are minimally invasive in-office procedures with less pain, early ambulation, and less recovery time. In this chapter, we review techniques for endovenous laser and endovenous radiofrequency treatments.

Endovenous Laser Therapy[1-7]

In January 2002, an 810-nm diode laser (Diomed Inc., Andover, MA) received Federal Drug Administration (FDA) clearance for use in endovenous laser therapy. This procedure can be done in-office under local anesthesia. After vein treatment, patients are able to walk immediately and most individuals are able to return to work the next day. The mechanism of action is the ablation of the target vein through delivery of laser energy. Since then, several wavelengths have been used in endovenous laser therapy (810, 940, 980, 1,319, 1320, and 1470 nm). Shorter wavelengths (810, 940, and 980 nm) are absorbed by deoxygenated hemoglobin and transmit heat to the vein wall. The extent of thermal injury when using shorter wavelengths depends on the energy settings, pulse duration, presence of blood in the lumen, pullback rate, and amount of tumescent anesthesia. Since the hemoglobin is the target, endothelial destruction and thrombotic vein occlusions can occur. Thrombus may progress into the deep venous system creating a deep vein thrombosis (DVT), which is usually asymptomatic. The likelihood of DVT is less than 1%.[6] With longer wavelengths (1319, 1320, and 1470 nm), heat is generated when the laser energy is absorbed by the intracellular water of the vein wall and the water content of the blood. Heat is produced endoluminally and eccentrically distributed. This leads to vascular contraction, venous wall (especially tunica intima) destruction, inflammation, and ultimately, fibrosis. Some reports have suggested that this direct heating of the vein wall tends to be more effective, less painful, and results in less incidence of vessel perforation. The reported rates of great saphenous vein (GSV) occlusion from endovenous laser treatments range from 84 to 100%. Recanalization is rare, but may occur as early as 1 week after treatment.[5] The mechanisms of recanalization remain unclear; however, some postulated factors include improper performance, laser fluence, anticoagulant or antiplatelet medication use during the perioperative period, and patients with body mass index greater than 35 kg/m^2. Some commercially available endovenous lasers are provided in Table 22.1.

M. Alam and M. Pongprutthipan (eds.), *Body Rejuvenation*,
DOI 10.1007/978-1-4419-1093-6_22, © Springer Science+Business Media, LLC 2010

Table 22.1 Some commercially available endovenous lasers

	Device type	Energy output (W)	Fiber	Target
Endovenous laser treatment (EVLT™) Delta laser *Diomed, Andover, MA* http://www.evlt.com	810 nm diode laser	Available in 15 and 30	600 μm. EVLT® Laser fiber with SiteMarks™	Hemoglobin
Vari-lase *Vascular solution, Minneapolis, MN* http://www.vascularsolutions.com	810 nm solid-state diode laser	Up to 30	600 μm. Flex catheter and ceramic distal tip fiber (Bright Tip Fiber™)	Hemoglobin
Pro-V *Sciton, Palo Alto, CA* http://www.sciton.com	1319 nm Nd:YAG laser	Up to 12	600 μm, optical fiber	Water
Cooltouch endovenous (CTEV™) *Cooltouch, Roseville, CA* http://www.cooltouch.com/ varicoseveins.aspx	1320 nm Nd:YAG laser	Up to 10	600 μm, optical fiber, available with single-use fiber or reusable fiber with automated pullback system	Water
Endo lase vein system painless (ELVeS™ PL) *Biolitec AG, Jena, Germany* http://www.biolitec.com	1470 nm diode laser	Up to 15	ELVeS™ Radial fiber (homogenous circumferential energy emission)	Water

Endovenous Radiofrequency Ablation[3,6,8]

Endovenous radiofrequency (RF) ablation (Closure® procedure, VNUS Medical Technologies, Inc., San Jose, California) was FDA approved for the treatment of the great saphenous vein (GSV) in 1999. This is a minimally invasive, in-office treatment using local anesthesia with 1–2 days of downtime. Eighty-five percent of patients return to normal activity within 1 day. Instead of using optical fibers, VNUS technology applies RF energy directly to the vein walls through a endoluminal catheter fitted with metal electrodes at the tip. Radiofrequency generators (VNUS RFG*plus*™) create a temperature-controlled delivery of heat endoluminally (85°C by ClosurePLUS fiber or 120°C by ClosureFAST fiber) (Fig. 22.1(a,b) and Fig. 22.2(a,b)) to optimize endothelial denudation, collagen contraction, and vein wall thickening for fibrotic vein occlusion. The consistency of endoluminal temperature may be a safety advantage over laser techniques. Several studies use thermocouple monitors to show lower mean peak perivascular tissue temperature in comparison to endovenous laser treatments, suggesting less risk of damage to the perivascular tissue and the skin above. The ClosureFAST fiber (Fig. 22.2(b)) is the newest generation of this technology to shorten procedure times from around 24 min to less than 5 min by applying segmental ablation instead of full length

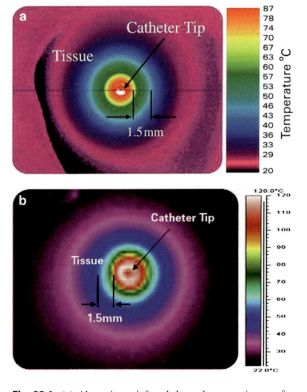

Fig. 22.1 (**a**) Above is an infrared thermal camera image of a ClosurePLUS catheter heating a vein inside a block of tissue. Note uniformity and limited depth of heating; temperature decreases from 85 to 43°C at 1.5 mm radial distance from intima. Image Copyright@ VNUS Medical Technologies,Inc. Used with permission. (**b**) Above is an infrared thermal camera image of the ClosureFAST™ catheter heating a vein inside a block of tissue. Note uniformity and limited depth of heating; temperature decreases from 95° C to 43° C at 1.5 mm radial distance from intima. (Image Copyright@VNUS Medical Technologies, Inc. Used with permission.)

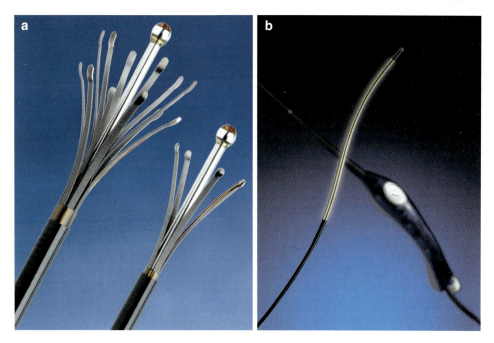

Fig. 22.2 (**a**) ClosurePLUS™ and (**b**) ClosureFAST™ (Image Copyright@VNUS Medical Technologies, Inc. Used with permission.)

continuous ablation. This eliminates the pullback speed variability, shortens the operating time, and simplifies the procedure. Recently, the ClosurePLUS fiber is no longer manufactured or distributed. Recurrence rates of VNUS have been reported to be comparable or better than endovenous laser techniques, varying from 0.5 to 2.8% during the following 2 years.

Table 22.2 CEAP classification: clinical class score (C)

	Class description
C_0	No visible or palpable signs of venous disease
C_1	Telangiectases, reticular veins, malleolar flare
C_2	Varicose veins, distinguished from reticular veins by a diameter of 3 mm or more.
C_3	Edema
C_4	Skin changes ascribed to venous disease
	C_{4a} Pigmentation or eczema
	C_{4b} Lipodermatosclerosis or atrophie blanche
C_5	Skin changes in conjunction with healed ulceration
C_6	Skin changes in conjunction with active ulceration

Indications for Endovenous Ablation

- Reflux of the GSVs or SFJ, reflux of small saphenous veins (SSV) or saphenopopliteal junction (SPJ), and accessory saphenous branches.
- Varicose veins should have a Clinical Etiology Anatomy Pathophysiology (CEAP) classification score of 2–6 in the Clinical Signs category (Table 22.2).
- Preference for vessels that are at least 2.0 mm in diameter, as measured with the patient in the supine position.
- Preference for vessels that are at least 1 cm deep from the surface of the skin (with tumescence).

Contraindications

- Thrombus in the vein segment to be treated
- Severe arterial occlusive disease, as evidence by an Ankle–Brachial Index of less than 0.5
- Inability to ambulate
- Large tortuous vein which catheter cannot pass through
- Allergic to anesthetics
- Seriously ill patients (e.g., cardiovascular compromised, pulmonary compromised)
- Recent deep vein thrombosis
- Infection in the treatment area
- Pregnancy

Relative Contraindications

- Aneurismal section in the vein segment to be treated
- Hypercoagulable states

Clinical Examination and Patient History

Preoperative Evaluation

Patient history and physical examination should be properly taken to include any allergic reaction to medications, anesthetic agents, or antiseptics. Before the procedure, perform a duplex ultrasound examination to document reflux in the system to be treated. Patency of the entire lower extremity venous system (deep, superficial, and perforator) should be explored. Once the initial evaluation process is complete, preoperative planning is initiated, and the target vein is identified. In general, the most proximal site of reflux should be treated first. This may be the SFJ followed by the tributary branches, or it may be the SPJ followed by the SSV, then the branches. Routine hematologic or other laboratory studies should be completed if indicated by the patient history (i.e., anticoagulation therapy, pregnancy testing for women within reproductive age).

Treatment Application

Procedural Protocol

- Supplies and equipment needed
  - Tilt table
  - Duplex ultrasound scanner with sterile ultrasound gel and sterile ultrasound transducer cover
  - Tumescent anesthesia preparation: anesthetic fluid, tumescent infiltration device, 20 or 22G, 3.5 in. spinal needle for fluid infiltration, and Klein infusion pump
  - Protective eyewear
  - Surgical gown
  - Disposable face mask and sterile gloves
  - Trays set up includes: (The manufacturers also provide preassembled kits)

    - Surgical drapes: 80×120 in. Split Drape (patient leg), 60×44 in. Half Drape (patient torso)
    - 500-cc Plastic Bowl
    - 20 pieces of 4×4 in. 12 ply Gauze Sponges
    - Syringe (3 cc, 10 cc, 20 cc)
    - 25 Gauge, 5/8 in. and 1.5 in. needle
    - No.11 Scalpel blade
    - Skin preparation solution (i.e., iodine, etc.)
    - Surgical skin marker
    - 4 sterile towels
  - Sterile Esmarch bandage (optional)
  - Graduated compression stockings (20–30 mmHg)
  - For endovenous laser treatment: Laser unit (Fig. 22.3 (b and c)), laser safety goggles, micropuncture vascular access kit, introducer sheath set, guidewire and standard J-wire, and laser fiber
  - For endovenous radiofrequency treatment: VNUS RFGplus™ Radiofrequency generator (Fig. 22.3(a)), micropuncture vascular access kit(18-G thin-walled or 19-G ultrathin-walled needle), introducer sheath set and Closure® catheter with guidewire

- Technique
  The following pertains to the treatment of the GSV. For SSV, the technique will need to be modified.

1. Venous marking
   Position the patient in reverse Trendelenburg position (5–10°) to dilate the venous system, thus a tilting table is recommended. Slightly flex the hip and knee, and externally rotate it to facilitate access to the saphenous vein along the medial leg. After sterile preparation and draping the treatment area, GSV is marked, mapped, and measured with Duplex ultrasound sonography. For better vessel visualization, use a probe frequency of 7.5 MHz or greater.

2. Venous access
   Vascular access is generally accomplished at the knee level for the GSV and just above the ankle for the SSV. Administer local anesthesia at the vein access site. Micropuncture is performed, or insert a 19-G needle into the GSV. Place a guidewire (e.g., J-tipped guidewire) into the needle, remove the needle, and place the introducer sheath that has been flushed with heparinized saline over the wire guided by an ultrasound. Then remove the guidewire.

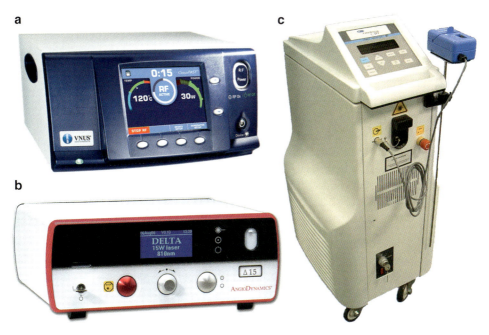

Fig. 22.3 (**a**) RF generator VNUS RFG*plus*™ (Image Copyright@VNUS Medical Technologies, Inc. Used with permission.) (**b**) DELTA laser 810 nm (Copyright ©2009 AngioDynamics) (**c**) CoolTouch CTEV™ 1320 nm laser and automatic pullback device. (Photograph provided by CoolTouch Inc.)

3. Catheter advancement

   If the saphenous vein develops vasospasm prior to cannulation, adjunctive techniques include application of a tourniquet proximal to the site of cannulation, placement of the leg in a more dependent position, and/or placement of towels moistened with warm saline along the course of the saphenous vein to enhance vein dilation.[1]

For endovenous laser ablation:

Place a laser fiber through the introducer sheath. Connect the laser fiber to the laser device and verify the energy setting. The available modes of laser delivery include pulsed and continuous. The dose of laser energy delivered can be expressed as a Joule (J/cm), sometimes called linear endovenous energy density (LEED). LEED is the amount of laser energy delivered for a given surface area (J/cm²) to achieve the optimal setting for an individual patient. Calculating LEED requires estimation of the cross sectional area of the vein.[9] Varying settings are recommended by several studies either by fluence or LEED depending on the type of laser and extent of surgeon experience. For example, when using 810-nm diode laser, the recommended setting is 65–70 J/cm per length of treated GSV and SSV.[10,11] With the optimal setting, recanalization and recurrence rates were reduced and had the highest overall success rate. Mark the laser fiber 3 cm longer than its sheath. Gently advance the laser fiber/sheath into the vein. Confirm that the tip of the laser fiber is positioned at least 2 cm distal from the SFJ or SPJ and distal to the inferior epigastric vein.[2] After withdrawing the sheath to the marked site to reveal the laser tip, lock the laser fiber and its sheath together. Mark the point on the skin at which the laser treatment can be stopped. Carefully remove the introducer sheath.

For endovenous radiofrequency ablation:

When venous access is established, the patient remains in the reverse Trendelenburg position. Flush and fill the radiofrequency ablation catheter lumen with sterile, normal saline. Wipe the outer surface of the catheter with normal saline. Check the electrode impedance in sterile normal saline solution, typically 100–150 Ω for 6 Fr catheter and 40–70 Ω for 8 Fr catheter.[11] Advance the catheter to the SFJ. If difficulties manifest when advancing the catheter due to excessive tortuosity of the vein or prior phlebitis, take caution because of the increased risk of dislodging emboli or causing perforation. The "skin stretch maneuver" may be performed by straightening the vein with external compression.[3] Longitudinal imaging with the ultrasound probe will best define the location of the epigastric vein and SFJ in relation to the catheter tip. For GSV ablation, the tip of the catheter is placed distal to the SFJ (5–10 mm for ClosurePLUS and 15–20 mm for ClosureFAST) and distal to the inferior epigastric. For SSV ablation, the tip of the catheter is placed at 20 mm distal to the SPJ. Check the impedance again; the expected impedance for 6 Fr catheter is $>200\,\Omega$ and $>150\,\Omega$ for 8 Fr catheter.[12]

4. Anesthesia

Tumescent anesthesia is preferred for endovenous treatment for several reasons. It provides compression of the vein to achieve better contact between the endothelium and catheter prongs or laser fiber, adds space between the catheter tip and skin surface to prevent skin burn, and protect the perivascular tissues from the thermal effects of intravascular energy. The technique involves infiltration of the subcutaneous fat compartment by using an irrigation pump with 0.05–0.1% lidocaine solution. Position the 22-gauge spinal needle in the perivascular tissue and infiltrate, guided by ultrasound imaging to achieve circumferentially compression of the vein (distribute anesthetic fluid approximately 10 ml/cm vein or 300 mL/limb). Separate the skin and catheter by at least 10 mm.

5. Catheter withdraw and ablation

For endovenous laser ablation:

Before catheter withdrawal, have the patient shift to Trendelenburg position, so that the leg is above the heart to facilitate vein collapse, apposition, and exsanguination. Confirm the location of the device tip by ultrasonography and visualization of the red indicator light through the skin. Turn on the device and withdraw relatively rapidly and continuously pull back at about 1–5 mm/s, depending on the laser wavelength, mode of operation (continuous or pulse), and power (i.e., 3 mm/s for 810 nm when using the DELTA laser, 1 mm/s for 1320 nm when using the Cooltouch CTEV™ laser with automatic pullback). The amount of energy delivered during endovenous laser therapy is an important parameter in achieving successful ablation of the GSV. Manual compression of the vein aids with obliteration of the lumen and facilitates venous closure. For safety, when you finish the treatment, turn the laser into "standby mode" then remove the fiber/sheath from the vein. Record necessary information, including watts, laser on-time, total joules, and length of the treated vein. Energy used per length of the treated vein should be calculated.

For endovenous radiofrequency ablation:

Place the patient in the Trendelenburg position. Confirm the location of the device tip by ultrasonography. When using the ClosurePLUS catheter, the outcome is determined by the withdrawal rate, total energy delivery, and amount of contact surface due to its "umbrella catheter" and continuous energy delivery. While energy is being delivered, monitor the probe temperature, impedance, generator output, and elapsed time on the screen to guide the rate of withdrawal. The newer RF generator also delivers an audio tone to indicate withdrawal speed. The unit will automatically adjust the minimum power necessary to maintain the desired electrode temperature. The impedance may rapidly rise in case of coagulum formation on the electrodes; the programmed RF generator will automatically shut off. The recommended withdrawal rate for 85°C probe temperature is 2–3 cm/min. If probe temperature reaches 90°C, withdrawal rate should be 4–6 cm/min. During the treatment, the expected impedance for 6 Fr catheter is $>150\,\Omega$ and $>100\,\Omega$ for 8 Fr catheter.[11] Common problems causing lower and higher impedance are usually from poor contact between the electrode and vein wall, and coagulum formation at the thermocouple tip, respectively.[12] Stop the treatment when the catheter tip enters the introducer sheath.

The ClosureFAST catheter has a 7 cm long heater element that reaches 120°C in 20 s. By conductive heat transfer, the vein wall segment in contact with the catheter heating element reaches a temperature of 100–110°C. The catheter is then moved distally in 6.5 cm increments (0.5 cm overlapping surface), and the cycle is repeated.[3] This catheter tip provides ease of use, no required saline drip, increased efficacy, and faster operative time.

For larger vessels, adjunctive strategies to improve outcome include increasing tumescent fluid volume, manual compression using an Esmarch bandage, and placing the patient in extreme Trendelenburg position.

Precaution:

• Appropriate laser safety goggles must be worn by the patient and all operating personnel to protect from direct and reflected laser energy.

- The integrity of the fiber and/or sheath may be compromised when using excessive energy, and may result in embolization of device components.
- When the laser fiber or RF catheter is inserted, it should be manipulated under ultrasound visualization.
- After the catheter is moved out of the treatment zone, it should not be re-advanced into a recently treated area.
- Do not advance the catheter or guide the wire against resistance–vein perforation may occur.

6. Postoperative ultrasound

At the completion of the procedure, return the patient to a horizontal position. Perform an ultrasonography to evaluate a successful closure and to assess patency of the deep venous system. With successful occlusion, ultrasound imaging will show a thickened vein wall with the absence of a flow in the lumen. If there is still spontaneous flow, the procedure can be repeated. If the second attempt fails to close the vein, surgical ligation should be performed.

7. Compression bandage

After the procedure, cover access site(s) with a sterile bandage. Apply waist high 20–30 mmHg compression stockings.

Postoperative Instructions

For the first 24 h after the procedure, encourage ambulation of all patients to minimize potential thromboembolic complications and continue ambulation at least 1 h daily for 1 week. Perform a follow-up Duplex ultrasound scan 3–5 days after the procedure to confirm procedural success, and ensure no thrombus into the femoral vein has occurred. Compression stockings should be continuously applied during the day and evening for the following week. Patients may experience a "string-like" pulling sensation, pain, inflammation, and bruising. Generally, varicosity symptoms reduce rapidly in a few days following the procedure; however, some patients may experience persistent symptoms for up to 6 weeks. Clinical improvement in the appearance of varicosities is typically observed within 4–6 weeks.

Alternative Treatment Methods

Ambulatory phlebectomy, ultrasound-guided foam sclerotherapy and venous stripping and ligation are the alternative treatments for GSV and SSV varicosities. These techniques are preferred in previously treated varicosities, recurrent veins after surgery (i.e., neovascularization), or perforator veins. They may be performed in combination with endovenous radiofrequency/laser ablation (Fig. 22.4), or after the failure of an endovenous treatment.

Complications

The most common complaint of endovenous therapy (up to 90%) is the report of a "string-like" pulling

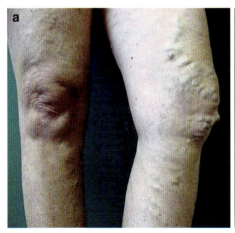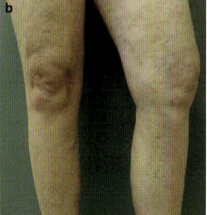

Fig. 22.4 Leg veins treated by CTEV™ combined with ambulatory phlebectomy (**a**) before and (**b**) 6 months after treatment. (Courtesy of Girish Munavalli, MD)

sensation along the course of the ablated vein that may persist for 1–2 months. Other common complaints are erythema, superficial and deep thrombophlebitis, vessel perforation, ecchymosis, hematoma, and hyperpigmentation. Skin burns are less common when using tumescent anesthesia and when practicing caution when the laser approaches the puncture site. There are a few reported cases of arteriovenous fistula causing recanulization in patients who underwent endovenous laser treatments. Reports of thromboembolic events include deep vein thrombosis, common femoral vein clot extension, and pulmonary embolism. Prophylaxis with low molecular weight heparin before surgery in patients with a history of DVT or other risk factors for the development of DVT is controversial. Nerve injuries may occur and cause paresthesia and dysesthesia. The sural nerve is prone to injury when endovenous laser therapy is used for SSV ablation. To reduce the possibility of nerve injury, perform the procedure guided by ultrasound imaging near the knee, and provide good circumferential tumescent anesthesia around the target vein are suggested. Complications depend not just on the methods and tools used, but the experience of the surgeon.

Pearls

- Tumescent anesthesia is a key to improve efficacy and safety.
- Avoid treating small tortuous vein. With this vessel type, endovenous treatment may increase the risk of perforation and unsuccessful surgery.
- Managing patient expectation and counseling for additional treatment.

Conclusion

Endovascular ablation has many advantages over the traditional high ligation and stripping procedures for the treatment of GSV and SSV varicosity. This minimally invasive office-based technique has been shown to have a high technical success rate, low morbidity rate, and high patient satisfaction. Short- and long-term success rates are equivalent or better than traditional vein ligation and stripping; however, the cost of endovenous approach may be higher when compared with other procedures. Discussion of advantages and disadvantages of each procedure should be discussed with the patient prior to treatment selection.

References

1. Johnson CM, McLafferty RB. Endovenous laser ablation of varicose veins: review of current technologies and clinical outcome. *Vascular*. 2007;15(5):250-254.
2. Singh M, Sura C. Endovenous saphenous and perforator vein ablation. *Oper Tech Gen Surg*. 2008;10(3):131-135.
3. Weiss RA, Munavalli G. Endovenous ablation of truncal veins. *Semin Cutan Med Surg*. 2005;24(4):193-199.
4. Gibson KD, Ferris BL, Pepper D. Endovenous laser treatment of varicose veins. *Surg Clin North Am*. 2007;87(5):1253-1265.
5. Proebstle TM, Gül D, Lehr HA, Kargl A, Knop J. Infrequent early recanalization of greater saphenous vein after endovenous laser treatment. *J Vasc Surg*. 2003;38(3):511-516.
6. Nijsten T, van den Bos RR, Goldman MP, et al. Minimally invasive techniques in the treatment of saphenous varicose veins. *J Am Acad Dermatol*. 2009;60(1):110-119.
7. Mundy L, Merlin TL, Fitridge RA, Hiller JE. Systematic review of endovenous laser treatment for varicose veins. *Br J Surg*. 2005;92(10):1189-1194.
8. Dietzek AM. Endovenous radiofrequency ablation for the treatment of varicose veins. *Vascular*. 2007;15(5):255-261.
9. Darwood RJ, Gough MJ. Endovenous laser treatment for uncomplicated varicose vein. *Phlebology* 2009;24 supple 1:50-61.
10. Theivacumar NS, Darwood R, Gough MJ. Neovascularisation and recurrence 2 years after varicose vein treatment for Sapheno-Femoral and Great Saphenous Vein Reflux: a comparison of surgery and endovenous laser ablation. *Eur J Vasc Endovasc Surg*. 2009;38(2):234-236.
11. Hamel-Desnos C, Gérard JL, Desnos P. Endovenous laser procedure in a clinic room: feasibility and side effects study of 1700 cases. *Phlebology*. 2009;24(3):125-130.
12. Zimmet SE. Endovenous ablation. In: Ngyugen T, Alam M, eds. *Procedures in Cosmetic Dermatology Series- Leg Veins*. London: Elsevier; 2006:147-163.

Chapter 23
Noninvasive Body Rejuvenation

Amy Forman Taub

Introduction

Noninvasive body rejuvenation is a nascent area of aesthetic medicine. Dominant past invasive procedures include liposuction, body lifts, and tummy tucks. The success of tissue tightening on the face in the past 5 years has led practitioners and researchers to explore this new frontier of body shaping. The main focus of body shaping is fat, whereas the focus of facial contouring is dermal. Thus, body shaping presents unique technical challenges that have not been encountered before. In addition, cellulite is a different pathophysiologic entity (Fig. 23.1) than either laxity or excess fat and cannot be addressed in the same fashion.

Most of the published literature on body shaping has focused on demonstration of increased compactness of an extremity, abdomen, or buttocks via circumferential reduction. Difficulty is encountered in objective photographic assessment of subtle topographical changes (Fig. 23.2).

The literature reveals a range of 0.8–3.5 cm circumferential reduction per thigh with a device utilizing infrared light, suction, and bipolar radiofrequency.[1–5] The second-generation device (Velashape, Syneron Corp.) (Fig. 23.3) was the first to achieve FDA clearance for circumferential reduction of body areas (Fig. 23.4). In a study comparing the latter with a device utilizing diode laser, suction, and massage in a split thigh study, there was no significant difference in efficacy although more bruising was associated with the former.[6] In a study looking at a dual wavelength laser with suction and massage, 80% of patients experienced improvement as measure by high-frequency ultrasound imaging of treated thighs (Fig. 23.5).[7]

Focused ultrasound has been shown to reduce circumference of abdomen and thigh an average of 1.9 cm 12 weeks after one treatment[8] (Fig. 23.6), whereas after three treatments, the mean was up to 3.95 cm.[9]

Reports of tissue tightening of body areas have been limited to case reports and anecdotal reports, except for one large multicenter study on upper arm laxity and monopolar radiofrequency, with the TC tip revealing 56% of patients achieving positive results[10] (Fig. 23.7). Another study utilizing unipolar radiofrequency for the buttocks and thighs revealed a 20% volume reduction as measured by real-time ultrasound after two treatments (Fig. 23.8),[11] and an average of 2.45 cm thigh circumference reduction and suggested that skin tightening was responsible for the improvement.[12]

Patient History and Clinical Examination

Historically, important factors to note would be recent weight changes, prior surgery or liposuction in the proposed treatment area, presence of scars and/or hernias, and history of mastectomy if arm rejuvenation is considered.

When approaching a patient for examination for body rejuvenation, there are four factors to consider: cellulite, contour, laxity, and excess fat. Body rejuvenation is focused on noninvasive three-dimensional changes that include circumferential reduction (shaping), improvement in topography/cellulite (smoothing), reduction of laxity (tightening), and reduction of fat (Table 23.1).

The anatomical areas that are commonly treated are the abdomen, thighs, arms, and buttocks.

Physical Examination:

Abdomen (Figs. 23.9 and 23.10). Most common unwanted features of the abdomen include striae, laxity,

M. Alam and M. Pongprutthipan (eds.), *Body Rejuvenation*,
DOI 10.1007/978-1-4419-1093-6_23, © Springer Science+Business Media, LLC 2010

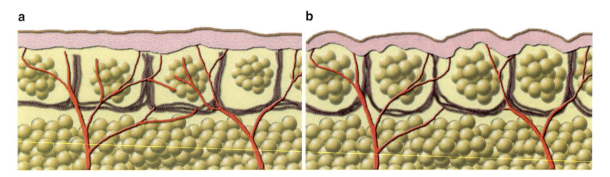

Fig. 23.1 Diagram of normal fat architecture (**a**) and cellulite architecture (**b**). Note in the normal (**a**) architecture the surface is flat and the fat globules are positioned well below the surface. In the cellulite architecture (**b**), the surface is irregular due to fat globules protruding into a more superficial area of skin. Schematic courtesy of Syneron Corp

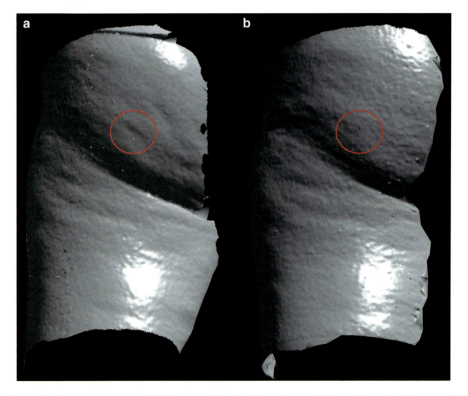

Fig. 23.2 Before and after one treatment with Thermage CL tip. Photo taken with three-dimensional image (Vectra, Canfield Scientific Corp, New Jersey), in order to better capture changes in the topography of the skin

and excess adiposity. Data would include degree of laxity, area(s) of laxity, presence or absence and degree of striae and contour.

Thighs and buttocks (Figs. 23.11 and 23.12). Common problems in these areas include cellulite, irregular contour (either genetic or postliposuction), fat pockets, and large diameter. Cellulite has four grades: (1) not present, (2) dimples present only when standing and

pinching the skin, (3) dimples present on standing at rest, and (4) dimples present when laying flat and at rest (Fig. 23.13). Ask the patient to stand with their back to you and clench their buttocks in order to grade appropriately.

Arms. The arms are usually a combination of skin laxity overall and surface wrinkles with atrophic skin and excess fat. Examination should be in the frontal

Fig. 23.3 Velashape device. Photograph courtesy Syneron Corp

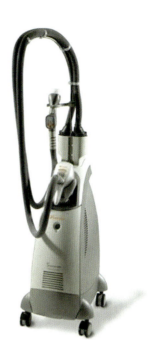

Fig. 23.4 Graph showing circumferential reduction at follow-up of subjects after 5 weekly treatments with Velashape. Areas treated included abdomen, thighs, and buttocks. Data courtesy Syneron Corp

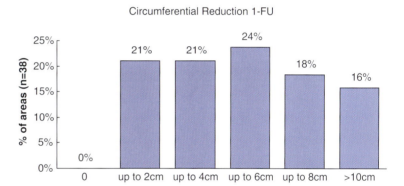

Circumferential Reduction 1-FU

% of areas (n=38)

25%
20%
15%
10%
5%
0%

0 — 0%
up to 2cm — 21%
up to 4cm — 21%
up to 6cm — 24%
up to 8cm — 18%
>10cm — 16%

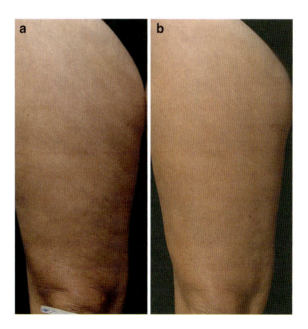

Fig. 23.5 Before (**a**) and (**b**) 12 weeks after 10 treatments with Smoothshapes dual wavelength laser device. Photo courtesy Elemé Medical

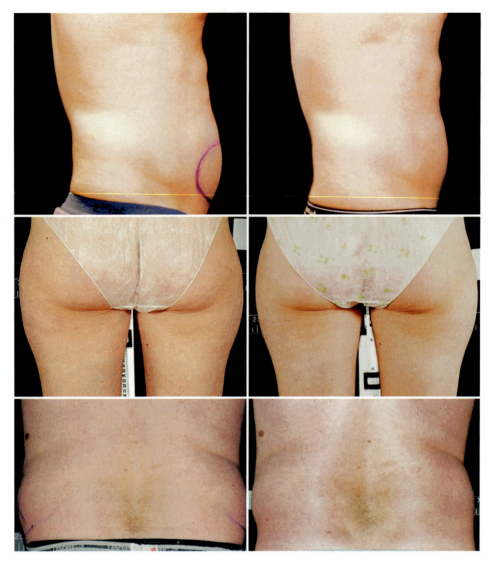

Fig. 23.6 Clinical responses to a single Contour I treatment in three cases. Reprinted with permission from: Teitelbaum SA, Burns JL, Kubota J, Matsuda H, Otto MJ, Shirakabe Y, Suzuki Y, Brown SA. Noninvasive body contouring by focused ultrasound: safety and efficacy of the Contour I device in a multicenter, controlled, clinical study. *Plast Reconstr Surg.* 2007; 120(3):779-789; discussion 790

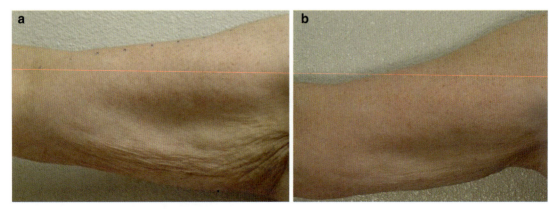

Fig. 23.7 Pre (**a**) and 2 months post 1 Thermage treatment of the upper arm (**b**). Photo courtesy of Martin Safko, MD and Thermage Corp

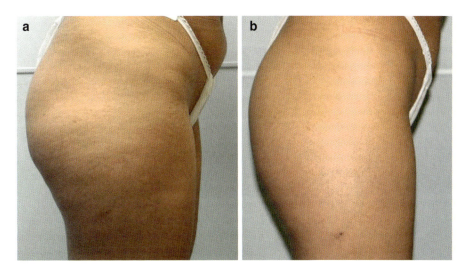

Fig. 23.8 Pre (**a**) and 15 days after one treatment (**b**). Parameters: unipolar, three passes at 150–160 W. Photo courtesy Emilia del Pino, MD and Ramon Rosado MD and Alma Corp

Table 23.1 Categorization of methods of body contouring according to components

	Cellulite	Laxity	Excess adiposity	Irregular contour
Suction massage [Endermologie (LPG, valence, France)]	+	−	−	+
Liposuction	−	+/−	+[a]	+
Chemical lipolysis (Mesotherapy)	−	−	+[a]	+
Laser lipolysis [SmartLipo (SmartLipo, Deka, Florence, Italy), CoolLipo (CoolTouch Corp., Roseville, CA), Lipotherme, Osyris, Lille, France]	−	+	+[a]	+
Combo suction, rollers, IR light, bipolar RF (Velasmooth)	+	+/−	−	+
Diode laser+suction massage [Triactive (Cynosure, Inc. Westford, MA, USA)]	+	+/−	−	+
Velashape (Syneron medical Ltd, Yokneam, Israel)	+	+	+[b]	+
Focused ultrasound (Ultrashape)	−	+/−	+[a]	+
Tissue tightening [Thermage, Titan, Lux IR (Palomar medical technologies, Burlington, MA, USA), ReFirme (Syneron Medical Ltd.), Accent (Alma Lasers, Buffalo Grove, IL, USA)]	− (+ for Thermage CL tip)	+	−	+

[a]Physical reduction of fat quantity
[b]Redistribution of fat quantity

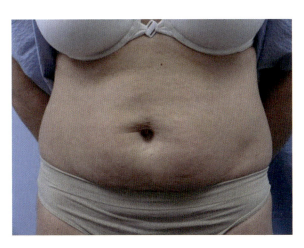

Fig. 23.9 This abdomen needs contouring and fat reduction. Photograph courtesy Thermage Corp

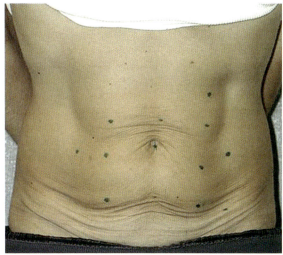

Fig. 23.10 This abdomen needing skin tightening only. Photograph courtesy Thermage Corp

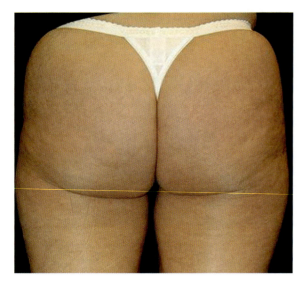

Fig. 23.11 Thighs and buttocks in need of circumferential reduction and shaping. Photo courtesy Thermage Corp

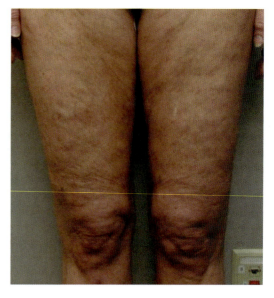

Fig. 23.12 Thighs in need of cellulite reduction. Photograph courtesy Thermage Corp

Gynoid Lipodystrophy Scale (GLD)

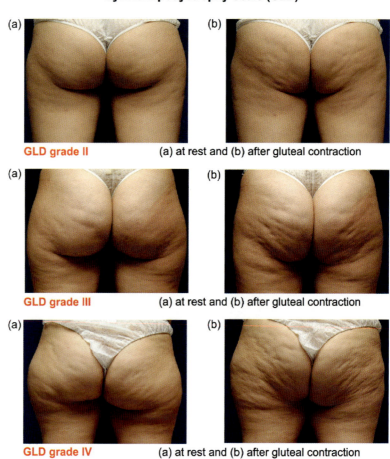

Fig. 23.13 Grading scale for cellulite or gynoid lipodystrophy. Photo Courtesy Thermage Corp

standing position with arms outstretched perpendicular to the body. Note preexisting scars.

Method of Device or Treatment Application

Dosages and Settings

Dose and setting selections vary by make of equipment and method of action. These would also vary depending on body area being treated (arms, abdomen, thighs, buttocks). Therefore, only a range of settings/doses for each instrument will be given, based on their brand names. Number of recommended treatments and mechanism of action are listed in Table 23.2.

Treatment Techniques by Device

Velashape (Syneron Medical Ltd, Yokneam, Israel). An area is treated that is 25–40 cm^2 on each side. Fifty percent overlap of pulses treating in the direction of lymphatic drainage and doing a total of 10 min on each side, with extra pulses for problem areas, vectors or to create symmetry.

Smoothshapes (Elemé Medical, Merrimack, NH, USA) (Fig. 23.14). Passing motions with the handpiece are made over the area in the direction of lymphatic drainage. Approximately 10 min of repetitions of this are included per area.

Thermage (Solta Medical Inc., Hayward, CA, USA). After applying the grounding cable and grid, areas of directional laxity or excess tissue are marked with the

Table 23.2 Categorization of methods of body contouring according to technology, mechanism of action, number of treatment and frequency

	No. of treatments (frequency)	Type of energy	Mechanism of action	Need for maintenance therapy
Suction massage (Endermologie)	14+(2×/week)	Vacuum and mechanical manipulation	Redistribution of fluids	Yes
Liposuction	1	Heating from ultrasound, suction, human exertion	Removal of fat	No
Chemical lipolysis (Mesotherapy)	4–6 (every 3 weeks)	Heat from chemical reaction	Necrosis of fat cells	No
Laser lipolysis (Smart Lipo, Cool Lipo)	1	Laser fiber induced heating	Ablation of fat	No
Combo suction, rollers, IR light, bipolar RF (Velasmooth)	12–16 (biweekly)	Vacuum, mechanical manipulation, broadband infrared light, bipolar radiofrequency	Redistribution of fluid, alteration of fibrous tissue, increased metabolism of fat cells	Yes
Diode laser + Suction massage (Triactive)	10–14	Diode laser, mechanical manipulation and vacuum	Redistribution of fluid, alteration of fibrous tissue	Yes
IR light, suction, massage, bipolar RF (Velashape)	4–6	Same as Velasmooth	Same as Velasmooth	Yes
Focused ultrasound (Ultrashape)	1–2	Focused ultrasound	Photoacoustic lipolysis	No
Tissue Tightening (Thermage, Titan, Lux IR, ReFirme, Accent)	1–5	Monopolar, bipolar or unipolar radiofrequency, broadband infrared light, combination infrared light and bipolar radiofrequency	Alteration of connective tissue	No
Photomology (Smoothshape)	8	Dual wavelength laser light (630 and 900 nm), suction, massage	"Photomology," laser induced release of lipids from fat cells, liquification of fat, redistribution of fluid, tightening	Yes

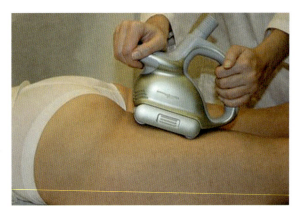

Fig. 23.14 Application of Smoothshapes handpiece. Photo courtesy Eleme Corp

patient standing up (Fig. 23.15). Treat entire grid with staggered passes (Fig. 23.16) 2–3 times, then treat vectors and problems areas with 1–4 passes. Treat distal to proximal and medial to lateral (legs or arms). Treatments are performed (Fig. 23.17) to visual tightening/smoothing (typically 900–1200 pulses, depending on area utilizing the TC, CL, or DC tip, or 300 pulses with the 16.0 tip).

Titan (Cutera Inc, Brisbane, CA, USA). Same as Thermage except for no placement of grid or grounding cable. Treatments are more effective if an area the size of approximately two decks of cards are treated at one time, which decreases the number of pulses necessary to bring a given area to temperature yielding tissue conformational change. Ultrasound gel is

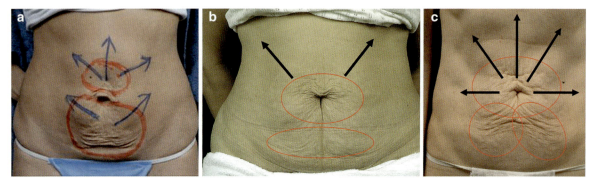

Fig. 23.15 Designing appropriate and different treatment approaches to three different abdomens for tissue tightening. Photo courtesy Thermage Corp

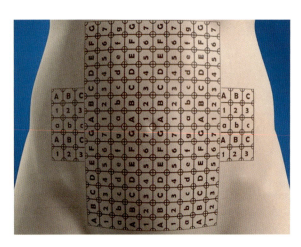

Fig. 23.16 Staggered passes design for abdominal treatment with Thermage. Photo courtesy Thermage Corp

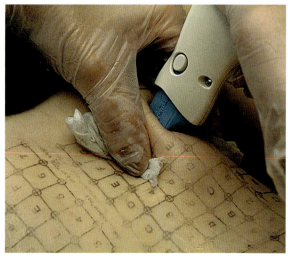

Fig. 23.17 Application of Thermage handpiece to patient. Photo Courtesy Thermage Corp

necessary. Two to four treatments over 2–5 months are performed.

Refirme (Syneron Medical Ltd, Yokneam, Israel). Essentially the same as Titan.

Accent RF (Alma Lasers Ltd, Caesarea, Israel). Utilizing the monopolar handpiece that has a rolling ball, an area on the skin the size of the dorsal hand is continuously contacted using circular motions. The area is treated until the external temperature (monitored with a radar temperature gun) reaches 40–42°C, and then the next area is heated in like fashion.

Ultrashape (UltraShape Ltd., Tel Aviv, Israel). (Fig. 23.18). During treatment, a video camera captures the treatment area and the transducer in real time and guides the user, by means of graphic overlays displayed on the system monitor, to place the transducer on the next treatment spot ("node"). The nodes homogeneously cover the treatment area, which is detected by the system, without overlap and without extension beyond the marked boundaries of the treatment area. Any area where the fat compartment is more superficial than 2 cm is not appropriate for treatment with this device.

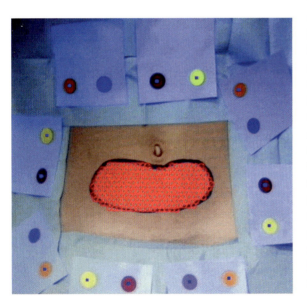

Fig. 23.18 Ultrashape treatment area (abdomen) homogeneously covered by individual treatment nodes, as guided by the Contour I real-time video monitoring and guidance system as it appears at the completion of treatment. Reprinted with permission from: Teitelbaum SA, Burns JL, Kubota J, Matsuda H, Otto MJ, Shirakabe Y, Suzuki Y, Brown SA. Noninvasive body contouring by focused ultrasound: safety and efficacy of the Contour I device in a multicenter, controlled, clinical study. *Plast Reconstr Surg.* 2007; 120(3):779-789; discussion 790

Postoperative Care

None of the noninvasive procedures discussed in this chapter require postoperative care, unless there is a complication.

Management of Adverse Events

Most adverse events with these devices are mild and/or transient. These could include discomfort during or after the procedure which is short-lived, erythema, and/or radiating heat from the area which can last minutes to hours. Blisters require conservative care and usually heal without incident. The main cause of adverse events is excessive heating of an area or lack of adequate coverage with medium (such as gel or conductive fluid, if required). It is important to discontinue any treatment that causes excessive discomfort or severe heat sensation and to immediately discontinue the procedure and/or increase cooling. If overheating were severe enough, a first or second degree burn could occur with subsequent hypo- or hyperpigmentation and/or scarring. If pulses are stacked in tissue tightening procedures, or an area is significantly overheated, fat necrosis and permanent concavity could occur. This type of result is less common with newer protocols of more frequent passes and moderate temperatures. Bruising can also occur with devices, which include mechanical manipulation and/or suction. This is usually managed via discontinuation of any blood thinning medications if not necessary, and/or time. Many of the early studies of these devices found no perturbations of serum lipids or liver function tests. However, in devices that utilize suction and massage, increased frequency of urination and defecation without known metabolic or infectious abnormalities have been not uncommonly reported.

Conclusion

Body shaping technologies are in their infancy. Focused ultrasound is not approved for use in the US, whereas tissue tightening devices such as uni and monopolar radiofrequency move forward with second-generation devices (Accent XL, Velashape II, Thermage NXT) or new tips (DC and CL and 16.0 tips on the Thermage) (Figs. 23.19 and 23.20) and combination therapies have added increased energy and utility (Velashape) (Fig. 23.21), while new devices (Smoothshapes) are being introduced. These devices will continue to become more specific for fat reduction, utilize lesser treatments and result in greater improvements as technological advances continue. Combination therapies

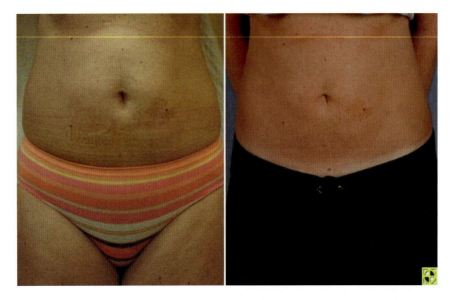

Fig. 23.19 Before and 2 months after two treatments with the Thermage DC tip. Photo courtesy Amy Forman Taub MD

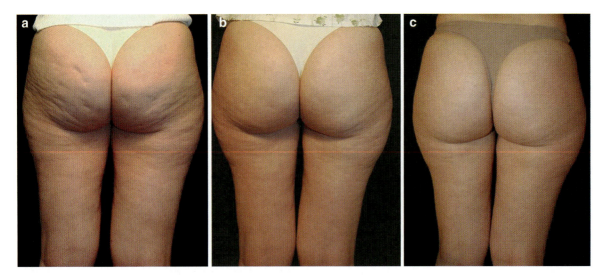

Fig. 23.20 Pre (**a**), 6 months after one treatment with Thermage CL tip (**b**) and 14 months after treatment (**c**). Photo courtesy Silvia Cuevas, MD and Thermage Corporation. postcellulitethermage14mossilviacuevas.jpg

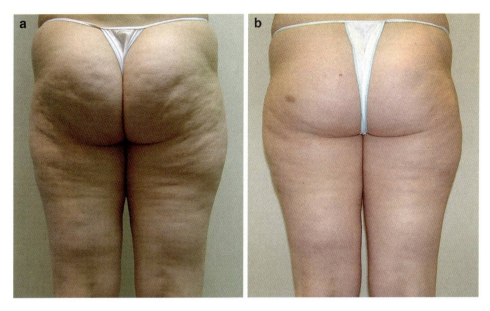

Fig. 23.21 Before (**a**) and after four treatments with the Velashape device (**b**). Photo courtesy Gerald Boey, MD and Syneron Corp

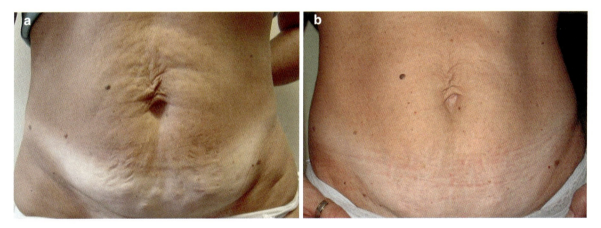

Fig. 23.22 "Velafirme" – before (**a**) and after four treatments with both Velasmooth and Refirme (**b**). Photo courtesy B. Niemann, MD and Syneron Corporation

are being explored to create synergistic changes (Fig. 23.22). Noninvasive body contouring and shaping is the new frontier for aesthetic medicine.

References

1. Wanitphakdeedecha R, Manuskiatti W. Treatment of cellulite with bipolar radiofrequency, infrared heat, and pulsatile suction device: a pilot study. *J Cosmet Dermatol*. 2006;5(4):284-288.

2. Sadick N, Margo C. A study evaluating the safety and efficacy of the VelaSmooth system in the treatment of cellulite. *J Cosmet Laser Ther*. 2007;9(1):15-20.

3. Kulick M. Evaluation of the combination of radiofrequency, infrared energy and mechanical rollers with suction to improve skin surface irregularities (cellulite) in a limited treatment area. *J Cosmet Laser Ther*. 2006;8:185-190.

4. Boey G. Cellulite treatment with a radiofrequency, infrared light, and tissue manipulation combination device. Abstract. American Society of Dermatologic Surgery Annual Meeting, Oct. 2006.

5. Alster TS, Tanzi EL. Cellulite treatment using a novel combination radiofrequency, infrared light, and mechanical tissue manipulation device. *J Cosmet Laser Ther*. 2005;7(2):81-85.

6. Nootheti PK, Magpantay A, Yosowitz G, Calderon S, Goldman MP. A single center, randomized, comparative, prospective clinical study to determine the efficacy of the VelaSmooth system versus the Triactive system for the treatment of cellulite. *Lasers Surg Med.* 2006;38(10):908-912.

7. Khatri KA, Stol ML, et al. Effectiveness of Smoothshapes cellulite treatment as monitored with high-frequency ultrasound laser. Presented at the American Society of Laser Medicine and Surgery 2008 Annual Meeting, Orlando, FL.

8. Teitelbaum SA, Burns JL, Kubota J, et al. Noninvasive body contouring by focused ultrasound: safety and efficacy of the contour I device in a multicenter, controlled, clinical study. *Plast Reconstr Surg.* 2007;120(3):779-789. discussion 790.

9. Moreno-Moraga J, Valero-Altes T, Riquelme AM, Isarria-Marcosy MI, de la Torre JR. Body contouring by non-invasive transdermal focused ultrasound. *Lasers Surg Med.* 2007;39(4): 315-323.

10. Atkin D, Goldberg D, Kilmer S, et al. A multicenter study to assess the effectiveness of monopolar radioFrequency energy on the upper arm. *Poster World Congr Dermatol.* 2007.

11. del Pino Emilia M, Rosado RH, Azuela A, et al. Effect of controlled volumetric tissue heating with radiofrequency on cellulite and the subcutaneous tissue of the buttocks and thighs. *J Drugs Dermatol.* 2006;5(8):714-722.

12. Goldberg DJ, Fazeli A, Berlin AL. Clinical laboratory, and MRI analysis of cellulite treatment with a unipolar radiofrequency device. *Dermatol Surg.* 2008;34(2):204-209.

Chapter 24
Reduction of Cellulite with Subcision®

Doris Hexsel, Taciana Dal' Forno, Mariana Soirefmann, and Camile Luiza Hexsel

Introduction: Evidence from Literature

Subcision® is a simple surgical technique used for the treatment of cutaneous depressions. It was originally described by Orentreich and Orentreich for the treatment of cutaneous scars and wrinkles in 1995.[1] (level of evidence *C) Subsequently, Subcision® was reported for the treatment of cellulite and liposuction sequella by Hexsel and Mazzuco in two series of cases with 46[2] (*C) and 232[3] (*C) patients.[3] Subcision® has also been reported for the treatment of atrophic depressed scars[4] (*C), acne scars[5] (*C), stretch marks[6] (*B), and auricular deformities in rabbits[7] (*C).

The most frequent cellulite lesions are depressions in the cutaneous surface of the affected areas. These lesions are related to the subcutaneous septa, which pull the skin down[8] (*C). Interestingly, a study demonstrated that significantly thicker subcutaneous fibrous septa are present in areas with cellulite compared to areas without cellulite.[9]

Subcision® works for specific degrees of cellulite by a multistep process. The first mechanism is the section of the fibrous dermal and subcutaneous septa with the purpose of releasing traction to the skin.[1] The subsequent hematoma formation is followed by secondary connective tissue deposition, which fills the depression.[1]

> ### *Levels of Evidence
>
> A. Literature on randomized and meta-analyses of clinical trials
> B. Well-designed clinical and observational studies
> C. Reports and case series
> D. Publications based on consensus and opinions of specialists

Clinical Examination and Patient Selection

The ideal candidates for Subcision® are healthy patients who present one or more evident depressed lesions of cellulite on the buttocks and/or upper thighs. According to the current classification of cellulite (Gynoid Lipodystrophy Scale), ideal candidates are those presenting 2nd and/or 3rd degree of cellulite (Table 24.1).[3]

Patients should be evaluated in a standing position with relaxed muscles, and only the evident depressed lesions are selected for the treatment. This means that lesions should be independently visible of pinch test or muscular contraction. Lesions up to 3 cm in diameter or less, or even parts of larger lesions, are eligible for the procedure.[3] A light source in a downward position is helpful to visualize and mark the lesions to be treated.[10]

Contraindications

The following conditions are contraindications for the treatment of cellulite with Subcision®:

- Relative contraindications: history of hyperthophic or keloid scars, active local or systemic infections, and use of drugs that interfere with coagulation or with local anesthetics.
- Absolute contraindications: pregnancy, 1st degree of cellulite, cottage cheese or orange peel lesions, coagulation disorders, severe illnesses, and patients who will be unable to follow postoperative recommendations or with unrealistic expectations.[3]

M. Alam and M. Pongprutthipan (eds.), *Body Rejuvenation*,
DOI 10.1007/978-1-4419-1093-6_24, © Springer Science+Business Media, LLC 2010

Table 24.1 Classification of cellulite on the basis of clinical criteria

Degree or stage	Clinical characteristics
0 (zero)	There is no alteration to the skin surface
I	The skin of the affected area is smooth while the subject is standing or lying, but the alterations to the skin surface can be seen by pinching the skin or with muscle contraction
II	The orange skin or mattress appearance is evident when standing, without the use of any manipulation (skin pinching or muscle contraction)
III	The alterations described in degree or stage II, are present together with raised areas and nodules

Method of Device and Treatment Application

Preoperative Recommendations

The preoperative care for Subcision® includes coagulation studies. The following recommendations are given to the patients undergoing to the procedure:

1. Seven days prior to the procedure, discontinuation of drugs that may interfere with blood coagulation, such as anticoagulants, analgesics, and anti-inflammatories;
2. Discontinuation of iron supplements one month prior to the procedure;
3. Prophylactic antimicrobial therapy with ciprofloxacin 500 mg should be started 6 h prior to the procedure;
4. Identify the patients who are in use of any drug that may interfere with the results of the procedure (e.g., beta-blockers, immunosuppressants, neuroleptics, and oral isotretinoin).

Treatment of Cellulite with Subcision® Technique

After marking the lesions, the following steps are recommended:

- Antisepsis of the skin with 70% alcohol;
- Infiltrative local anesthesia with 2% lidocaine plus a vasoconstrictor agent (epinephrine or phenylephrine); local anesthetics are injected beyond the limits of

the marked area, and an intradermic anesthetic button should be left in the locations where the Subcision® needle will perforate the skin;

- After the maximum vasoconstriction (Fig. 24.1), the skin should be punctured using an 18-G BD Nokor Needle or a common needle. The needle is inserted into the subcutaneous tissue to a depth of 1.5 or 2 cm, and then parallel to the cutaneous surface;
- At the subcutaneous level, it is possible to press the needle against the septa, facilitating the detection of the septa responsible for the skin depression. Only septa responsible for depressions to the skin surface should be cut. Subsequently, the needle is pressed against the septa and the cut is made in the same direction in which the needle will be withdrawn (Fig. 24.2).
- A gentle pinching of the skin helps to determine the presence of residual septa which still pull the skin;

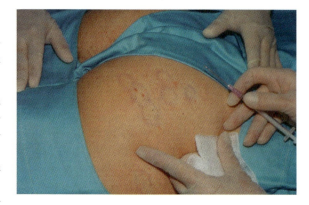

Fig. 24.1 A patient during Subcision® showing paleness and hair erection due to vasoconstriction after local anesthesia

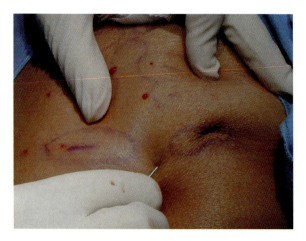

Fig. 24.2 The needle is pressed against the septa during the Subcision®

if that is present, the needle can be reinserted to cut these specific septa;

- The blood vessels that accompany the septa are also bisected, promoting the formation of hematomas;
- Compression of the treated areas with specifically designed pillows, weighing around 10 pounds for 5–10 min and wrapped in a sterile sheet guarantees a homogeneous compression, hemostasis, and control of the size of the hematomas formed by the procedure.
- The procedure is finalized with the application of micropore bandages and compressive garments.

Postoperative Recommendations

Ciprofloxacin 500 mg should be taken twice a day during the first 3 days. Moreover, patients may take acetaminophen 750 mg once every 6 h, as needed for pain. Compressive garments are recommended to be worn both day and night and encouraged during the day for 30 days. Light physical activity is allowed in the first 30 days.

Results

The final result can be observed 30–60 days after the procedure, when the hematomas have completely resolved (Figs. 24.3 and 24.4, 24.5 and 24.6). If further

intervention is necessary, the procedure can be repeated, as long as there are no sequelae from the previous procedure, after an interval of two or more months.[9] The number of procedures necessary to correct a specific depression or lesion will depend on the size, depth, and location of the defect as well as the ability of the individual's body to form and deposit the necessary amount of collagen to fill the depression.

Complications, Postoperative Care, and Management of Adverse Events

If the procedure has been accurately carried out, complications resulting from the treatment with Subcision® are rare and easily treated.[2,3] These complications are described as follows:

- The resulting hematomas and ecchymosis are expected and needed for the formation of the new connective tissue, acting as an autologous filling (Fig. 24.7); they tend to regress spontaneously within a period varying from 30 to 60 days. If the surgical area has been sufficiently compressed by the recommended compressive garments, the hematomas will have a better evolution;
- Seromas can occur in some treated lesions. They usually appear as hardened nodules that are sensitive to the touch. They tend to regress spontaneously in 3–4 months;

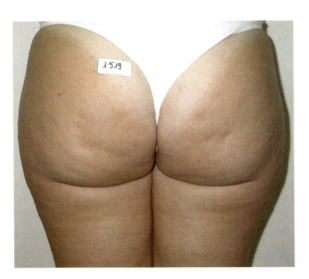

Fig. 24.3 Patient showing cellulite depressions on buttocks before Subcision®

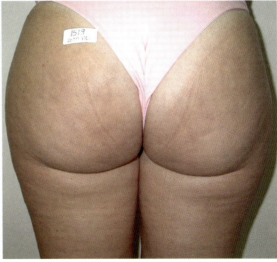

Fig. 24.4 Same patient as in Fig. 24.3, 20 days after Subcision®

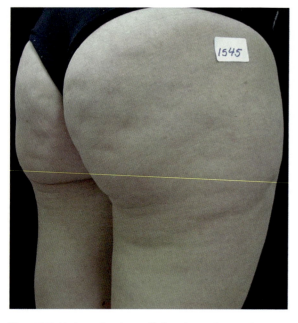

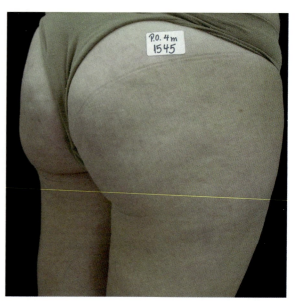

Fig. 24.6 Same patient as in Fig. 24.5, 4 months after Subcision®

Fig. 24.5 Patient showing cellulite depression on buttocks before Subcision®

- Pain may occur during the first days of the postoperative period. It can be controlled with common analgesics such as acetaminophen;
- Infections can be prevented by a careful clinical exam and by administration of prophylactic antibiotics. If an infection occurs, treatment is recommended;
- Brownish spots may occur in the areas of the hematomas due to iron deposition, which is more intense and persistent in patients who had ingested large amount of iron in medicines or diet or patients with high baseline hemoglobin. These spots may take over one year to fade. Restriction in iron intake from diet or supplements one month prior to the procedure, as well as other measures mentioned before is quite efficient in preventing this complication;
- Suboptimal response may occur, but a new intervention can be done as long as there are no sequelae from the previous procedure;
- Excessive response may occur in 5–10% of all cases. A true excessive response is due to formation of excessive fibrosis resulting from the procedure. This condition can be treated with intralesional triamcinolone;
- A false excessive response may also occur.[3] This is due to herniating of the fat, causing by cutting unnecessary additional septa and causing detachment of a fat layer and projection of the fat to the skin surface

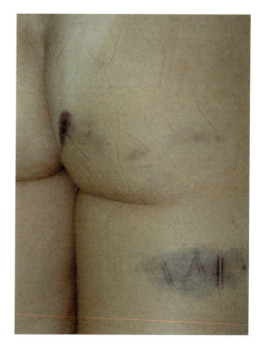

Fig. 24.7 Hematomas in the third postoperative day of Subcision®

in the treated area. This particular condition can be prevented by avoiding Subcision® over large lesions or extensive areas and concomitant section of all septa. It is important to keep in mind that some of the septa that are not exerting excessive skin retraction should remain intact;

- Although formation of keloid scars has not been observed in our experience of the treatment of more than 2,000 patients, this may happen, as their occurrence is related to individual factors.

Conclusion

Subcision® is a useful technique for the correction of depressed alterations and lesions of the skin, including cellulite, liposuction sequela, scars, and other alternations in the skin relief. It is an outpatient surgical intervention that produces long-lasting results.

References

1. Orentreich DS, Orentreich N. Subcutaneous incisionless (subcision) surgery for the correction of depressed scars and wrinkles. *Dermatol Surg*. 1995;21(6):543-549.
2. Hexsel DM, Mazzuco R. Subcision: Uma alternativa cirúrgica para a lipodistrofia ginoide ("celulite") e outras alterações do relevo corporal. *An Bras Dermatol*. 1997;72: 27-32.
3. Hexsel DM, Mazzuco R. Subcision: a treatment for cellulite. *Int J Dermatol*. 2000;39(7):539-544.
4. Goodman GJ. Therapeutic undermining of scars (Subcision). *Australas J Dermatol*. 2001;42(2):114-117.
5. Alam M, Omura N, Kaminer MS. Subcision for acne scarring: technique and outcomes in 40 patients. *Dermatol Surg*. 2005;31(3):310-317; discussion 317.
6. Luis-Montoya P, Pichardo-Velázquez P, et al. Evaluation of subcision as a treatment for cutaneous striae. *J Drugs Dermatol*. 2005;4(3):346-350.
7. Karacalar A, Demir A, Yildiz L. Subcision surgery for the correction of ear deformities. *Aesthetic Plast Surg*. 2004; 28(4):239-244.
8. Nürnberger F, Müller G. So-called cellulite: an invented disease. *J Dermatol Surg Oncol*. 1978;4(3):221-229.
9. Hexsel D, Soirefmann M, Rodrigues TC, Lima MM. Anatomy of subcutaneous structures in areas with and without cellulite by magnetic resonance images. (Poster – 66th Annual Meeting – American Academy of Dermatology, San Antonio, February 1-5, 2008).
10. Hexsel D, Mazzuco R. Subcision. In: Goldman, Hexsel, Baccci, Leibashoff, eds. *Cellulite: Pathophysiology and Treatment*. Marcel Dekker, Inc. New York.

Chapter 25
Body Contouring with Tumescent Liposuction

Carolyn I. Jacob

Introduction

Liposuction is the aesthetic removal of undesirable, localized collections of subcutaneous adipose tissue.[1] An individual may be near his or her ideal body weight, yet still have disproportionate, localized adipose deposition. Such a patient is an ideal candidate for tumescent liposuction. This technique of infiltrating large volumes of dilute lidocaine and epinephrine obviated the need for general anesthesia, virtually eliminated the need for blood transfusions, and decreased patient recovery time.[2–4] Lidocaine toxicity is the most significant factor that limits the amount of anesthesia used in tumescent liposuction. Using the tumescent technique, lidocaine dosages up to 55 mg/kg can be used with minimal risk of lidocaine toxicity.[5]

Clinical Examination and Patient History

The physician should take the patient's wishes into consideration, as well as the overall proportions of the patient. Not only is proportion important, but contour, flow, and symmetry of body lines are an essential part of liposuction planning. Patients with localized irregular contours or localized fat deposits are superb candidates for liposuction. Identify those body areas that can be contoured with liposuction to create an overall aesthetic and contour improvement.

For some patients, skin laxity, muscle flaccidity or location of fat pads deeper than the subcutis (i.e., intra-abdominal) may not make them good liposuction candidates. One judges skin laxity by the "snap test." To perform this test, the surgeon pinches 1–3 cm of skin, retracts and releases. Slow recoil or excess laxity may be an indicator that the patient will have redundant skin folds or surface irregularities after liposuction. In some cases, a combination of procedures may enable the patient to obtain results they were anticipating. Locations that are at particular risk for poor skin retraction (in the patient with poor skin tone) are the neck, upper arms, lower abdomen, and inner and outer thighs. I refer to patients with less than optimal skin elasticity as having *soft skin*. This can be recognized as the preoperative appearance of cellulite and dimples on the outer thigh, ridges or folds on the abdomen, hanging neck skin, or wrinkled inner thigh skin. Patients with soft skin must be treated with caution, and they should be counseled as to the expected outcome of surgery. However, even patients with good skin tone and elasticity can experience poor skin retraction, most commonly on the upper abdomen, distal anterior thighs, and the anterior axillae.

A thorough medical history is essential to evaluate undue risk of bleeding, infection, emboli, thrombophlebitis, edema, and a history of past surgeries, which may complicate the technique.[1] Patients should be screened for concomitant use of medications, which are known as P450 CYP3A4 inhibitors, such as erythromycin, ketoconazole, or serotonin reuptake inhibitors.[6] These medications should be avoided 2 weeks prior to the procedure (Appendix A), and patients should be given information regarding what to expect on the day of the procedure. This helps alleviate anxiety and minimize confusion. Not only should current medications and medication allergies be recorded but also any history of hepatitis, hepatotoxic chemotherapy, and use of birth control pills or cytochrome P450 competitors. A complete skin examination includes adipose distribution, quality of skin tone, and elasticity as previously mentioned (i.e., snap test). All treatment sites should be evaluated for preexisting hernias, varicosities, scars,

Box 25.1

Liver function tests

Hepatitis profile
Electrolytes
Complete blood count
Prothrombin time
Partial thromboplastin time
Pregnancy test for premenopausal women
Other tests may include urinalysis, bleeding
    time, or infectious disease studies such as
    for the human immunodeficiency virus[1]

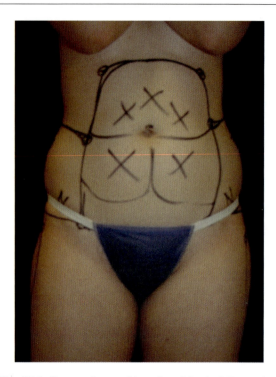

Fig. 25.1 Preoperative markings for abdominal liposuction. Note use of flow lines and markings (large "X" to denote areas of adipose concentration) to aide surgeon intraoperatively

asymmetry, or other findings. Laboratory studies are done to screen patients for general health, bleeding disorders, and underlying disorders, which may affect the metabolism of medications used throughout the procedure. Typical studies are shown in Box 25.1.

To minimize local bacterial flora, some physicians have the patient wash at home with antibacterial soap (Hibiclens, Zeneca Pharmaceuticals, Wilmington, DE) prior to the procedure.[8]

Before surgery, laboratory examinations should be reviewed and confirmed, and informed operative consent signed and last minute questions answered. The initiation of preoperative antibiotics as well as the discontinuation of medications that can promote bleeding (Appendix B) should be confirmed. The patient's weight should be obtained on the day of surgery, and used both as a reference for postoperative visits as well as to calculate maximum lidocaine dosage for the procedure. If preoperative calculations are performed by nursing staff or assistants, the surgeon should be certain to verify calculations, including the conversion of pounds to kilograms and the calculation of lidocaine dosage.

Method of Treatment

A set of preoperative photographs should be taken from at least two angles of the area being treated. While the patient is alert, and utilizing a standing position, the physician should mark the treatment areas. The physician needs to be able to clearly denote areas to be aggressively treated, areas not to be treated, and areas to be "feathered" or lightly treated (Fig. 25.1). Use a fine point black

Sharpie (Sanford, Bellwood, IL) pen as it works well, does not come off during the procedure, and fades during the following few days. Because the marking procedure relies on the patient being cognitively alert, the treatment zones are delineated and confirmed with the patient.

The patient is prepped in a sterile manner with a surgical scrub (Betadine®, Purdue Fredrick Co., Norwalk, CT or Hibiclens®, Zeneca Pharmaceuticals, Wilmington, DE) to minimize skin flora and risk of infection. Areas not to be treated are covered with sterile drapes, exposing only the treatment area(s). Many patients become chilled during the procedure, so it is helpful to have a table heating device in place under the patient (Gaymar hydrocollator heating pad, George Tieman Co., New York, or the Bear Hugger Warmer, Augustine Medical Inc., Minnesota), as well as careful control of room temperature. Additional options are stocking caps to contain body heat and prevent loss through the scalp, warm socks, and the LipoSat infusion device (LaserPoint AG, Nordkirchen, Germany), which allows heating of the tumescent solution to 37°C for patient comfort. Warm solution has also been shown to be more comfortable during infusion.

The equipment used for tumescent liposuction varies greatly between practitioners, depending on style, training, treatment site, patient factors, and desired aggressiveness of liposuction. Common items are an infusion mechanism and cannula for infusion of the tumescent anesthetic solution, suction apparatus, and suction cannulas of specified diameters and tip designs. Some cannulas are coated with zirconium nitride or polytetrafluoroethylene to enhance slickness and reduce resistance. Tip shapes vary and include blunt, bullet, spatula, and "V" shapes. Standard cannula lengths range from 10 to 35 cm. The length of the cannula should be sufficient to effectively cover the entire area to be treated. This is necessary to ensure proper feathering of edges, and allow for complete triangulation of the treated area. Suction cannulas vary in length, diameter, tipstyle, and orifice placement. All of these components factor into the aggressiveness of the suction cannula. More aggressive cannulas are wider in diameter, shorter, have an open or pointed tip rather than blunt tip, and have more and larger orifices for aspiration. Nearly all cannulas are designed to be used with the suction holes directed away from the underside of the dermis (Box 25.2 and Table 25.1) (Fig. 25.2a–c).

Box 25.2   Cannulas

Aggressive – large diameter, numerous holes, holes placed toward tip of cannula

Keel Cobra	3–3.7 mm
Capistrano	10–12 gauge
Mercedes	10–12 gauge
Pinto	10–12 gauge
Toledo	10–12 gauge

Intermediate – medium diameter, distal holes oriented away from dermis

Accelerator/triport	3 mm
3-Port radial or standard	3 mm
Pyramid	3 mm
Klein (dual port)	12 gauge
Capistrano	14 gauge
Keel Cobra	2.5 mm
Texas	2.5 mm
Dual port standard	2.5 mm
Fournier	2.5 mm
Sattler	2 mm

(continued)

Box 25.2   (continued)

Least aggressive – small diameter, distal holes oriented away from dermis

Capistrano	16 gauge
Klein (dual port)	14–16 gauge
Spatula	2–3 mm
1-Hole standard	2 mm

Table 25.1   Gauge-Millimeter equivalents for liposuction cannulas

Gauge	Equivalent
8	4.2 mm
10	3.4 mm
12	2.8 mm
14	2.2 mm

Cannulas may be purchased with or without handles. Those without handles use either standard luer lock or deluxe luer-lock tip bases to fasten them to the handles. A recent study evaluated the variety of cannula handles available, testing them for ergonomic ease. The most ergonomic was found to be the biplane handle, whose construction allows a full two plane grip with a trap of the two planes allowing a more relaxed grip (Fig. 25.3a and b).[9]

Many infusion devices and aspirators are available for use (Box 25.3) (Fig. 25.4a–e).

Saline is used as the foundation for liposuction anesthesia, and when placed in the subcutaneous space, it is absorbed slowly into the microvasculature. This form of volume replacement, known as hypodermoclysis, is the mechanism for volume replacement during tumescent liposuction surgery. Since the fluid is absorbed slowly over hours and not minutes (as with intravenous fluids), it allows the patient to mobilize and excrete fluids at a rate controlled by normal homeostatic mechanisms. This allows for long term hydration of the patient over the immediate postoperative period, yet virtually eliminates the risk of fluid overload.

Epinephrine has a threefold importance for tumescent liposuction. It provides excellent hemostasis, slows the rate of lidocaine absorption, and prolongs local analgesia. Unlike lidocaine, there is no described limitation for epinephrine dosing.[7] When utilizing the tumescent technique for liposuction, total epinephrine

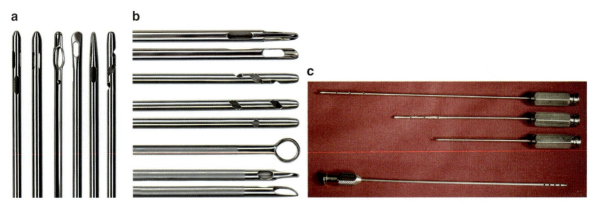

Fig. 25.2 (**a–c**) Cannula varieties

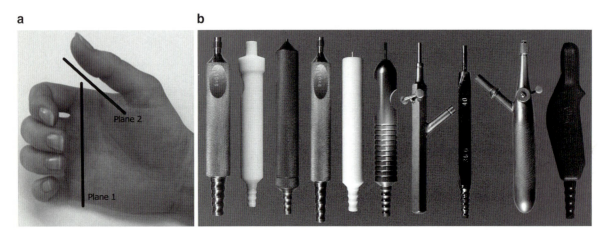

Fig. 25.3 (**a** and **b**) Cannula handles and the biplanar grip. The handle furthest right has the most ergonomic biplanar hold

Box 25.3 Commonly Used Infusion and Aspiration Pumps

Wells Johnson Single or Dual Infusion Pump (Wells Johnson, Tuscon, AZ)
HK Infusion pump (HK Surgical, San Juan Capistrano, CA)
Hercules aspirator (Wells Johnson, Tuscon, AZ)
Reliance aspirator (Bernsco, Hauppauge, NY)
Byron Psi-Tec III (Byron Medical, Tuscon, AZ)
LipoSat (LaserPoint AG, Nordkirchen, Germany)
Titan (Miller Medical, Mesa, AZ)

doses as high as 10 mg have been used without adverse effects.[7] The author recommends limiting total epinephrine dose to 5 mg to avoid toxicity. Without the addition of sodium bicarbonate, the tumescent solution will be acidic, which may cause burning during infusion. The tumescent solution is also buffered because sodium bicarbonate added to lidocaine in vitro augments the bacteriocidal activity of lidocaine.[10] In dilutions of 0.05%, lidocaine is bacteriostatic for staphlococcus aureus.[11] Therefore, when tumescent anesthesia is used, infection is a rare complication.[12]

A higher concentration of lidocaine (0.1%) is used for more sensitive areas, such as the abdomen, lateral thighs, knees, inner thighs, periumbilical area, neck, flanks and back.[5,13] When treating a large area, one may use a 0.075% solution, which retains much of the anesthetic activity of the 0.1% solution but with 25% less lidocaine, allowing the areas to be treated in one session.

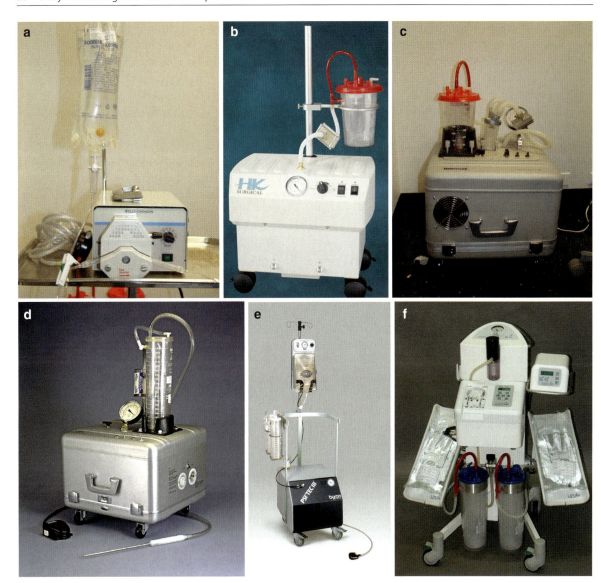

Fig. 25.4 (**a**) Wells Johnson infusion pump. (**b**) HK aspirator. (**c**) Wells Johnson Hercules aspirator. (**d**) Reliance aspirator. (**e**) Psitec III infusion pump and aspirator. (**f**) LipoSat infusion and aspiration pump

Table 25.2 Tumescent anesthetic solution

Strength	0.1%	0.075%	0.05%
2% Lidocaine	50 cc	37.5 cc	25 cc
0.9% Normal saline	1 L	1 L	1 L
Epinephrine 1:1,000	1 mg	1 mg	1 mg
Sodium bicarbonate 8.45%	12.5 mL	12.5 mL	12.5 mL
Triamcinolone 10 mg/cc	1 cc	1 cc	1 cc

The following table (Table 25.2) lists the standard tumescent anesthetic preparations.

There are many ways to deliver the tumescent anesthesia. Peristaltic mechanical pumps are able to deliver up to 5–6 l of fluid in 15–20 min. However, a rate of less than 100 cc/min is commonly used.[4] Tumescent anesthesia fluid is delivered by blunt-tipped, 6–12 in., small diameter cannulas (12–14 gauge). These are less traumatic than conventional sharp-tipped needles and preserve the neurovascular structures.[14] They also minimize risk for penetrating deeper structures. In skilled hands, 18–20 gauge spinal needles can also be used for infusion. Appropriate incision sites should be planned to account for the length of the liposuction cannula to be used, to provide adequate access to all treatment areas, and to facilitate draining of the tumescent fluid during the postoperative period. The surgeon can maximize the use of anatomic landmarks during this phase of the procedure, such as hiding an incision adjacent to the umbilicus.

Using a 30 gauge needle with a 3 cc syringe, each cannula incision site should be anesthetized. Some physicians use buffered 1% lidocaine with epinephrine, but I prefer to use the same solution as that will be used to provide tumescent anesthesia. A 3–4 mm incision with a No. 11 blade serves as a cannula insertion site.[4] Insert the No. 11 blade only partially and at an angle to avoid trauma to deeper tissues. The blunt-tipped small diameter infusion cannula is inserted, attached to either the peristaltic motorized pump, pressurized infusion bag, or other delivery system. As discussed earlier, the infusion rate may vary and is titrated to the comfort of the patient, most commonly less than 100 cc/min (a setting of 2–3 on the Klein Pump).

Varying combinations of sedatives and analgesics are given (Box 25.4), however, each patient will respond to and metabolize medication at varying rates. Therefore, dosages and choice of medications used should be titrated to each patient individually.

It is best to criss cross paths of anesthetizing both horizontally and vertically within the depth of the adipose tissue to ensure complete anesthesia. The infusion cannula is moved slowly within the subcutaneous space to thoroughly anesthetize each region. Areas closer to the infusion incision are anesthetized first to allow the cannula to move comfortably to distal regions. The anesthetic fluid also serves to hydrodissect the tissue

creating a plane for the cannula to move in.[4] Trying to change directions, or angling the cannula while in mid-stoke should be avoided. A change in cannula direction during its motion can cause tenting or dimpling of the overlying skin. This can be particularly problematic during the suctioning phase and produce contour irregularities.

The endpoint for infusion is reached when the tissue becomes firm to hard, and indurated. For both infusing tumescent anesthesia fluid and suctioning, one hand moves the cannula and the other serves as a "smart hand" to guide and feel the cannula position. This usually nondominant hand lies on the skin and palpates, constantly assessing the movement of the cannula, depth in the tissue, and degree of tissue induration. This same hand can be used to massage the areas as the anesthesia is infused, thereby decreasing discomfort via distraction. The endpoint for infusion can also be assessed by blanching as a result of vasoconstriction. The amount of tumescent anesthesia fluid infiltrated will depend on the anatomic location (Table 25.3). The surgeon must be cautioned that there is no absolute rule as to how much anesthesia is required to fully treat an area. Factors that can affect volumes of infiltration include body weight and the amount of fat in a particular anatomic area, and the amounts listed in Table 25.3 represent averages based on the author's experience.

A minimum of 30–45 min is required to establish the profound anesthesia that is essential for performing adequate and careful suctioning. The areas anesthetized should extend beyond the border of the intended liposuction sites to prevent tenderness at the periphery, and allow for feathering.

The concept of liposculpture is evolving as physicians treat not just one cosmetic unit but adjacent cosmetic

---

Box 25.4 Commonly Used Sedatives and Analgesics[15]

Diazepam (5–15 mg PO)

Lorazepam (1–2 mg PO)

Triaxzolam (Halcion: 0.25 mg PO)

Hydroxyzine Hydrochloride (Vistaril 25–50 mg IV or IM)

Midazolam Hydrochloride (Versed: 2.5–5 mg IV or IM)

Promethazine Hydrochloide (Phenergan: 25 mg IV or IM)

Meperidine Hydrochloide (Demerol: 50–75 mg IV or IM)

Table 25.3 Approximate volume of anesthesia used according to body site

Site	Volume (liters)
Neck	0.4
Arms	1.0 per side
Upper abdomen	0.75
Lower abdomen	1.0
Hips	0.75 per side
Love handles	1.0 per side
Flanks	0.75 per side
Outer thighs	1.0 per side
Inner thighs	0.75 per side
Knees	0.5 per side
Calves and ankles	1.0 per side

units (Box 25.5), blending the treatment sites to result in a more natural symmetry of proportions. Preoperative markings help the surgeon to delineate areas to be treated, with an improvement in the overall aesthetic appearance as the goal of surgery. However, it is the intraoperative technique that ultimately determines the final result. The surgeon must pinch, feel, inspect, move, and contour the subcutaneous tissue in a manner that will produce an improved skin contour. As liposuction surgeons, we rely on the skin's remarkable ability to contract and drape over the underlying soft tissue. It is imperative to keep the patient's unique physical characteristics and skin type in mind while suctioning. Skin that has poor elasticity as well as skin with good tone will not recontour without good suction technique, and this is part of the art of liposuction/liposculpture. The surgeon factors in all of these issues to determine just how much fat to remove and from which areas, to produce the final result.

The physician should use all sides of the operative table to examine and treat the patient, accessing areas from a minimum of two directions, preferably three. I refer to this method of suctioning as *triangulation*. Patient position should also be changed during surgery if the physician needs to access the fat. An advantage of tumescent liposuction surgery is that the patient is awake and therefore able to follow commands. The patient can be asked to change body position during the procedure to make it easier for the surgeon to treat an area of the body. The central premise is that the surgeon must be certain to treat all marked areas in a manner that will yield smooth contours. If an area is suctioned from one direction, it is possible to leave ridges, as small areas of fat between the cannula tunnels remain. Suctioning from two directions helps to reduce this risk, but the third vector dramatically reduces the appearance and feel of residual fat and ridges.

The nondominant smart hand is one of the most important elements of liposuction surgery. This hand is used to guide the cannula as well as assess cannula position and depth within the fat, bring fat into the cannula path, stretch or stabilize skin, and in general, serve as the sensory input from the patient back to the physician. Visual clues are also extremely helpful for liposuction contouring, but the smart hand is an invaluable link between the surgeon and patient. A surgeon's mastery of the smart hand concept is likely to improve liposuction results significantly.

With the use of tumescent anesthesia, blood loss is minimal. The physician should continuously be monitoring the aspirate for quantity and quality of adipose.

Adequate tumescent anesthesia should make the procedure nearly painless. The use of large cannulas initially takes advantage of the period of maximal anesthesia. Smaller cannulas cause less pain as they are advanced through the adipose tissue and offer more options for fine-tuning and removing the remaining adipose tissue (Box 25.6).

Box 25.5 Liposuction Cosmetic Units

Neck, submental region, and jowls
Posterior upper arm
Posterior axillary line and upper back
Upper abdomen
Lower abdomen
Hip or Love Handles
Waistline and mid back
Outer thigh
Inner thigh extending to knee
Anterior thigh
Posterior thigh
Calve and ankle
Breast

Box 25.6 Anatomic Sites and Liposuction Aggressiveness[17]

Aggressive	Love handles
80–100% removed	Back/flank
	Male breast
	Medial knee
	Upper and lower abdomen
Moderate	Hips
50–80% removed	Arms
	Outer thighs
	Buttock
	Inner thighs
	Calves/ankles
	Neck
	Jawline
Light	Mid inner thigh
Less than 50% removed	Jowls
	Anterior distal thigh and knee
	Posterior knee

Liposuction of the Arms

Liposuction of the arms is performed almost exclusively on women, with the posterior and posterolateral aspects of the arm involved more often than the anterior and medial upper arms. On occasion, a localized fat deposit on the ulnar side of the proximal forearm requires treatment as well. Conservative but thorough fat extraction is obtainable without undue trauma due to the soft quality of the fat in the area. In some patients, radiofrequency skin tightening can be a useful adjunct to upper arm fat removal.

The patient is evaluated in a standing position with arms extended horizontally with the thumb pointing up, or elbows bent, to maximize the laxity of the posterior and posterolateral compartments. If skin tone is poor preoperatively, the patient may still achieve significant skin contraction if thorough fat removal is performed, but texture will often not improve. For some patients, concurrent treatment of the upper back and anterior/posterior axillary regions is performed as well.

At least two incision sites are needed for infusion of 0.1% tumescent anesthesia. For infiltration of the posterior and posterolateral arm, incision sites are just proximal to the elbow and at the apex of the posterior axillary line. Pinching, lifting, and downward pressure from the smart hand is not necessary in this area, and may increase the risk for subdermal fibrosis, adhesions, puckering, and indentations. The 3 mm Accelerator (Eliminator) or 12 gauge Klein cannulas have a relatively nonaggressive tip, and with their recessed openings placed away from the dermis, they are ideal for fat removal of the arms. Particular attention must be paid to thoroughly treat the proximal upper arm and fat overlying the medial epicondyle, as incomplete treatment of these areas are the most common causes of patient dissatisfaction. An incision site just distal to the fat overlying the medial epicondyle provides access to that area as well as the more fibrous fat just proximal to the elbow. Postoperative pain of the arms is minimal compared to other areas, and increase with poorly fitting compression garments (Fig. 25.5a–d).

Liposuction of the Trunk

Upper and Lower Abdomen

Prior to suctioning, the patient must be evaluated for abdominal hernias and scars. Ventral hernias including umbilical, postsurgical, and Spigelian (lateral rectus sheath)

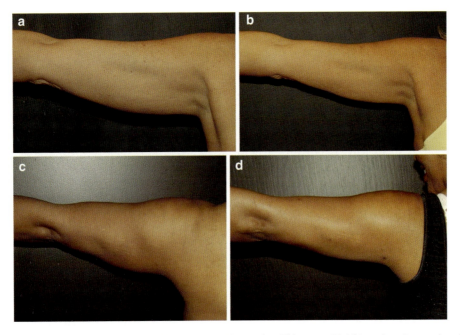

Fig. 25.5 Forty-two year old female (**a**) before and (**b**) after arm liposuction. Fifty year old African American patient (**c**) before and (**d**) 6 months after arm liposuction

should be ruled out through clinical exam. Preoperative markings should reflect the extent of suctioning, areas to be suctioned, and localized collections of adipose tissue. The lower abdomen, when suctioned alone, is often clearly demarcated and easily outlined. When the lower and upper abdomen are to be treated together, the extent of suctioning extends from under the breasts to the suprapubic region.

Anesthesia is obtained through two incisions placed along the suprapubic region, as well as from mid-abdominal sites along the lateral aspect of the area to be treated. Anesthesia is placed in the mid-subcutaneous space, and allowed to sit for a minimum of 30 min prior to suctioning. Tumescent 0.075–0.1% lidocaine anesthesia is used for the upper abdomen, especially the areas over the costal margin. Suctioning is performed with the 3.7 mm swan neck Keel Cobra cannula for debulking larger patients. The 3 mm Accelerator cannula can be used to debulk smaller patients. The 12 gauge Klein cannula is used to feather treatment sites and ensure maximal smooth fat removal.

It is essential to thoroughly suction the periumbilical region as well as the deep fat of the upper and lower abdomen. Many patients will have well-defined adipose collections that lie on the rectus sheath deep to Camper's and Scarpa's fascia, both superior to the umbilicus and inferior/lateral to the umbilicus. Suctioning of these areas is essential to produce a flat abdomen (Fig. 25.6). It is often necessary to lift the skin with the smart hand and carefully advance the cannula into a deep adipose plane to access this fat. Clearly, caution is needed to prevent subrectus suctioning. I have found it helpful to use short cannula strokes, and avoid any cannula motion lateral to the rectus sheath when attempting this deep fat maneuver. By avoiding cannula motion lateral to the rectus, it reduces the chances of becoming subrectus with cannula position. It is also imperative that cannula position be superficial when crossing the costal margin to prevent injury in that location.

Hips

The hips are either treated alone or in combination with the upper back and waistline. Some women will also have the outer thighs treated in combination

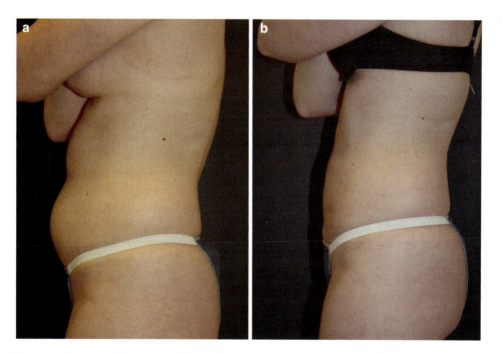

Fig. 25.6 Forty year old female (**a**) before and (**b**) 6 months after upper and lower abdominal liposuction

with the hips to recontour the lateral silhouette (Fig. 25.7). Correction of the *double-bulge violin deformity* of the hips and outer thighs can have a profound impact on body shape. The hip is outlined bilaterally with the patient in the standing position. The inferior border of the area to be treated is often

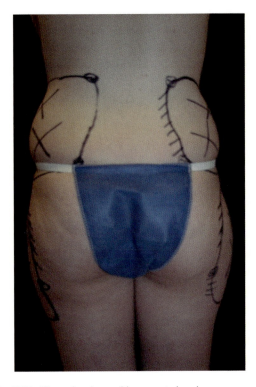

Fig. 25.7 Hip and waist markings, posterior view

easily recognized as a distinct junction between hip and upper lateral thigh. This pseudo-groove should not be treated, even when combining hip and lateral thigh liposuction, since this can produce disfiguring depressions. The anterior and posterior hip are also usually distinct, and the surgeon can feel for the boundaries of the hip with the pinch technique. Typically, the amount of fat one can pinch diminishes substantially as you move away from the central area of hip adipose tissue. The superior hip can have an indistinct border, and it is for this reason that hip liposuction is often combined with treatment of the waistline. When treating the hip alone, it is important to feather suctioning up into the waistline.

The right hip is anesthetized (and suctioned) with the patient lying on the left side, and vice versa for the left hip. Initial debulking can be performed with the 12 gauge Klein or 3 mm Accelerator cannulas. Final blending is done with the 12 gauge Klein cannula. Sufficient fat is removed to achieve this result, and can vary significantly. For most patients, 50–80% fat removal from the hip is adequate. Occasionally, near 100% fat removal is needed to obtain the desired contour (Fig. 25.8a and b).

Mid-lower Back and Waistline

Contouring of the waist can produce beautiful aesthetic results, and a shapely waistline is one of the things appreciated most by patients after their liposuction surgery.

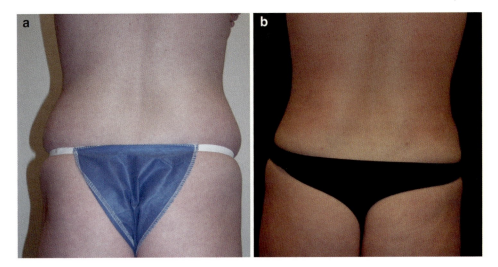

Fig. 25.8 Thirty-five year old female (**a**) before and (**b**) after hip liposuction

The patient is marked in the standing position, with vectors of suctioning clearly marked. It is important to suction along intended vectors of skin retraction to promote skin redraping postoperatively. The surgeon can pinch the lower back fat to localize it, and this area is marked. Incisions along the mid-waist, posterior mid-back, and under the lateral breast are used for anesthesia and suctioning. Additional incisions are placed as needed at the inferior zone of treatment to promote triangulation and facilitate drainage. Anesthesia is obtained with 0.075–0.1% lidocaine and allowed to sit for 40–45 min. It is advisable to allow the tumescent solution in this region to sit for slightly longer than other areas to provide maximal anesthesia. The waistline and mid-lower back can be a particularly sensitive area to treat due to the very fibrous nature of the fat. Some surgeons prefer to use external ultrasound in this area (and other areas with fibrous fat) to make fat removal easier, but I have found this to be cumbersome and unnecessary.[15,16]

The goal of waistline and upper back suctioning is near 100% fat removal. Initial debulking is performed with either the 3.7 mm Keel Cobra or 3 mm Accelerator cannulas. The surgeon must be certain to suction the very deep fat that lies just superficial to the muscular fascia, similar to the technique for the upper and lower abdomen deep fat. The smart hand is sometimes used to lift the skin of the waistline to allow the cannula to access the deeper fat. Final blending and contouring can be done with a 12 gauge Klein cannula, but for many patients, the 3 mm Accelerator is adequate for this task. It must be emphasized that triangulation and aggressive suctioning are needed to fully contour the waistline. A few extra minutes of attention to detail in this region can produce dramatic improvements in results.

Liposuction of the Buttock

The goal here is to treat the buttock so that it fits in harmony with the shape and silhouette of the patient. For these reasons, treatment of the buttock is often combined with treatment of the hips and lateral thighs, considering this to be an extended cosmetic liposuction unit. Caution must be used to avoid the inferomedial buttock in the vicinity of the sciatic nerve as well as the medial buttock near the gluteal cleft. In addition, suctioning and cannula motion should never cross the

inferior gluteal crease where the buttock meets the upper posterior thigh. Suctioning of the inferior buttock/upper thigh crease can disturb the fibrous junction in that region and lead to an unnatural ptosis of the buttock. Oversuctioning can produce a flattened buttock with irregular contours, which is not desirable.

The patient is often positioned in the prone position for anesthesia, occasionally rocking gently onto one hip to allow anesthesia of the contralateral buttock. Incision sites should be placed in the lateral infragluteal crease, the upper medial buttock, and the upper lateral buttock to promote triangulation. Anesthesia is placed predominantly in the mid and deep fat of the buttock.

Caution must be used to remain in the mid and deep fat of the buttock, avoiding superficial suctioning. Treatment of the superficial fat can quickly lead to contour irregularities in this very technique-sensitive region. The main theme that should guide the surgeon is to retain the contour and convexity of the buttock while decreasing size and improving contours. Mid and deep fat liposuction are essential tools for the physician. Initial gentle debulking can be done with a 3 mm Accelerator cannula in most patients, while larger patients can be treated with the more aggressive 3.0 or 3.7 mm Keel Cobra cannula. Following debulking, the mid-fat is contoured with a 12 gauge Klein cannula (Fig. 25.9a and b).

Liposuction of the Legs

Localized adipose deposits of the legs are particularly well-suited to liposuction surgery. Although some people (usually women) have diffusely large legs with abundant adipose tissue, many have well shaped legs with discrete collections of fat. It is for these women that liposuction is ideal. Thorough contouring of these localized fat deposits can dramatically change the shape and flow of leg lines. Clothing fits better, and the patient usually feels much more comfortable with their shape in general. As opposed to truncal obesity, many women struggle with the shape of their thighs for years, even when close to their ideal body weight. Genetics plays a significant role in determining leg shape.

Women with generalized leg obesity can be improved with liposuction surgery, but many have underlying bone and muscle anatomy that will not support the appearance of a thin, shapely leg. These women must

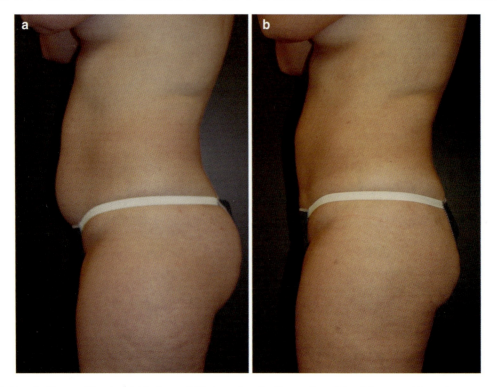

Fig. 25.9 Female 43 year old patient (**a**) before and (**b**) 6 months after liposuction of the abdomen and buttocks

be counseled preoperatively that although liposuction can alter leg contours and perhaps thin their legs, it is unlikely that they will convert from someone with an obese leg to one with a thin leg. Naturally, there are exceptions to this rule, but we have found this to be true in general. Also, there is a subset of women who have *soft skin*. This term refers to women who have abundant cellulite in the setting of a relatively obese leg. The limiting factor for women with soft skin is that overaggressive suctioning can produce rapid and dramatic skin depressions. Caution, and if anything undertreatment, are the rules for such patients.

It is useful to think of the leg as having discrete cosmetic liposuction units. These include the (1) outer thigh, (2) inner thigh extending down to and including the knee, (3) anterior thigh, (4) posterior thigh, and (5) the calves/ankles. With lidocaine toxicity as the limiting factor, the surgeon must factor in anatomy, patient desires, and surgical reality in determining which cosmetic units to treat. The outer thighs, inner thigh, and knee are commonly treated in one session together. Occasionally, the outer thigh is treated alone in the absence of other leg obesity, but in many cases, the outer thigh and hip are treated together.

Outer Thighs

The goal of therapy is creating a flow of skin that allows the outer leg to blend naturally with the hip, buttock, and trunk. Suctioning of the outer thigh must be approached with caution, as taking too little fat will yield a disappointed patient and taking too much a disfigured patient. The outer thigh is a landmark area, one that is used as a reference point by those casually observing a woman's shape to determine overall body type, thinness, and aesthetic contour. When the outer thigh is large or unnatural in shape, it tends to stand out and be noticeable to the eye. Therefore, improvement in outer thigh contours can have a profound effect on body shape and patient self-image.

The patient is marked in the standing position (Fig. 25.10). Anesthesia is obtained with 0.075 or 0.1% lidocaine and allowed to sit for 30 min. Each leg is anesthetized and treated with the patient lying on the contralateral thigh. Three to four incisions are used, the most common in the lateral aspect of the gluteal crease. The other incisions are placed at 2, 8, and 10 o'clock around the typical oval drawn to mark the outer thigh.

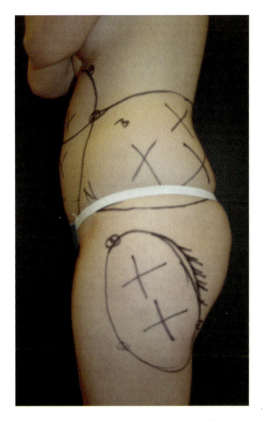

Fig. 25.10 Preoperative markings of the waist, hip, and outer thighs

Initial debulking is performed with the 3 mm Accelerator cannula in most individuals, but with the 12 gauge Klein in thin women. The 12 gauge Klein is then used to suction more superficially and to perform final blending and triangulation. Although relatively superficial liposuction is performed, it is advisable to leave a narrow zone of intact subdermal fat to retain optimal contours.

Areas to be cautious include the upper lateral thigh, distal lateral thigh, and Gasparotti's point.[17] The upper lateral and distal lateral thigh are susceptible to oversuctioning and ridging or dimpling, particularly around cannula insertion holes. It is important to move the cannula from one insertion hole to the next with regularity to avoid oversuctioning through one incision and creating a dimple under that incision. Gasparotti's point is just posterior to the greater trochanter, and depressions in this location result from aggressive suctioning of the deep fat (Fig. 25.11a and b). Abduction and internal rotation of the leg are useful to drop the greater trochanter out of the surgical field, and thus protect against a Gasparotti point depression. Numerous devices are available, including the triangular wedge pillow (Wells Johnson, Tuscon, AZ), which promote this leg position and aid the surgeon. The author prefers to have an assistant abduct the leg.

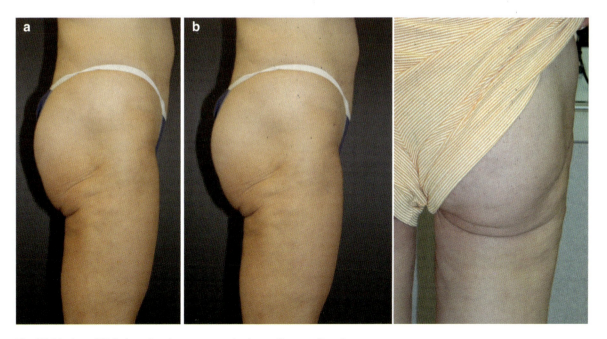

Fig. 25.11 (**a** and **b**) Indentation due to oversuctioning at Gasparotti's point

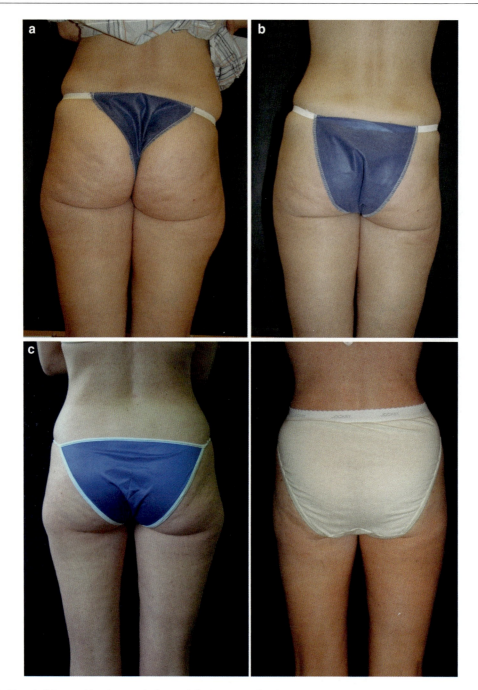

Fig. 25.12 Female 35 year old patient (**a**) before and (**b**) 3 months after liposuction of the outer thighs

The endpoint for outer thigh liposuction is subjective. Contour and flow are the most important concerns, and the smart hand pinch technique is invaluable. The surgeon pinches other areas of the leg that appear to be well contoured, and determines how many finger-widths (using the index finger) of skin is contained in the pinch. This becomes the set-point of the leg, and is often 1–1.5 finger-widths. The goal of outer thigh suctioning becomes bringing the outer thigh pinch test to match that 1–1.5 finger-widths. But the surgeon must use the pinch test in conjunction with visual and other tactile clues to determine the optimal liposculpture endpoint (Fig. 25.12a and b).

Inner Thighs and Knees

For many women, the inner thigh region is a difficult place to lose weight and improve contours. Diet and exercise programs can have some limited success, but liposuction is a superb treatment option for this anatomic region. When evaluating the inner thigh and knee, the surgeon must determine both the amount of fat removal to be performed as well as the extent of surface area to treat. Specifically, a decision must be made to either treat the entire inner thigh and knee region as one unit, or to treat the upper inner thigh and/ or knee as separate cosmetic units.

The difficulty with treating the inner thigh or knee as distinct entities is that the risk of contour irregularities and step-offs increases. Blending of the knee or inner thigh with the mid-thigh can be challenging, and the amount of fat that can be removed from these regions is limited if the surgeon must prevent a line of demarcation at the junction with the mid-thigh. Suboptimal cosmetic results can be more frequent when the mid thigh is not treated.

For these reasons, the author has developed a preferred method for treating the entire inner thigh and knee as one cosmetic unit, extending from the inguinal crease down to the superomedial calf. Very gentle suctioning of the mid-thigh region allows more thorough fat removal from the upper inner thigh and knee, improves blending and feathering into the mid-thigh, and increases patient satisfaction by contouring and debulking the entire medial upper leg.

The patient is marked in the standing position with the knee fully extended, the leg advanced forward (a modified lunge position), and externally rotated. The fat pads of the medial knee and upper inner thigh are identified and delineated, as is the inguinal crease. Markings should include the proximal medial calf as treatment of this area helps to define knee contours and improve the flow of skin lines. The surgeon should be certain to mark and identify the posterior knee and posterior upper thigh fat pockets, as failure to treat these areas will lead to less than optimal postoperative contours. Adequate contouring of these posterior adipose collections is essential since these fibrous areas will dominate the postoperative appearance if not removed. Also, reduction of these compartments allows the remainder of the inner thigh and knee skin to *fall* into position after suctioning rather than being tented by these posterior fibrous adipose collections. The anterior and posterior borders of the region to be treated should also be marked, and are loosely used as feathering guides into the anterior and posterior thigh. Careful feathering is essential to maintain normal thigh contours and flow.

Anesthesia is obtained with 0.075–0.1% tumescent lidocaine anesthesia through multiple incision sites. Incision sites below the knee should be avoided since they often heal less well than those above the knee. Thorough anesthesia of the fibrous posterior knee and inner thigh regions is helpful for improving patient comfort. Anesthesia should be placed 2–3 cm beyond the anterior and posterior markings to allow for feathering. Anesthesia should sit for a minimum of 30 min prior to suctioning.

The knee is suctioned first, with the patient in the frog-leg position and slightly rotated onto the side being treated. The degree of convexity of the medial femoral condyle and the tibial plateau may create a pseudo-lipodystrophy in an area devoid of fat. Palpation upon physical examination will differentiate the depth of the fat pad from the underlying bony prominences. A 12 gauge Klein cannula is used to treat the knee, with near complete fat removal as the goal. The surgeon should feather this treatment area into the proximal calf and the mid-thigh. It is useful to perform the feather maneuvers during the initial phases of suctioning, as this can allow for more thorough and even fat removal from the knee and upper inner thigh. Early feathering tends to improve the surgeon's feel during the procedure, often eliminating the need to "chase" a persistent ridge or depression. Treatment of the posterior fibrous knee fat is performed with the 12 gauge Klein cannula, but in some patients, a more aggressive cannula such as the 12 or 14 gauge Capistrano cannula is needed to debulk this area.

The proximal inner thigh is initially gently debulked in the deep fat with the Capistrano cannula. The 12 gauge Capistrano is used for most patients, but thinner patients can be debulked with the 14 gauge. Caution is a must when using the Capistrano cannula in this region. Its benefit is that it can quickly and thoroughly debulk the upper inner thigh, including the very fibrous and resistant posterior inner thigh fat. However, overzealous or superficial use of this cannula can produce persistent ridges and contour irregularities. The surgeon should limit the number of cannula strokes performed from any single incision with the Capistrano cannula, so triangulation is essential with this instrument. The upper thigh is then fine-tuned with the 12 gauge Klein cannula, with blending and feathering into the mid-thigh. Fat removal from the upper inner thigh should not be 100%, but more in the 50–80% range. This is one area where *flow* and the surgeon's aesthetic sense are essential determinants of the end point of treatment.

The mid-thigh is the medial region located between the upper inner thigh and the knee. It should be viewed as a connector, essentially a bridge between the upper and lower inner thigh region. For this reason, treatment of the mid-thigh helps the surgeon to blend and contour the inner leg. The overall contour changes of the inner leg come from suctioning of the upper inner thigh and knee, but the mid-thigh is the *glue* that holds the cosmetic unit together. Suctioning of the mid-thigh should be performed gently in the mid-fat with a 12 gauge Klein cannula, taking only what comes very easily. The endpoint of treatment is when the upper thigh and knee blend smoothly with the mid thigh, as well as when the entire inner thigh blends smoothly with the anterior and posterior thigh. Caution should be exercised in the vicinity of Hunter's canal and the femoral artery, since aggressive suctioning in this area can produce a very unnatural postoperative fullness (lump) in the area. Final blending with the upper inner thigh, posterior upper thigh, and knee is performed during the final stages of mid-thigh suctioning. The rule of thumb is that it is better to remove too little rather than too much fat from the mid thigh.

It is useful for the surgeon to think of the inner leg as an entire cosmetic unit during the final stages of suctioning. Taking a literal step back to view the flow and contours of this region can help the surgeon see areas that require further treatment and blending. Post operative compression of the upper inner thigh is especially important, and the surgeon should be certain to choose garments that provide adequate support in this area (Fig. 25.13a–d).

Love Handles and Abdomen on Men

Fat removal from the abdomen and love handles should be thorough for men. Most male patients desire and benefit from near 100% fat removal in these areas. However, adipose tissue in these areas is quite fibrous, and aggressive suctioning is indicated.

Careful treatment of the superficial fat compartment is often essential in these regions, as failure to remove this tissue can lead to persistent fullness.

The love handles can be treated alone, or combined with treatment of the upper and lower abdomen. Evaluation for hernias is essential preoperatively (*see* section on liposuction of the female abdomen). Many men have intraabdominal fat that causes a protuberant abdomen. It is essential to identify this during the initial consultation and educate patients about the location of their adipose tissue. Fat that is deep to the rectus muscle cannot be treated with liposuction. Patients who have fat superficial and deep to the rectus will often be disappointed with their results if they are not counseled preoperatively as to the limitations of treatment. The ideal patient has little to no intraabdominal fat and well-defined adipose collections superficial to the rectus and oblique muscles.

Multiple incision sites are used, hiding them in the suprapubic, periumbilical, and hair bearing regions when possible. Initial suctioning can be performed with the 3.0 or 3.7 mm Keel Cobra cannula in larger individuals, as well as 10–12 gauge Capistrano cannulas. Caution must be used to prevent ridging when using these aggressive instruments despite the fact that men tend to have resilient skin. Further suctioning is performed with the 3 mm Accelerator cannula, and superficial fat removed with either the Accelerator or 12 gauge Klein cannulas.

The abdomen is treated with the patient in the flat supine position. Caution should be used when crossing the costal margins. Each love handle is best treated with the patient lying on his contralateral side. Very aggressive suctioning of the deep fat in the love handles is essential for contouring. Many men have firm, fibrous fat in the posterior love handle/lower back region, and this can be a challenge to maximally debulk (Fig. 25.14a and b). Use of aggressive cannulas such as the 10–12 gauge Capistrano can be useful.

Postoperative compression is obtained with 9 or 12 in. elastic abdominal binders. Male patients are encouraged to wear these garments as much as possible to compress and contour the treated areas. Lycra bicycle shorts may also be beneficial for the first 1–3 days to prevent fluid collections in the scrotal area.

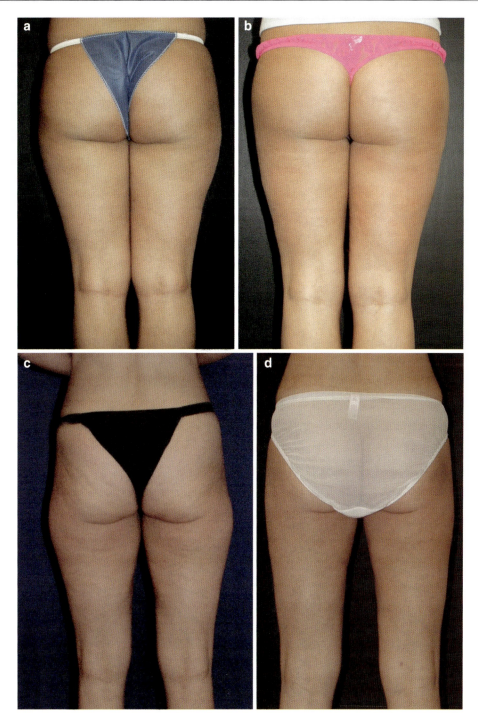

Fig. 25.13 Nineteen year old female (**a**) before and (**b**) 6 months after inner thigh, knee, and outer thigh liposuction. Forty year old female (**c**) before and (**d**) after inner thigh, knee, and outer thigh liposuction

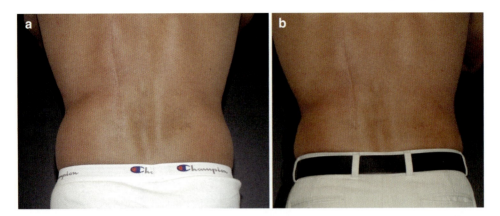

Fig. 25.14 Forty year old male (**a**) before and (**b**) 6 months after liposuction of the love handles. Note the persistence of some subdermal adipose

Postoperative Clinical Considerations

Patients may be greatly distressed by the quantity of drainage during the postoperative period unless they have been adequately prepared by the medical team. Placement and changing schedules for the various pads and support garments may be easily confused by the sedated patient, and should be provided in writing. Any instructions regarding medications (antibiotics and analgesics), and continued avoidance of certain products, should also be provided in writing.

Most patients' post operative pain is well-controlled with acetaminophen, requiring acetaminophen with codeine or other narcotics only the first few days, if at all.

Support garments applied by the medical team in the operating room will facilitate drainage of the tumescent fluid, provide significant pain control, improve final outcomes and contours, and reduce the risk of seroma formation. These garments should compress all surgical areas; multiple garments may be needed. A compression level between 17 and 21 mm of mercury is desired.[18] Adequate circulation and perfusion must be ensured before the patient is discharged. These garments should not be removed by the patient for the first 24 h. The patient is instructed to return to the office on the first postoperative day where the medical team assists them with removing the garments for the first time. This is best done with the patient supine, and they should be closely monitored for hypotension as the pressure garment is removed.

Incision sites are not sutured postoperatively, and therefore tend to drain copious amounts of fluid. Super absorbent pads are applied over incision sites under the support garment. Additional pads may be placed over the garment to facilitate changing by the patient. These may be changed as frequently as necessary to absorb discharge. Some patients have found sleeping the first two nights on a plastic mattress cover facilitates clean-up.

The patient is asked to wear the compression garment for 23–24 h a day for the first 7 postoperative days, removing it to shower when needed. After the first week, the patient is instructed to wear the compression garments for 8–10 h a day for the following 3–4 weeks. Compression is particularly important for the neck, upper arms, upper inner thighs, and the abdomen.

If preoperative antibiotics were initiated, they are usually continued for 5–7 days postoperatively. The patient is instructed not to shower for the first 24–48 h to decrease the risk of infection. For the same reason, they should not bathe in a tub or sit in a jacuzzi until all incision sites have healed. They should be informed of the signs of possible infection, such as fever, chills, increased pain or redness and told to notify the physician immediately if there is concern.

Since the lidocaine plasma peak level may actually occur after the patient has left the office, it is imperative that the patient also be aware of the signs of lidocaine toxicity: difficulty speaking, ringing in the ears, tremors or tingling around the mouth, and confusion. I prefer to have the patient in the company of another person for 12–24 h after surgery so they are not left unattended. Epinephrine toxicity is initially manifest by patient anxiety, agitation, or palpitations.

With increased levels, hypertension, tachycardia, or arrhythmias may occur. A study of twenty patients undergoing liposuction, monitored at 3-, 12- and 23-h after tumescent fluid infiltration, demonstrated the peak serum epinephrine levels to occur at 3-h. The majority had returned to normal at 12 h. The only reported side-effect was anxiety.[7]

The patients are asked to not drink alcohol for 3 days after surgery, refrain from smoking for as long as possible, and to avoid strenuous activity for 1 week. They are encouraged to drink fluids and have a soft diet for the first 24 h, after which they may resume their regular diet.

Edema, ecchymosis, dysesthesia, fatigue, and soreness are common complaints that improve with time. Wearing the compression garments will also improve these symptoms. For this reason, some patients will choose to wear their garments for many weeks after the procedure. Areas that become firm to the touch can be gently massaged, twice a day for 10–15 min until they resolve. This usually occurs between weeks 2–4. Dysesthesia of the overlying skin tends to resolve over 1–3 months, and some patients may complain of an "itchy" sensation. It is important to inform the patient that this is a normal phenomenon. Some degree of entry site scars should be expected by the patient, and followed clinically for improvements over a year. After the initial dressing change on postoperative day 1, patients are seen again 1 week postoperatively to assess healing and effectiveness of garments. Modifications can be made to the postoperative plan as indicated, and patients are routinely seen 1 month postoperatively and then again at 3–6 months.

Conclusion

Liposuction is a challenging surgical procedure that can produce superb aesthetic results when performed properly. Careful suctioning, use of the smart hand, triangulation, and fluid management are all important parts of the liposuction procedure. Final outcomes depend on both the skill of the surgeon and the healing response of the patient. However, it is the responsibility of the surgeon to have thorough knowledge and training in the procedure to minimize the possibility that surgical technique is the contributing factor to less than optimal results. It is the blend of physician skill and artistry that ultimately determines outcomes, and the surgeon can create beautiful contours by managing the interplay of skin healing dynamics, cannula motion and position, thoroughness of fat removal, and body shape.

Appendix A: Medications Which Inhibit Cytochrome P450

Drug	Generic name (Trade name)
Generic name (Trade name)	Miconazole (Micatin)
Acebutolol (Sectral)	Midazolam (Versed)
Acetazolamide	Nadolol (Corzide)
Alprazolam (Xanax)	Naringenin (grapefruit juice)
Amiodarone (Cordarone)	
Anastrazole (Arimidex)	Nefazodone (Serzone)
Atenolol (Tenoretic)	Nelfinavir (Viracept)
Cannabinoids	Nevirapine (Viramune)
Carbamazepine (Tegretol)	Nicardipine (Cardene)
Cimetidine (Tagamet)	Nifedipine (Procardia)
Chloramphenicol	Omeprazole (Prilosec)
Clarithromycin (Biaxin)	Paroxetine (Paxil)
Cyclosporin (Neoral)	Pentoxifylline (Trental)
Danazol (Danocrine)	Pindolol
Dexamethasone (Decadron)	Propranolol (Inderal)
Diltiazem (Cardiazam)	Propofol (Diprivan)
Diazepam (Valium)	Quinidine (Quinaglute)
Erythromycin	Remacemide
Esmolol (Brevibloc)	Ritonavir (Norvir)
Fluconazole (Diflucan)	Saquinavir (Invirase)
Fluoxetine (Prozac)	Sertinadole
Fluvoxamine (Luvox)	Sertraline (Zoloft)
Norfluoxetine	Stiripentol
Flurazepam	Tetracycline (Achromycin, Sumycin)
Indinivir (Crixivan)	
Isoniazid (Rifamate)	Terfenadine (Seldane) (not available)
Itraconazole (Sporanox)	
Ketoconazole (Nizoral)	Thyroxine
Labetolol (Normodyne, Trandate)	Timolol (Blocadren, Cosopt, Timolide)
Methadone	Triazolam (Halcion)
Methylprednisolone (Solu-Medrol, Depo-Medrol)	Troglitazon (Rezulin)
	Troleandomycin (Tao)
Metroprolol (Toprol-XL)	Valproic Acid (Depakote)
Metronidazole (Flagyl)	Verapamil (Calan)
Mibefradil (Posicor)	Zafirlukast (Accolate)
	Zileuton (Zyflo)

Modified from Shiffman M. Medication potentially causing lidocaine toxicity. *Am J Cosmet Surg.* 1998:227-229. McEvoy GK, ed. AHFS drug information. Bethesda, MD: 2000. Gelman CR, Rumack BH, Hess AJ, eds. Drugdex R. System. Englewood, CO: Micromedex Inc; 2000.

Appendix B: Medications that May Affect Bleeding

Patient to avoid use of these agents 2 weeks prior to liposuction

Accutane-Alert MD	Ecotrin
Advil	Empirin
Alka-Seltzer Tablets	Emperin with Codeine
Alka-Seltzer Plus Cold Medicine	Emprazil-C Tablets
Anacin Capsules and Tablets	Equagesic
Anacin Maximum Strength Capsules/Tabs	Excedrin
APC Tablets	Fiorinal with Codeine
APC with Codeine, Tabloyd Brand	Four (4)-Way Cold Tablets
Arthritis Formula by the makers of Anacin Tablets	Gemnisyn
	Goody's Headache Powders
Ascodeen-30	Ibuprofen
Ascriptin	Indocin
Aspirin	Measurin
Aspergum	Midol
Aspirin Suppositories	Momentum Muscular Backpain Formula
Anarox	Monacet with Codeine
Bayer Aspirin	Motrin
Bayer Children's Chewable Aspirin	Naprosyn
Bayer Children's Cold Tablets	Norgesic/Norgesic Forte
Bayer Timed-Released Aspirin	Norwich Aspirin
BC Powders	Pabirin Buffered Tablets
Buff-a Comp Tablets	Panalgesic/Percodan/ Percodan Demi tabs
Buffadyne	Persistin
Bufferin	Quiet World Analgesic/ Sleeping Aid
Bufferin Feldene	Robaxisal Tablets
Butalbital	Salsalate
Cama Inlay Tablets	SK-65 Compound
Cetased, Improved	St. Joseph's Aspirin for Children
Cheracol Capsules	Sine-Aid
Clinoril	Sine-Off Sinus Medicine/ Aspirin Formula
Congespirin	Stendin
Cope	Stero-Darvon with Aspirin
Coricidin D Decongestant Tablets	Sulindac
Coricidin Medilets Tablets for Children	Supac
Darvon	Synalgos Capsules
Darvon with Aspirin	Tolectin
Darvon-N with Aspirin	Triamcinilin

Dristan Decongestant Tablets/ Capsules	Verin
Duragesic	Viromed Tablets
	Vitamin E

References

1. Coldiron B, Coleman WP III, Cox SE, et al. ASDS Guidelines of care for tumesent liposuction. *Dermatol Surg.* 2006;32: 709-716.
2. Klein JA. Tumescent technique for liposuction surgery. *Am J Cosmetic Surg.* 1987;4:263.
3. Lillis PJ. Liposuction surgery under local anesthsia: limited blood loss and minimal lidocaine absorption. *J Dermatol Surg Ondol.* 1988;14:1145.
4. Narins RS, Coleman WP. Minimizing pain for liposuction anesthesia. *Dermaol Surg.* 1997;23(12):1137-1140.
5. Hanke CW, Bernstein G, Bullock S. Safety of tumescent liposuction in 15, 336 patients. *Dermatolo Surg.* 1995;21:459-462.
6. Klein JA, Kassarjdian N. Lidocaine toxicity with tumescent liposuction: a case report of probable drug interactions. *Dermatol Surg.* 1997;23:1169-1174.
7. Hanke W, Cox SE, Kuznets N, Coleman WP III. Tumescent liposuction report performance measurement initiative: national survey results. *Dermatol Surg.* 2004;30(7):967-977.
8. Coldiron B, Fisher AH, Adelman E, et al. Adverse event reporting: lessons learned from 4 years of Florida office data. *Dermatol Surg.* 2005;31(9 Pt 1):1079-1092.
9. Coleman WP III. Liposuction and anesthesia. *J Dermatol Surg Oncol.* 1987;13:1295.
10. Klein JA. Tumescent technique for regional anesthesia permits lidocaine doses of 35 mg/kg for liposuction. *J Dermatol Surg Oncol.* 1990;16:248-263.
11. Ostad A, Kageyama N, Moy R. Tumescent anesthesia with a lidocaine dose of 55 mg/kg is safe for liposuction. *Dermatol Surg.* 1996;22:921-927.
12. deJong RH. *Local Anesthetics.* St. Louis, MO: Mosby-Year Book Inc., 1994.
13. Covino BG. Clinical pharmacology of local anesthetic agents. In: Cousins MJ, Bridenbough PO, eds. *Neural Blockade.* Philadelphia: Lippincott; 1988.
14. Tucker GT, Boas RA. Pharmacolkinetic aspects of intravenous regional anesthesia. *Anesthesiology.* 1971;34:538-542.
15. Grazer FM. Complications of the tumescent formula for liposuction. *Plast Reconstr Surg.* 1997;11(7):1893-1896.
16. Burk RW, Guzman-Stein G, Vasconez LO. Lidocaine and epinephrine levels in tumescent technique liposuction. *Plast Reconstr Surg.* 1996;97(7):1379-1384.
17. Sifton DW, ed. *Epipen. Physician's Desk Reference*, 54th edn., Napa CA: Dey; 2000:958.
18. Bouloux P, Perett D, Besser GM. Methodological considerations in the determination of plasma catecholamines by high-performance liquid chromatography with electrochemical detection. *Ann Clin Biochem.* 1985;22:194.

Chapter 26
Skin Tightening Off the Face with Radiofrequency and Broadband Light

Douglas Fife and Anthony Petelin

Introduction

Radiofrequency (RF) devices and infrared broadband light (IBBL) are nonablative energy sources designed to volumetrically heat the dermis and subcutaneous tissue with the goal of skin tightening or girth reduction. They have been used successfully and safely in all skin types on the large areas of the body listed in Table 26.1. IBBL devices (wavelength 850–1350 nm or 1100–1800 nm) penetrate deeply to bulk-heat the dermis without melanin absorption. RF generates heat via the tissue resistance to an electric current passed through the skin, which causes tightening through presumed collagen remodeling. Unipolar (also called monopolar) RF systems use a ground electrode applied to an area of the body away from the current source and create a high power area at the electrode tip. Bipolar RF systems rely on two electrodes located within the handpiece.

Depending on the device, RF and IBBL can be a one-time treatment or multiple-treatment course that may produce immediate and delayed improvement without the need for anesthesia.[1] Compared to the face, the response to RF and IBBL on the body is less predictable and often less appreciable, possibly due to differences in tissue characteristics (skin thickness, gravity, underlying fat/muscle, pathogenesis of laxity) in certain areas of the body. Proper patient selection and expectations are of paramount importance when using these modalities off of the face.

Clinical Examination/Patient Selection

The ideal patient is one who is within 15–20 lbs of their ideal weight, has mild-to-moderate skin laxity or increased girth, has disposable income, and understands that the results are unpredictable and possibly unnoticeable. Few contraindications to the treatment exist (Table 26.2). During the initial visit, patients identify their treatment goals and anatomical areas of concern, which are photographed and measured. The physician examines these areas for firmness, mobility, and thickness, while anticipating the direction of desired contraction. Circling problem areas and drawing treatment vectors may assist in visualization during the procedure (Figs. 26.1–26.3). The likely outcome of mild-to-moderate improvement in laxity, girth, or cellulite[2] should be discussed, including the possibility that no appreciable results may be achieved (Fig. 26.4). Reduction in girth is more commonly seen with unipolar devices compared to bipolar RF or IBBL devices, which do not heat as deeply (Table 26.3).

Method of Device/Treatment Application

Dose/Setting Selection

For both RF and IBBL, the settings vary considerably by device (Table 26.3). In general, higher energies can be tolerated on the body compared to the face. Lower energies are necessary when treating over a bony prominence such as the knees or elbows or when treating thin or sensitive skin such as the area around the rib cage, epigastrium, above the pubis, adjacent to the umbilicus, inner arms, inner thighs, and sides of the abdomen, due to increased pain. Topical anesthesia is not usually helpful as pain is usually perceived in the deeper tissue, which the anesthesia will not reach.[1,3]

M. Alam and M. Pongprutthipan (eds.), *Body Rejuvenation*,
DOI 10.1007/978-1-4419-1093-6_26, © Springer Science+Business Media, LLC 2010

Table 26.1 Body areas that may be treated by RF and IBBL

- Inner and outer arms
- Abdomen
- Hips
- Buttocks
- "Love handles"
- Back
- Inner and outer thighs
- Knees
- Dorsal Hands

Table 26.2 Contraindications to treatment with RF and IBBL

Absolute contraindications:
- Implanted electrical device such as a pacemaker, defibrillator, cochlear implant, or other (this applies to RF only)
- Pregnancy (not well studied)

Relative contraindications:
- Body mass index (BMI) >30
- Unrealistic expectations expressed by the patient
- Excessive skin laxity, significant diastasis, or striations (plastic surgery candidates)

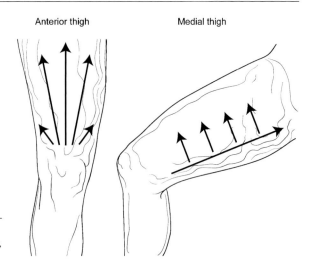

Fig. 26.1 Vectors when treating skin laxity on the legs. (Illustration by Alice Y. Chen)

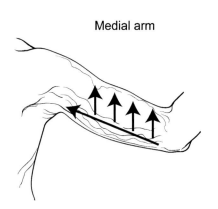
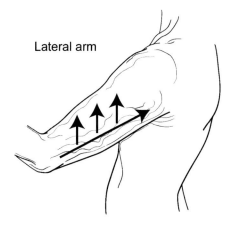

Fig. 26.2 Vectors when treating skin laxity on the arms. (Illustration by Alice Y. Chen)

Oral narcotic analgesics and mild anxiolytics may be administered in small doses if needed.

When using RF, treatment energies vary by body site. If using ThermaCool® devices (Thermage, Solta Medical Inc., Hayward, CA), the 3.0-cm² ThermaTip™ DC is used for volume reduction of larger areas for so-called "deep contouring." The conventional tips are used to tighten areas of skin laxity not requiring volume reduction. Similar to RF on the face, energy levels are titrated based on pain feedback, where a 2–2.5 out of 4 pain rating is desirable (Fig. 26.5). When treating sensitive areas, heat sensation may be reduced by

pinching the skin and treating between the elevated area without having to adjust the treatment setting. The generally accepted method of using lower energy settings with multiple passes is used for RF on the body.[4]

For the IBBL devices, thicker skin on most areas of the body compared to the face allows for higher energies to be used. With the LuxDeepIR™ (Palomar Medical Technologies Inc., Burlington, MA), for example, a patient may tolerate 70–80 J/cm² on the arms while only being able to tolerate 50–60 J/cm² on the face or 45 J/cm² on the neck. The patients should feel warmth but minimal pain.

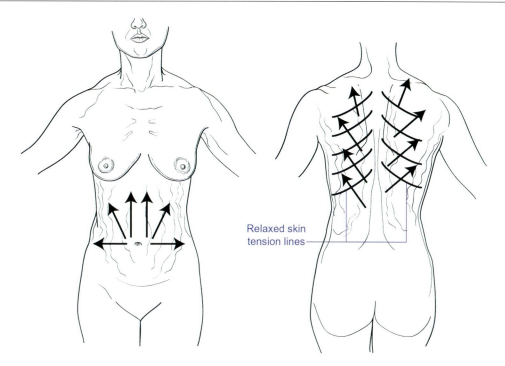

Fig. 26.3   Vectors when treating skin laxity on the abdomen and back. (Illustration by Alice Y. Chen)

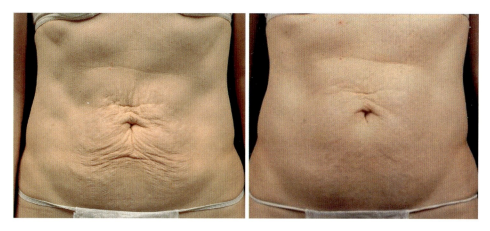

Fig. 26.4   Before and 6 months after Thermage treatment of the abdomen. Note the improvement in skin laxity and striae. Treatment by Richard Asarch, M.D. Photo property of Thermage, Inc

Treatment Technique when using RF

No specific pretreatment requirements are necessary. The patient should remove all metallic jewelry and objects. Next, the appropriate treatment grid is applied to the skin, which allows pulses to be delivered uniformly with at most a 50% overlap (Fig. 26.6). Then, the current return pad is placed away from the treatment site on a large surface area, and a generous amount of coupling fluid is applied to the treatment area.

While treating on most areas of the body, it is advantageous to preposition the skin in the direction of

Table 26.3 Device Comparison Chart

Infrared broadband light sources

Wave Length nm	Device name (Manufacturer)	Fluence (J/cm^2)	Pulse Duration	Spot size (mm)	Additional features
800–1400	BBL SkinTyte™ (Sciton Inc., Palo Alto, CA)	up to 55	10 msec–15 sec	15 × 15 15 × 45	Dual-flashlamp, integrated thermoelectric cooling with sapphire contact plates, adjustable from 0 to 30°C
850–1350	LuxDeepIR (Palomar Medical Technologies Inc., Burlington, MA)	up to154	3–10 sec	12 × 28	Fractionated surface plate protects epidermis with integrated active contact cooling
1100–1800	Titan™ (Cutera, Brisbane, CA)	5–65	4–10 sec	10 × 15 (Titan V) 10 × 30 (Titan XL)	Integrated active contact cooling
Traditional IPL 500–1200	Various	Variable	msec to 1 sec	Variable	In order to bulk heat without damaging the epidermis the shorter wavelengths would have to be filtered out

Radiofrequency devices

Device Name (Manufacturer)	Technical Specifications	Additional features:
Aluma™ Skin Renewal System (Lumenis Inc., Santa Clara, CA)	Bipolar RF	– Vacuum apparatus allows current to flow more deeply through the dermis – Can be incorporated into the Lumenis One combination platform
Accent™ XL (Alma Lasers Inc., Caesarea, Israel)	Bipolar or Unipolar 200 W, 40.68 MHz	– Two separate handpieces that deliver unipolar or bipolar RF energy
ThermaCool™ NXT (Solta Medical Inc., Hayward, CA)	Unipolar RF 400 W, 6.78 MHz	– Thermatip™ capacitive coupling technology – Integrated handpiece control with the NXT system – Tips of different sizes, including the 3.0 cm^2 ThermaTip™ DC for deep contouring
Visage™ (ArthroCare Inc., Sunnyvale, CA)	Unipolar RF	– Ablative RF technology at cooler temperatures, "Coblation"
ReFirme™, VelaShape™ (Syneron Medical Ltd., Yokneam, Israel)	ELOS™ (Combined infrared light and Bipolar RF)	– Chilled sapphire contact tip – Dermal temperature monitoring system

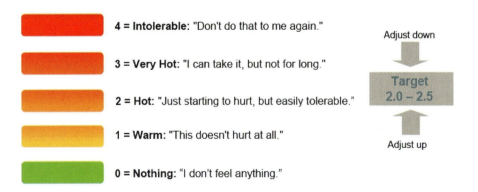

Fig. 26.5 Pain grading scale

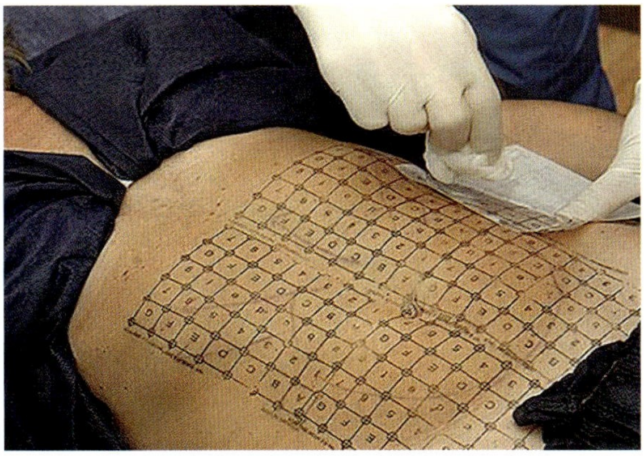

Fig. 26.6 Placement of treatment grid ensures uniform treatment and prevents no more than 50% overlap. Photo property of Solta Medical, Inc.

the desired placement vectors before administering the pulse, as this allows the skin to be tightened in the direction of desired skin contraction. Keeping the tip perpendicular to the skin, the first staggered pass is delivered in a caudal to cephalic, and medial to lateral direction using the standard "square then circle" progression until two full staggered passes have been completed over the entire grid. Tissue should be warm to touch, but not hot before retreating the same area. Vector and problem areas are then treated with repeated passes (2–8) in the direction of the vectors (see Figs. 26.1–26.3). The total number of pulses depends on the tissue response to treatment, the patient's goals, and the amount of pulses the tip can deliver. It is often more difficult to see a visual or palpable endpoint on the body compared to the face, so as many pulses are delivered as possible (average 600–900, but may require up to 1,200 or more).

When using the Aluma™ bipolar RF device, only one pass of adjacent pulses is delivered, and either the pulse time or pulse level can be adjusted to deliver the desired energy.

Treatment Technique when using IBBL

The skin is cleansed prior to treatment. For both the Titan™ and the LuxDeepIR™, a 2-second precool before each pulse is sufficient for most areas. A 3-second cool may be required for thicker skin on the body

treated with higher energies. Pulses are delivered adjacent to one another. Compared to treating the face, treating large areas of the body is more tedious and time-consuming and may require more concentration to appropriately cover all areas while at the same time avoiding overlapping. Initially, it may be helpful to draw a treatment grid on large areas of the body.

One or two complete passes are made over the entire treatment area. Similar to RF, vectors or problem areas can be treated with additional 1–8 passes. The skin is continually palpated and stretched to monitor for tightening or swelling/edema, both of which may be considered endpoints for treatment.

Care should be taken when treating thin skin or skin overlying bony prominences where the skin may more likely burn, possibly due to reflection of light off of the periosteum and the lack of a tissue "heat sink" below the treatment area. A good rule of thumb is to either decrease the energy by 20% or move the skin off to the side of the bony prominence while treating.

Postoperative Care

RF and IBBL treatments require little postprocedural care. The expected posttreatment reactions include mild-to-moderate redness, a warm sensation, and edema that usually resolve in 1–2 days. A bland emollient may be applied for comfort. A compression garment worn for 1–3 weeks posttreatment during the daytime may help to improve results. Some practitioners recommend avoidance of all external heat for the first 48 h and sunlight for the first 30 days. A record of the patient's weight and body measurements is essential to evaluate the improvement from the treatment. Effective and consistent photographs should be a part of the pre and postevaluation process (Figs. 26.7 and 26.8).

Number and Frequency of Treatments

Both RF and IBBL treatments cause an immediate and a delayed effect. This delayed effect, which may gradually improve the skin for up to 6 months, is thought to be due to continued "collagen remodeling"

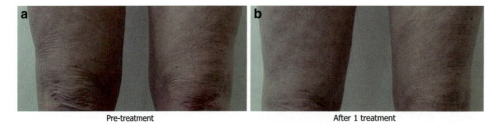

Fig. 26.7 Treatment of the anterior thighs and knees with the LuxDeepIR infrared handpiece (Palomar Medical Technologies, Inc). Photo Courtesy of Christine Dierickx, M.D.

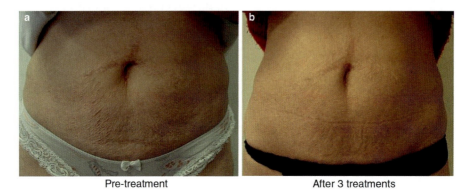

Fig. 26.8 Treatment of the abdomen with the LuxDeepIR infrared handpiece (Palomar Medical Technologies, Inc). Photo Courtesy of Christine Dierickx, M.D.

Table 26.4 Alternative treatment strategies for IBBL off of the face

1. Deliver one treatment now and assess the patient 3–4 months later (after a significant amount of "delayed tightening" has occurred) to determine whether another session is necessary
2. Deliver treatments every 4–6 weeks for a total of 3–4 treatments
3. Deliver one treatment now and a second and final treatment 2 months later

after the treatment. Thermage RF treatments are a one-session treatment. The Aluma™ device uses a multiple-session course of 6–8 treatments, each separated by 1–2 weeks.

The optimal number and frequency of IBBL treatments on the body is not well studied. Different treatment course strategies are listed in Table 26.4.

Management of Adverse Events

Side effects of RF are similar on the body and the face. The most common side effect is burning of the skin, seen as immediate erythema, crusting, or blistering. If burning occurs, immediate application of high potency steroids may minimize the reaction. Standard wound care techniques should follow. Skin indentations or contour irregularities occur rarely, are delayed phenomena, and tend to slowly resolve over time, but some may be permanent. Both burns and indentations can be prevented by using adequate amounts of contact gel/coupling fluid, by appropriately staggering pulses with at most a 50% overlap, and by using multiple lower-energy passes while titrating the energy according to the patient's pain.

Side effects of IBBL are rare, especially with newer devices with superior cooling and mechanisms, which prevent the delivery of pulses when the delivery plate is not in full contact with the skin. Burning of the skin may occur but is extremely rare when appropriate energies are used and the handpiece is kept in full contact with the skin.

Direction for the Future/Conclusion

Devices combining RF and IBBL into one delivery system have recently become available. One example is the VelaSmooth™ system (Syneron Medical Ltd., Yokneam, Israel), which combines bipolar RF with IBBL energy and a pulsatile vacuum suction into one hand-held applicator.[5,6] While some authors have shown this combination of heat effective in the treatment of cellulite,[1] further studies are warranted. Traditional intense pulsed light devices (wavelength 500–1200 nm) were not designed for skin tightening; however, newer devices with longer wavelengths and have higher cut-off filters may have a role. New ThermaCool® tips, including Thermage™ body tip 16.0 and Thermage™ cellulite tip 3.0 (CL), provide more options for treatment of the body.

"Pearls" for using either RF and IBBL on the body

- Select appropriate patients.
- Set realistic expectations. Improvement is less noticeable on the body compared to the face.
- Carefully identify and treat vectors and problem areas.
- Higher energies are required on most body areas compared to the face.
- Areas on the body with thicker skin may be harder to lift or tighten.
- Closely monitor patient's sensation of heat and discomfort. Stop the procedure if the patient is experiencing too much pain.
- Be aware of areas of thin of sensitive skin (abdomen, inner thighs, inner arms) where patients may experience more pain.

- Evaluate each patient and body area on a case-by-case approach, avoiding the "cookbook" approach.

Specific Pearls for RF treatment on the body:

- Avoid overlapping of pulses more than 50%.
- Use multiple pass-low energy technique.
- Unipolar RF more effective than bipolar at reducing girth.

Specific Pearls for IBBL treatment on the body:

- When treating over bony prominences lower fluence by 20% or move skin away to the side before delivering pulse.
- Always ensure adequate contact of handpiece to the skin to avoid burning.

Acknowledgments The authors would like to thank Nissan Pilest, M.D., Robert Weiss, M.D., E. Victor Ross, M.D., Michael Kaminer, M.D. and Amy F. Taub, M.D. for sharing their expertise in the preparation of this chapter.

References

1. Dierickx C. The role of deep heating for noninvasive skin rejuvination. *Lasers Surg Med* 2006;38:799-807.
2. Goldberg D, Fazeli A, Berlin A. Clinical, Laboratory, and MRI analysis of cellulite treatment with a unipolar radiofrequency device. *Dermatol Surg* 2007;34:1-6.
3. Kushikata N, Negishi K, Tezuka Y, Tezuka Y, Takeuchi K, Wakamatsu S. Is topical anesthesia useful in noninvasive skin tightening using radiofrequency? *Dermatol Surg* 2005;31: 526-533.
4. Kist D, Burns AJ, Sanner R, Counters J, Selickson B. Ultrastructural evaluation of multiple pass low energy versus single pass high energy radio-frequency treatment. *Lasers Surg Med* 2006;38:150-154.
5. Sadick N, Sorhaindo L. The radiofrequency fronteir: a review of radiofrequency and combined radiofrequency pulsed-light technology in aesthetic medicine. *Facial Plastic Surgery* 2005;21:131-138.
6. Sadick N, Magro C. A study evaluating the safety and efficacy of the velasmooth system in the treatment of cellulite. *J Cosmet Laser Ther.* 2007;9:15-20.

Chapter 27
Female Genital Surgery

Francesca De Lorenzi, Elena Mascolo, Francesca Albani, and Mario Sideri

Introduction

Our society attributes great importance to appearance and body image. In the recent past, cosmetic vulvar plastic surgery has been widely introduced in the western world. Modification of the cultural environment and increasing vulvar "visibility" have generated the erroneous identification of an ideally "normal" appearing vulva. The links between partner's relationship, sexuality, and body image have become more strict, and vulval morphology has become an important player in this complex scenario, especially at certain periods of the women's life, for example after delivery or during menopause, because of the changes and adaptations that the organs and the female genital system undergo normally. Cosmetic vulval surgery is therefore a natural evolution of our cultural environment. However, there are few papers addressing in detail this issue, indications, contraindications, and side effects. Clinicians who receive requests for cosmetic vulvar surgery should discuss with the patients the reasons for that request and perform an evaluation for any clinical signs or symptoms that may indicate the need for a surgical intervention. A patient's concern regarding the appearance of her genitalia may be alleviated by a frank discussion on the wide range of normal genitalia and reassurance that the appearance of external genitalia varies significantly from woman to woman and rarely is associated with functionality. On the contrary, any surgical intervention on the vulva can be the cause of worsening sexual function because of the scarring process, which is unpredictable in this area. Concerns regarding sexual gratification may be addressed by careful evaluation for any sexual dysfunction and an exploration of nonsurgical interventions, including counselling.

In this chapter, we will describe the technique of *labia minora reduction*, *Mons Pubis and labia majora enlargement*, and *vaginal rejuvenation*.

Functional and Aesthetic Labia Minora Reduction

Introduction and Definition

Enlarged or hypertrophic labia minora are characterized by different degrees of exposure between and beyond labia majora, whereas during childhood and in many adult virgins these cutaneous refolds are not outwardly visible. It can be functionally or psychologically bothersome. In the literature review, labia minora length exceeding 4 cm is considered for surgical reduction.

Clinical Examination and Patient History

Psycological concerns are the most important reason for women to have the size of their labia minora reduced. Protuberance of this genital structure is considered to be aesthetically and socially inconvenient, not only when the woman is naked but also when wearing tight-fitting clothes or swimsuit. Mechanical inconveniences may also be present in the personal history of these patients, with problems concerning difficulty in vaginal penetration, local irritation, problems of personal hygiene during menses, or after bowel movements, and pain or discomfort during cycling or sitting.

During medical consultation, possible reasons for hypertrophic labia minora are investigated although in the majority of cases congenital factors are responsible. Between them, mechanical irritation through excessive manipulation and intercourse, chronic irritation and inflammation as a consequence of local infections and dermatitis, exogenous androgen hormones, and stretching with weights.

During clinical examination, the redundancy of skin and mucosa of labia minora is assessed as well as skin laxity to determine the amount of tissue to be resected. All patients with labia minora length exceeding 4 cm are potential candidates for their reduction. Even after the patient has been assured that labia minora enlargement has no clinical significance and that variation in size is normal, many women remain dissatisfied and suffer psychological distress and therefore they ask for surgery.

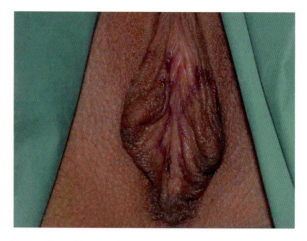

Fig. 27.2 Labia reduction. Straight amputation of the protuberant section of the labia minora and oversewing of the raw edge

Treatment Application

1. Local anesthesia.

Labium minus reduction is performed with the patient in the dorsal lithotomy position and under local anesthesia (1% lidocaine with 1:200,000 epinephrine).

2. Treatment technique and alternative methods

The simple and straight amputation of the protuberant segment and over-sewing the edge is usually performed (Figs. 27.1–27.3), but with this technique the labial edge is replaced by a stiff breakable suture line, potentially

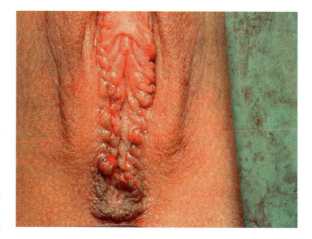

Fig. 27.3 Labia reduction. Straight amputation of the protuberant section of the labia minora and oversewing of the raw edge

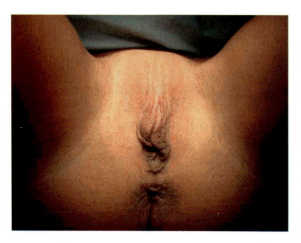

Fig. 27.1 Labia reduction. Straight amputation of the protuberant section of the labia minora and oversewing of the raw edge

associated to discomfort while walking and local irritation. Moreover, linear scar contraction can let to advancement of the posterior fourchette, resulting in the partial obliteration of the vaginal introitus and risk of painful intercourse. Alternative methods to overcome these undesirable outcomes include the running W-shaped resection with interdigitated suturing of the protuberant labia (zigzag technique, Fig. 27.4a; or wedge resections, Fig. 27.4b). In every case, the borders of the resection are directly approximated with interrupted absorbable sutures. Urinary catheterization is not necessary. Patients receive treatment with intravenous antibiotics and oral administration of antibiotics is continued until the third or fifth postoperative day.

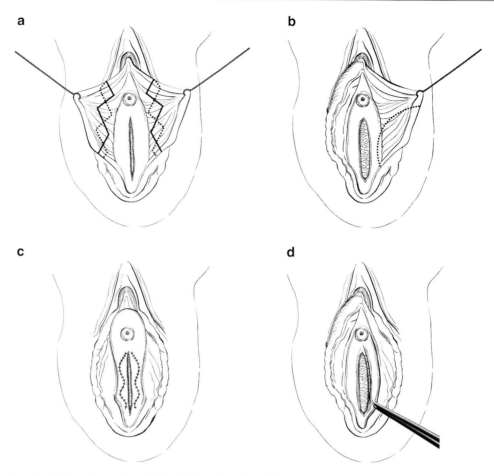

Fig. 27.4 Running W-shaped resection with interdigitated suturing of the protuberant labia. (Illustration by Alice Y. Chen)

They are discharged on the day of surgery or until the first postoperative day.

3. Postoperative care

Patient instructions include personal hygiene of the external genitalia after urinating, maintaining the vulva and the surgical wounds dry, topical application of iodine on the wounds, and placement of a dry sterile gauze to protect the suture line for approximately 10 days.

A medical examination of the vulvar region is required about 1 week after surgery to evaluate the healing process and exclude wound complications.

4. Management of adverse events

Adverse events are mainly correlated to wound healing problems and occur in the immediate postoperative period. Wound dehiscence of the surgical borders is the most common complication, it can be the only unfavorable event or can be caused by marginal necrosis of the surgical edges or hematomas. When the patient complies with postoperative recommendations, minimal dehiscence usually heals spontaneously and mucosa completely re-epithelializes within 2 weeks, resulting in unrestricted function and satisfactory appearance. Hematomas can drain spontaneously or mechanically. Infected wounds are treated with oral antibiotics with satisfactory outcomes.

Late complications such as sexual dysfunction, local pain, or skin retraction are rare, which can be avoided through an accurate selection of candidates, performing the zigzag technique or the wedge resections, and monitoring early wound healing problems which can impair the functional and aesthetic outcome.

Vulvar Reshaping and Vaginal Rejuvenation

Introduction and Definition

Under this section, we address two types of cosmetic and functional interventions: Mons veneris (mons pubis) and labia majora reshaping, and labia minora and vaginal rejuvenation.

The aim of Mons veneris (mons pubis) and labia majora *reshaping* is to preserve or increase turgidity, prominence, and elasticity. In contrast, the aim of labia minora and vaginal *rejuvenation* is to preserve or restore vaginal walls elasticity and hydration.

Clinical Examination and Patient History

Women might express a wish for rejuvenation on the basis of functional problems often mainly during menopause and in the postpartum period. With time Mons pubis and labia majora tend to atrophy. Vaginal walls tend to lose elasticity and hydration leading to a lower sensitivity and lubrication during coitus with a consequent dyspareunia and loss of sexual desire. These problems can influence the psychological sphere of women as well as that of their partner. Conversely, other patients wish their own ideal image to correspond with reality.

Following a thorough medical history evaluation as well as accurate clinical examinations the possible treatments are assessed, taking into consideration that these surgical techniques are invasive and may be the cause of side effects. Rejuvenation of the female genital mucosa means re-structuring, re-hydrating, and giving new turgescence not only for aesthetical purposes but also improving the functionality of the areas of interest. The procedures can affect sensitivity and lubrication during coitus and influence the psychological sphere of women as well as that of their partner.

Treatment Application

As in facial rejuvenation treatments, 1 ml syringes and 30.5-G needles are employed. The choice of the most appropriate material is at the surgeons' discretion. In the following, we shall suggest what is best for the female genital mucosal tissues, which are extremely delicate and sensitive.

On the basis of the areas to be treated, we ought to take into consideration that the aims could either be the increase in volume (mons veneris) or major tissue trophism or both. Therefore, the following substances will be chosen:

- Mixture of amino acids and Vitamin C, able to deeply restructure the tissues by means of fibroblast re-activation.
- Mixture of vitamins and hyaluronic acid, able to re-structure and moisture tissues through their water absorption action.
- Mere fillers, able to provide the desired volumes so that the treated areas become trophic again. They also have a water absorption action.

Volume Augmentation of the Mons Veneris and Labia Majora

Re-absorbable hyaluronic acid is an invaluable material. It is prepared in 0.5/0.8/1 ml preloaded sterile syringes, with 30.5-G and 27.5-G fine needles according to the density of the material chosen. (As an alternative, the surgeon can perform liposuction of adipose tissues removed from the abdomen or from the patient's fattier areas. The fatty tissue is then regrafted in the subcutaneous area to be hypertrophied. This is an outpatient surgical technique.)

Hyaluronic acid injections have to be performed in the medium or deep dermis – according to the parallel-arranged linear inoculation technique – in order to fill up the desired area, taking care to avoid injecting the vasal tissue (possible drawing). Small amounts of Hyaluronic acid should be injected in order to avoid vascular compression and necrosis in this highly vascularized area. It is advisable to use 0.5 ml pre-loaded syringes. The treated area needs to be massaged after administering the injection so that the substance is homogeneously and thoroughly distributed.

With this type of treatment, as with the fillers used in facial rejuvenation treatment, following an initial hyaluronic acid injection which the patient finds satisfactory, the surgeon will need to reassess and if necessary re-inoculated additional hyaluronic acid every 4–6 months, at least for the first 18 months. Subsequent hyaluronic acid re-inoculations could be performed every 6–12 months, according to the patient's local tissue metabolism.

Contraindications: There are surely more contraindications with respect to the re-structuring technique with the above-mentioned substances. Hyaluronic acids are mere fillers, surgeons need to take the same precautions as for facial rejuvenation treatments. These substances should not be used in patients who tend to develop hypertrophic scars, in patients with streptococcal infections, who have previously suffered from autoimmune diseases, or who have a known hypersensitivity to hyaluronic acid during pregnancy or breast-feeding. In case of valvular prolapse or prostheses, patients need to be prescribed an antibiotic prophylaxis (penicillin-type antibiotics are highly recommended, as is the case in surgical operations). Moreover, in the 2 weeks following treatment, patients are strongly recommended not to expose themselves either to temperatures below $0°$ or to saunas or Turkish baths. Also, the surgeon is required to inform patients (and to have them sign the informed consent) regarding possible early or late side effects, which may arise such as:

• Inflammatory reactions (rash, edema, erythema), itching, pain when exerting pressure on the treated areas (for a maximum duration of 1 week).
• Hardening or nodules where the injections were administered.
• Pigmentation of the treated area.
• Low treatment efficacy or low filling effect.

As regards facial inoculations, contraindications/side effects such as necroses, abscesses, or granulomas are referred to in the literature, which the surgeon should take into consideration.

Re-structuring, Hydration, and Turgescence of Vulvo-vaginal Mucosae

A commercial mix (vitamins, hyaluronic acid) used for facial rejuvenation, amino acids with a small diaphragm made of ascorbic acid and lidocaine, hyaluronic acid and vitamins, hyaluronic acid having a heavier molecular weight in order to more deeply re-hydrate the tissues. Doses will be proportional to the extent of the tissues

to be treated. Yet, the essential difference lies in the fact that genital organs are more delicate and that also special psychological care should be taken when treating these areas. Moreover, in some cases, local anesthetics (lidocaine) are mixed with active principles or injected subcutaneously in variable dosages (though lower than 1 ml) according to the patient's sensitivity.

We suggest positioning an ice pack before treating the areas as cooling reduces tissue sensitivity to pain.

Each area requires a treatment time which varies from approximately 15–30 min, patient cooperation permitting. Treatment frequency is based on the reaction and on the desired results. As regards restructuring, weekly treatments are generally necessary for the first 3–4 weeks, subsequently treatments can be performed every month or two.

Contraindications: There are no particular contraindications except for hypersensitivity to Vitamin C in some subjects. Therefore, Omega-3 and acetyl-salicylic acid assumption is highly recommended during treatment because of the lower platelet aggregation.

Also, the prescription of preparations based on *Arnica Montana* is recommended, to be administered a couple of days before and after inoculations in order to diminish the traumatic effect caused by needle penetration. Nevertheless, small ecchymoses might appear; these will spontaneously resolve within 2–3 days.

References

1. Lloyd J, Crouch NS, Minto CL, et al. Female genital appearance: "normality" unfolds. *BJOG*. 2005;112(5):643-646.
2. ACOG Committee Opinion No 378:. Vaginal Rejuvenation and Aesthetic Vaginal Procedures. *Obstet & Gynecol*. 2007;110: 737-738.
3. Maas SM, Hage JJ. Functional and aesthetic labia minora reduction. *Plast Reconstr Surg*. 2000;105(4):1453-1456.
4. Giraldo F, Gonzalez C, de Haro F. Central wedge nymphectomy with a 90-degree Z-plasty for aesthetic reduction of the labia minora. *Plast Reconstr Surg*. 2004;113(6): 1820-1825.
5. Munhoz AM, Filassi JR, Ricci MD, et al. Aesthetic labia minora reduction with inferior wedge resection and superior pedicle flap reconstruction. *Plast Reconstr Surg*. 2006;118(5): 1237-1247.
6. Likes WM, Sideri M, Haefner H, et al. Aesthetic practice of labial reduction. *J Lower Fem Gen Tract*. 2008;12(3): 210-216.

Chapter 28
Reduction of Excess Abdominal Skin via Liposuction and Surgical Excision

Emil Bisaccia, Liliana Saap, and Dwight Scarborough

Introduction

Since the inception of liposuction by Ilouz in 1977,[1] many modifications have been done to liposuction to increase its margin of safety and improve upon the cosmetic results, including the Klein technique of tumescent anesthesia.[2] For many patients who have good skin tone, abdominal liposuction alone can give good to excellent results.[3] However, there is a subset of patients who have small amounts of skin laxity of the lower abdomen that can benefit from a skin tightening procedure.[4] These patients have excess lower abdominal skin while still maintaining good abdominal muscle tone underneath making them excellent candidates for a "miniabdominoplasty" using a combination of tumescent liposuction and limited skin resection.[4] The good underlying muscle tone and minimal diastasis of the musculoaponeurotic wall obviate the need for a more extensive abdominoplasty.[4–13] For example, a young multiparous woman who has lower abdominal skin laxity and striae but still maintains minimal or mild lower abdominal musculofascial looseness is an excellent candidate for this procedure.

Clinical Examination and Patient History

Proper selection is paramount to a successful procedure. First, one must assess what is the underlying physical deficiency, and what specific procedures can provide satisfactory results, as well as what are the patients' expectations and preferences concerning the degree of skin tightening, scarring, and morbidity.

A general assessment of health and risk factors needs to be reviewed. Patients who smoke , have a history of thrombophlebitis, are morbidly obese, or have moderate to severe upper abdominal laxity and lower abdomen flaccidity are not good candidates for these procedures as they are at increased risk for complications and less than satisfactory results. Among the principal factors that need to be assessed are the degree of centripetal adiposity, the amount of skin laxity over the abdomen, and the degree of flaccidity of the abdominal wall musculofascial system. This is best done by examining the patient in the supine, upright, and bent forward position into the diver's position.[4] As the patient is in the upright position, the pinch test (between thumb and index finger) is done to measure the subcutaneous fat. If there is good skin tone, no overhanging redundant skin, and a pinch test of more than 1 in., liposuction alone is all that is needed. When the patient bends in the diver's position, the weakened abdominal muscles will bulge. The patient is then asked to contract the abdominal muscles, providing further testing of muscle tone and indication of any hernias. The patient then lies supine and raises the head and shoulders to tighten the muscles. This allows the surgeon to again check the musculoaponeurotic system for weakness, hernias, and diastasis of the rectus muscles.

The ideal patient for the miniabdominoplasty has poor lower abdominal skin tone with mild to moderate laxity, yet only minimal lower abdominal musculofascial looseness. If the patient has good skin tone and mild or no abdominal musculofascial looseness, then he/she may benefit from liposuction alone, while if musculofascial looseness is marked then he/she may benefit from a more extensive abdominoplasty (Table 28.1).[11–13] Finally, it is important to review with the patient the extent of improvement as well as limitations of the procedure as well as scarring.

M. Alam and M. Pongprutthipan (eds.), *Body Rejuvenation*,
DOI 10.1007/978-1-4419-1093-6_28, © Springer Science+Business Media, LLC 2010

Table 28.1 Decision making guide for abdominal recontouring

Physical findings	Treatment options
Lower abdominal adiposity only	Liposuction alone is treatment of choice
Abdominal adiposity combined with discrete skin laxity only	Combination liposuction with limited miniabdominoplasty
Abdominal adiposity combined with significant skin laxity and abdominal muscle flaccidity	Combination of liposuction with rectus muscle plication and miniabdominoplasty or standard abdominoplasty
Mild to moderate pannus formation	Two-stage liposuction procedure (Liposuction surgery followed by mini-abdominoplasty 3–6 months later)

Adapted from Bisaccia and Scarborough[11]

Method of Device and Treatment Application

First and foremost, the surgeon has to have requisite knowledge of the relevant anatomy. The abdominal wall is multilayered and has its principle blood supply originating superiorly and inferiorly. The blood supply to the skin of the abdomen is supplied by the direct cutaneous vessels and musculocutaneous perforating vessels.[4,10,15] These blood vessels are spared in liposuction by the use of tumescence and blunt tunneling. If these are disrupted sloughing of the skin and necrosis can occur. The innervation of the abdominal wall is routinely supplied from the lateral oblique direction and is derived from the roots of the nerves T7 to L4. The skin of the lower abdomen is more movable because it is less firmly attached, covering the soft areolar subcutaneous tissue. In the upper abdomen, the skin is usually less mobile and more firmly attached by the many retinacula to the deep fascia. This is the reason liposuction more easily removes the lower abdominal fat. More in depth anatomy review of the abdominal wall is beyond the scope of this chapter and can be obtained in other anatomy text books and articles.[14,15]

Tumescent liposuction is performed first, employing a standard tumescent technique,[3] via two small incisions just above the mons pubis (Fig. 28.1). This provides for debulking, while the dermatoadipose flap development is assisted by this pretunneling of the lower abdomen staying superficial to the abdominal musculoaponeurotic system. A transverse incision is then made with a 15-blade that connects the two liposuction

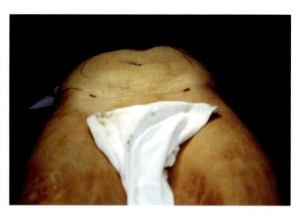

Fig. 28.1 Two standard incisions made above the mons pubis so that liposuction debulking can be done

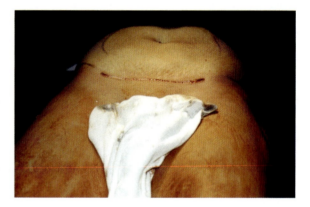

Fig. 28.2 Transverse incision is then made with a 15-blade that connects the two liposuction incisions

incisions (Fig. 28.2). The tunnels are horizontally connected using Metzenbaum scissors to a level midway to one-third below the umbilicus, depending on the extent of the skin resection desired (Fig. 28.3).

The excess skin is pulled inferiorly with an appropriate degree of tension and bifurcations are made to approximate the amount of redundant skin to be excised (Fig. 28.4). If additional skin needs to be removed, the incisions may be extended latero-superiorly in accord with the French-line method. The field is dried using unipolar electrocautery. In select cases, limited plication of the rectus muscle is then accomplished using non-absorbable monofilament suture. Multiple absorbable tacking sutures may be placed from the subcutaneous tissue to the musculofascial layer to help advance the flap downward, taking tension of the final closure line (Fig. 28.5). These sutures form attachments that change a large "dead space" into smaller compartments,

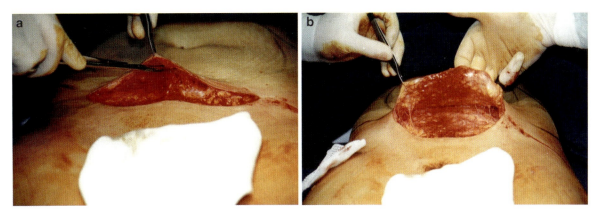

Fig. 28.3 (**a** and **b**) The tunnels are horizontally connected using Metzenbaum scissors to a level midway to one-third below the umbilicus

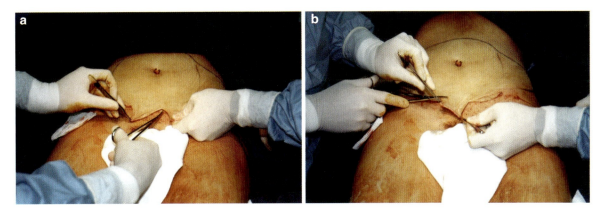

Fig. 28.4 (**a** and **b**) The excess skin is pulled inferiorly with an appropriate degree of tension and bifurcations are made to approximate the amount of redundant skin to be excised

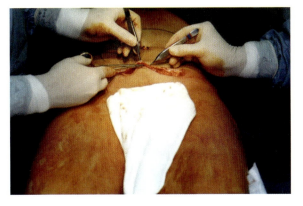

Fig. 28.5 Multiple absorbable tacking sutures are placed from the subcutaneous tissue to the musculofascial layer to help advance the flap downward, taking tension of the final closure line

which helps prevent seromas or hematomas. We routinely use no drains. Final closure includes subcutaneous closure with absorbable sutures and a subcuticular pullout suture on the skin, although in certain cases, small skin staples are used (Fig. 28.6). After completing the closure, sterile surgical tape strips cover the wound and an elastic binder provides support (Figs. 28.7–28.10).

Postoperative care

Patients are instructed to avoid aspirin or any non-steroidal anti-inflammatory drugs, such as ibuprofen and naproxen, for 2 weeks prior to the surgery and 2 weeks

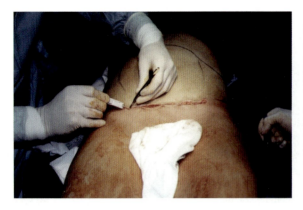

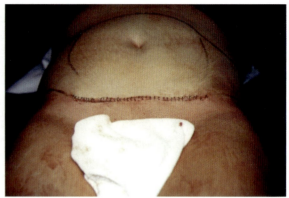

Fig. 28.6 Final closure includes subcutaneous closure with absorbable sutures and a subcuticular pull-out suture on the skin, although in this case, small skin staples were used

Fig. 28.7 Final closure with skin staples

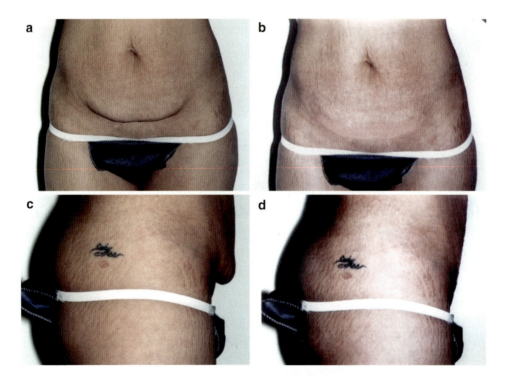

Fig. 28.8 Pre (**a,c**) and post-op (**b,d**) miniabdominoplasty and liposuction

postoperatively. Patients are also instructed to stop smoking, 2 weeks prior and 4 weeks after the procedure, and stop consuming alcoholic beverages for 24 h prior or 3 days after surgery. To minimize risk of infection, an appropriate antibiotic is given starting 24 h prior to surgery. Pain medications are prescribed prior to surgery, so patient can have them ready before leaving recovery. To optimize results of the procedure,

patients are instructed to begin a light exercise regimen of brisk walking for at least 1 h, 3–4 times a week starting at least 2 weeks before the procedure. Postoperatively, gentle normal activity is recommended for days 1–10, followed by increasing activity to walking at a gentle pace for 10–20 min a day from day 10 to 3 weeks. Between weeks 3 and 6 weeks moderate walking is recommended, with one mile per day

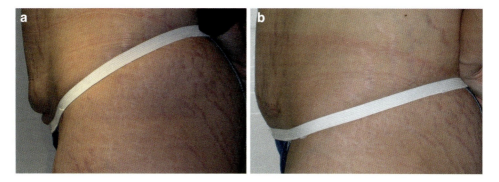

Fig. 28.9   Pre (**a**) and 7 weeks post-op (**b**) miniabdominoplasty without liposuction

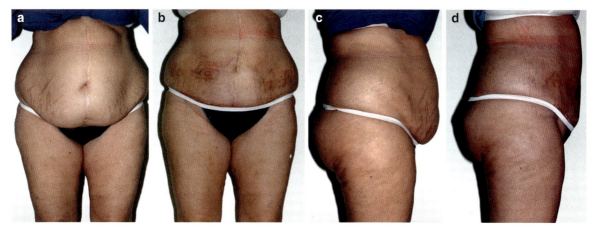

Fig. 28.10   Pre (**a,c**) and 8-week post-op (**b,d**) miniabdominoplasty and liposuction

and increasing to 30–40 min or 3 miles as day. After 6 weeks, full exercise and/or brisk daily walks are recommended in the amount of 40 min for a minimum of 6 months.

The garment that is applied immediately postoperatively should be worn for 72 h. After 72 h, it can be removed for a brief shower, and then put back on after wound care. Wound care consists of cleansing the wound with water in a cotton-tip applicator, applying an antibiotic ointment on a telfa pad, and applying tape to secure the telfa pad twice a day. At night, the tape can be omitted to minimize skin irritation. The binder is to be worn for 3–6 weeks, 24 h a day for the first 21 days, and then 12 h a day for the next 21 days. As the body shrinks, the binder may become loose, and if so patients are asked to purchase a second commercial girdle to account for a smaller size. Follow-up visits are scheduled at 3 days, 2–3 weeks, and 3 months after surgery. Sutures or surgical clips are removed at 14–21 days.

Possible Complications

In a study of all types of abdominoplasties, seromas (5%) were the most common complication followed by hematomas (3%), infection (3%), skin or fat necrosis (2.5%), and delayed healing (2%).[16] Late complications in this study included 'dog ears' (12%), localized fatty excess (10%), and unsatisfactory scars (8%). Pulmonary emboli and pancreatitis accounted for only 1 out of 278 patients each (0.3%).[16] Unfortunately, this study did not divide complications according to type of abdominoplasty performed, though only 65 of the 278 patients underwent a miniabdominoplasty and 206 underwent primary standard abdominoplasty.

The occurrence of seromas may be limited by using sequential tension sutures as described earlier[17] and limiting liposuction to the lower abdomen, as liposuction to both the upper and lower abdomen have increased risk of seroma formation. If seromas do form, these can be treated by aspirating and evacuating them with an 18-gauge needle. Hematomas are rare in our experience and can be prevented by appropriate use of tumescent anesthesia with blunt tunneling and suction, as well as adequate hemostasis before closing the flap. If they occur, the flap may need to be partly opened to allow for drainage, and appropriate antibiotics given to prevent infection. Meticulous attention to sterile perioperative technique as well as pre- and postoperative infection prophylaxis is the best approach to avoid infection. In the event of an infection, early recognition and treatment is paramount. Skin sloughs are very rare after modified abdominoplasty and seem to be more common in more extensive abdominoplasties. The recommended approach is to limit undermining only under the skin that is planned to be excised so as not to disturb the musculocutaneous perforators.[10] Dehiscence is possible with too much tension on the closure, a severe coughing spell, overexertion, or straining from constipation. Sequential tension sutures, as well as a regimen of fiber medication to decrease constipation that can be caused by pain medications are important. Just as with liposuction, other possible complications include transient hypesthesia, hyper or hypopigmentation, asymmetry or contour irregularities, and hypertrophic scarring in incision sites.

Pulmonary emboli are rare but the risk is increased in patients with a family history of PE, a history of deep venous thrombosis, malignancy, systemic lupus, protein C and S deficiency, nephrotic syndrome, and being on oral contraceptives. To minimize risk of pulmonary embolism, proper patient selection is paramount, as well as minimizing the duration of surgery and encouraging mild activity as outlined above. Fat emboli are a very rare but a possible complication. This risk is minimized using tumescent anesthesia.

Conclusion

Recent developments in abdominal contouring procedures have included the extensive use of liposuction and the use of modified or limited scars, producing a "downsizing" of the operative procedures for many patients. The use of minimally invasive techniques with liposuction alone, liposuction combined with the skin excisions and fascial plication can provide a comparable aesthetic result with less morbidity than traditional abdominoplasty in select patients.

References

1. Illouz YG. *A new technique for localized fat deposit*. Paris: Les Nouvelles Esthetiques; 1978.
2. Klein JA. The tumescent technique for liposuction surgery. *Am J Cosmet Surg*. 1987;4:263.
3. Bisaccia E, Scarborough DA. Syringe-assisted liposuction: a cosmetic surgeon's office technique. *J Dermatol Surg Oncol*. 1988;14(9):982-989.
4. Scarborough DA, Bisaccia E. Miniabdominoplasty using combination liposuction and limited skin resection. *Cosmetic Dermatol*. 1997;10(7):10-12.
5. Matarasso A. Minimal-access variations in abdominoplasty. *Ann Plast Surg*. 1995;34(3):255-263.
6. Eaves FF 3rd, Nahai F, Bostwick J 3rd. Endoscopic abdominoplasty and endoscopically assisted miniabdominoplasty. *Clin Plast Surg*. 1996;23(4):599-616; discussion 617.
7. Matarasso A. Liposuction as an adjunct to a full abdominoplasty. *Plast Reconstr Surg*. 1995;95(5):829-836.
8. Ribeiro L, Accorsi AJ, Buss A. Midiabdominoplasty: indications and technique *Aesth Plast Surg*. 1998;22:313-317.
9. Brauman D. Liposuction abdominoplasty: an evolving concept. *Plast Reconstr Surg*. 2003;112(1):288-298; discussion 299-301.
10. Avelar JM. Abdominoplasty combined with lipoplasty without panniculus undermining: abdominolipoplasty – a safe technique. *Clin Plast Surg*. 2006;33(1):79-90, vii.
11. Bisaccia E, Scarborough DA. Body analysis. In: *The Columbia manual of dermatologic cosmetic surgery*. New York: McGraw-Hill; 2002:85-94.
12. Matarasso A, Belsley K. Abdominal contour procedures: evaluating the options. *Dermatol Clin*. 2005;23(3):475-493, vi-vii. Review.
13. Sozer SO, Agullo FJ, Santillan AA, Wolf C. Decision making in abdominoplasty. *Aesthetic Plast Surg*. 2007;31(2):117-127.
14. Grevious MA, Cohen M, Shah SA, Rodriguez P. Structural and functional anatomy of the abdominal wall. *Clin Pastic Surg*. 2006;33:169-179.
15. Netter F. Abdomen: body wall. In: *The Atlas of Human Anatomy*. New Jersey: Ciba-Geigy Corporation; 1989:231-250.
16. Stewart KJ, Stewart DA, Coghlan B, Harrison DH, Jones BM, Waterhouse N. Complications of 278 consecutive abdominoplasties. *J Plast Reconstr Aesthet Surg*. 2006;59(11): 1152-1155.
17. Khan UD. Risk of seroma with simultaneous liposuction and abdominoplasty and the role of progressive tension sutures. *Aesthetic Plast Surg*. 2008;32(1):93-99.

Part VII
Advanced and General Topics

Chapter 29
Ablative Laser Resurfacing Off the Face

Richard Fitzpatrick and William Groff

Introduction

Though ablative laser resurfacing is generally considered to be the gold standard for the rejuvenation of facial photodamage and scarring, its use has declined dramatically because of its associated risk factors: postoperative infection, hypopigmentation, and scarring. To avoid these problems, it requires significant expertise and experience. When ablative laser procedures have been attempted off the face, the margin for error is much smaller, and the possibility of complications increases dramatically. In order to control these risks, the depth of resurfacing generally has to be limited to the epidermis, and the surface area must be significantly limited. Achieving dermal effects of tissue tightening, scar correction, rejuvenation of atrophic or wrinkled skin may not be realistic and must be approached with extreme caution. Any treatment on the legs becomes even more problematic because of the slow healing related to that area.

Ablative resurfacing of the chest and the lower 1/3 of the neck is particularly risky if depths extending deeper than the epidermis are attempted. When attempting to treat epidermal lesions that may extend into the dermis via rete ridges, such as seborrheic keratoses or actinic keratoses, particular care must be taken. Compound nevi are challenging as well because of the dermal component of the lesion. Failure to remove deep epidermal extensions of seborrheic keratoses, actinic keratoses, and compound nevi results in the regeneration of the lesions. On the other hand, ablation to depths of complete removal can result in significant dermal injury and often results in a hypopigmented scar.

Patient Selection

The conditions amenable to ablative treatment include the following:

- Neck and chest: photodamage and scarring of various etiologies as well as epidermal growths
- Hands and arms: photodamage, scarring, and epidermal growths
- Torso – hips: striae alba, scars, and epidermal growths
- Legs and feet: photodamage, scars, and epidermal growths

Photodamage includes dyschromia (permanent irregular hyperpigmentation, telangiectasia, lentigines, and ephelides), altered texture (atrophic skin with irregular crepey texture), skin laxity, and wrinkles. Epidermal growths are usually coexistent or a component of photodamage and include seborrheic keratoses, skin tags, actinic keratoses, and disseminated superficial actinic porokeratosis (DSAP). Scars are visible because of discoloration (red, brown, or white), shadowing secondary to their atrophic nature (with either smooth or sharp borders) or because of the elevation above the surface (hypertrophic).

Method of Device and Treatment Application

The advent of new technologies has revived interest in the use of ablative procedures off the face and has given physicians the tools to achieve excellent results

M. Alam and M. Pongprutthipan (eds.), *Body Rejuvenation*,
DOI 10.1007/978-1-4419-1093-6_29, © Springer Science+Business Media, LLC 2010

without significant risk. The new technologies to be discussed are Portrait® Plasma Skin Regeneration, fractional CO_2 resurfacing (Reliant Fraxel Re:pair will be discussed), and the adjunctive use of spot therapy with the conventional CO_2, erbium or alexandrite lasers with epidermal enzymes.

When using the Portrait® Plasma Skin Rejuvenation (Rhytec Inc., Waltham, MA) procedure on the neck, chest, hands, or arms, it is important to decrease the pulse energy according to the anatomic location. Achieving even, thorough epidermal coverage is important as well. Supplementing the procedure with alexandrite laser pretreatment of lentigines and seborrheic keratoses will result in a more significant clinical benefit. The Portrait® will achieve improvement in the epidermal components generally 50–90%, and may give mild improvement in some of the dermal features of photodamage and scarring, but more than one treatment session may be necessary. Dermal heating of collagen occurs down to approximately 300 μm at these parameters, so there is definitely stimulation of new collagen and this will result in some degree of smoothing of the skin's texture and skin tightening in

many patients. Pulse energies as high as 3.0 J may be used safely on the upper 1/3 of the neck, but the energy should be dropped to 2.0–2.5 J for the lower 2/3 of the neck. Repeat passes are necessary to assure complete and even coverage. For the hands and arms, pulse energies of 2.5–3.0 J may be used safely.

Lentigines and ephelides are pretreated with the Q-switched alexandrite laser using a 4 mm spot and 4.0–5.5 J/cm². Thick seborrheic keratoses located off the face are treated with a focused spot of CO_2 laser, pulse-stacking to create an epidermal–dermal blister to lift off the lesion precisely at the epidermal/dermal juncture (Fig. 29.1).

Fractional Resurfacing

The Fraxel Re:pair however allows much more aggressive and deeper treatment of these conditions off the face. Depths of treatment as great as 1600 μm can be used safely, but there must be close attention to density, or percent coverage. The primary area of

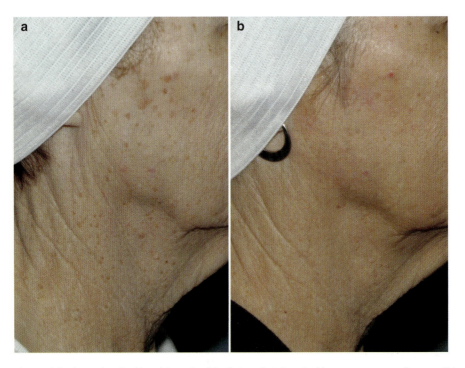

Fig. 29.1 (**a**)Before and (**b**) 3 months after Fraxel Re:pair of the face and neck and with spot treatment using a traditional CO_2 laser for seborrheic keratoses

concern off the face, as far as potential poor healing or scarring, is the lower neck. Densities greater than 20% should not be used in this area or on the chest. Although a single treatment with 25–30% coverage leaves 70–75% of the tissue untreated, we have seen infection occur at these settings that has resulted in scarring (Fig. 29.2). The ability of the lower neck to respond to any adverse event posttreatment appears to be severely compromised at these densities. When treating moderate to severe photodamage or scarring of the upper neck, we commonly use densities of 35% and pulse energies of 40–70 mJ. When treating mild to moderate photodamage or scarring, we generally drop the upper neck density to 20–35% and the pulse energy to 20–30 mJ. The lower neck and chest are treated at densities of 10–20% and pulse energies of 20–50 mJ. Repeat treatment sessions are likely to improve the overall response and these may be done at 1–6 months intervals.

As with the Portrait® procedure, we commonly use the Q-switched alexandrite laser as an adjunctive treatment when there are large numbers or large lesions of lentigines or seborrheic keratoses.

In a single treatment, we expect to see mild tightening (10–30%) (Fig. 29.3), mild improvement in lines and texture (15–40%), and significant improvement in dyschromia, including poikiloderma (usually >75%).

Treatment of the hands and arms is generally approached as a series of treatment, often combining the less-aggressive Fraxel Re:store for one or more of the anticipated four treatments in order to decrease the downtime of the patient. For the Fraxel Re:pair, we use densities of 10–30% and pulse energies of 20–50 mJ when treating photodamage. Isolated areas of traumatic or surgical scarring are usually treated with 70 mJ pulse. As with other procedures discussed, the alexandrite laser is used first to treat the most visible lentigines and seborrheic keratoses (Fig. 29.4). One lesion seen commonly on the forearms is hypopigmented flat seborrheic keratoses. These lesions are treated lightly with an erbium or CO_2 laser to help improve response, because of the lower densities generally being used with the Fraxel Re:pair.

When the Fraxel Re:store is used as a follow-up treatment, we will use pulse energies of 70 mJ and 32% coverage.

With this approach, we invariably see significant improvement in texture, lines, tissue laxity as well as more uniform color, with elimination of lentigines, seborrheic keratoses, and actinic keratoses. Lesions of DSAP do diminish somewhat, but in order to eliminate these persistent lesions, a more targeted approach is necessary, which will be discussed in the section on treatment of the legs.

Striae alba are very common findings on the lower abdomen after pregnancy and on the hips and upper lateral thighs secondary to adolescent growth spurts. There has never been a treatment that we have felt capable of giving significant improvement in the cosmetic appearance of these lesions. Not only are they visible because of the hypopigmentation and loss of natural skin texture lines, but many are also atro-

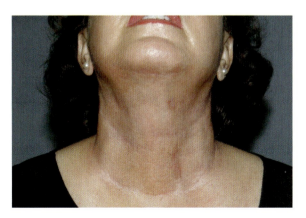

Fig. 29.2 Three months after treatment with Fraxel Re:pair. Patient had been treated at 30 mJ and 35% coverage on upper neck and 25% density on lower neck. Linear vertical scar corresponding to the medial edge of the platysma is present. More subtle scarring noted in horizontal plane secondary to wound infection during first week of postoperative recovery

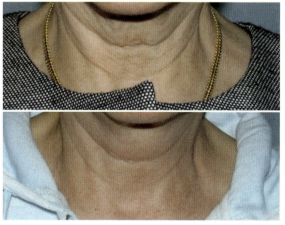

Fig. 29.3 Before and 1 month after treatment with the Fraxel Re:pair. Treatment setting were 20 mJ and 10% density

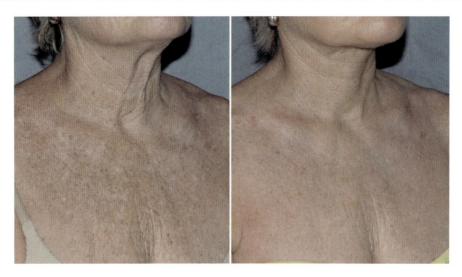

Fig. 29.4 Before and 5 months after treatment of lentigines and seborrheic keratoses with a Q-switched alexandrite laser

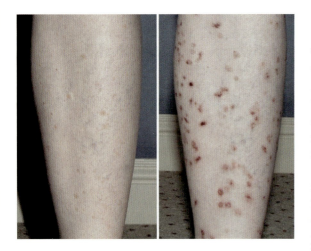

Fig. 29.5 Before and 1 week after treatment of seborrheic keratoses with erbium YAG laser in conjunction with enzymes

Treatment of Lesions on the Leg

Treatment of the legs has been confined at this time to targeting individual lesions of seborrheic keratoses, actinic keratoses, lentigines, and DSAP. The challenge with all of these lesions is to achieve complete epidermal/dermal separation throughout the lesion so that recurrence is limited and scarring or hypopigmentation is avoided.

Our approach is to use the erbium laser (Sciton, Inc. 25 μm ablation/25 μm coagulation and 3 mm spot size, 2–5 Hz) to ablate the stratum corneum and upper 50% of the epidermis (Fig. 29.4). Once this is accomplished, trypsin and papain are applied sequentially. These enzymes will not penetrate through the stratum corneum, so this layer must be fully ablated. Trypsin disrupts the protein bonds between the cells of the epidermis and papain disrupts the protein bonds between the basal cell layer and the dermis. Once the enzymes are applied, Saran Wrap is placed over the area to enhance penetration. When pinpoint bleeding is seen throughout the lesion, the treatment session is complete. If this is not seen (usually because of the thickness of the lesion), a second or third application of the enzymes is performed to reach the appropriate endpoint. Using this technique, we can achieve >75% improvement in elimination of these epidermal lesions without causing hyperpigmentation or scarring (Figs. 29.5 and 29.6).

phic. We have found in a small number of patients treated that each has had some degree of improvement, enough so that continued treatment is warranted. The treatment density used with Fraxel Re:pair has been 20–25% density and the pulse energy has varied from 20 to 40 mJ. With Fraxel Re:store, the recommended setting is 17–32% density at 40–70 mJ. When comparing between Fraxel Re:store and Fraxel Re:pair, the later has a higher likelihood of improvement at the expense of an extended recovery period up to 3 weeks.

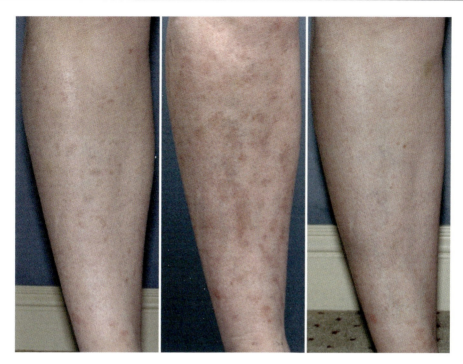

Fig. 29.6 DSAP present for 35 years and recalcitrant to numerous previous treatments, shows excellent improvement following treatment with erbium laser stratum corneum ablation followed by application of trypsin and papain

Chapter 30
Prepackaged Injectable Soft-Tissue Rejuvenation of the Hand and Other Nonfacial Areas

William Philip Werschler and Mariano Busso

Introduction

The presence of soft tissue fillers in aesthetic surgery has grown exponentially since the introduction of botulinum toxin A into the aesthetic environment in the early 1990s. Representative soft tissue fillers currently seen in clinician offices include collagens (Cosmoplast®, Zyderm®, Zyplast®), hyaluronic acid compounds (Captique®, HylaForm®, HylaForm Plus®, Juvederm®, Restylane®, Perlane®), poly-L-lactic acid (PLLA; Sculptra®), polymethylmethacrylate (PMMA; Artefill®), and calcium hydroxylapatite (CaHA; Radiesse®). The last filler mentioned here is a soft tissue filler increasingly referenced in the clinical literature and the one described in detail herein for the soft tissue augmentation of nonfacial areas.

Radiesse is a biphasic mixture of 30% CaHA microspheres (25–45 µm in diameter) and 70% carboxymethylcellulose carrier gel. The gel dissipates in vivo typically within 8–12 weeks, leaving the microspheres intact. In the soft tissue, they induce collagenesis so that a matrix forms around each of the microspheres. The duration of effect in soft tissue has been estimated from nearly a year up to 18 months.[1–3] Approved in late 2006 for treatment of moderate to severe wrinkles, such as nasolabial folds, and also for treatment of HIV-associated facial lipoatrophy, CaHA has also been used in several other off-label areas of the face. These include cheek augmentation, marionette lines, prejowl sulcus, and nasal defects.[1,4,5]

In addition to its use in facial areas, the use of CaHA in other parts of the body has begun to be explored by clinicians. For example, two articles published in early 2008 describe the application of CaHA for the treatment of the aging hand.[6,7] Experienced clinicians know that treatment of the hand poses challenges both in terms of efficacy and pain management. Autologous fat grafting, for example, requires multiple visits and ongoing management of pain in the innervated areas of the hand.[6] Combining CaHA with lidocaine mitigates much of the pain associated with injection into the hand, with results that are both immediate and long-lasting.

Other off-label areas of the body in which CaHA and other soft tissue fillers hold promise include the chest, the feet, the nipples, and other areas where soft tissue augmentation is desired, for example, following surgery or trauma. In this chapter, the authors provide instructions on how to combine the CaHA with anesthetic agents, how to approach treatment of the hand with CaHA, and suggest other nonfacial areas of treatment that might be pertinent in the future.

Clinical Examination

Prior to injection of any soft tissue filler, the patient should be counseled about the product itself, expected duration of effect, posttreatment self-care procedures, possible adverse events, pain management, and schedule for follow-up. Counseling may include a rationale for selection of one product over another, based on the needs of the patient at the time. Informed consent should be obtained in the same counseling session. Pretreatment photos, with standardized placement of the camera, can help the patient remember the appearance of the treated area in the moments, days, and weeks post injection.

Treatment Application

Administration of CaHA in the Hand

The treatment tray should be set up in advance of the first session so that the clinician has the necessary equipment for combining the soft tissue filler with lidocaine. Table 30.1 is a checklist for the procedure (courtesy of Dr. Busso).

Combining CaHA and lidocaine. To combine the CaHA and the lidocaine requires a 1.3 mL syringe of Radiesse (CaHA and gel), a "Luer-Lok" connector, and a second syringe also having a Luer-Lok connector and containing 0.15 mL of plain 2% lidocaine. The Radiesse syringe contents should be introduced to the anesthetic first, with the Luer-Lok connection. Push the Radiesse into the syringe containing 0.15 mL of 2% lidocaine. Then press the pusher of the lidocaine-containing syringe back into the Radiesse syringe. Ten "passes" of the Radiesse-lidocaine are sufficient for homogeneity.[7] Mixing the CaHA and the lidocaine lowers the viscosity and the extrusion force found in the original Radiesse formulation but does not compromise the properties of the CaHA. The particles remain suspended in the gel carrier so that the compound can be injected normally into the targeted area (Fig.30.1).[6]

(Author's note: Portions of this section previously appeared in the *Journal of Dermatologic Therapy.* Used by permission of the publisher.)

Identifying the area of treatment. The space that is injected is bound laterally by the fifth metacarpal, medially by the second metacarpal, proximally by the dorsal

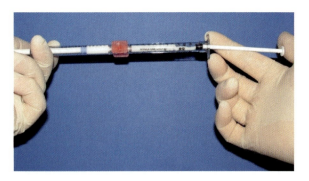

Fig. 30.1 Mixing CaHA with lidocaine, using a Luer-Lok connection. (All figures courtesy of Journal of Dermatologic Therapy; used with permission.)

wrist crease, and distally by the metacarpophalangeal joints. Approximately 1.3 mL of Radiesse fills this subcutaneous space of the dorsum of the one hand.

Isolating the area of treatment. Skin tenting is used to separate skin from vascular and tendinous structures by using the thumb and forefinger of the noninjecting hand to lift skin over the dorsal aspect of the hand being treated, as shown in Fig. 30.2a.

Injecting the mixture into the hand. Filler mixture is introduced as a bolus (0.5–1.4 mL) in the areolar plane between the subcutaneous layer and superficial fascia as shown in Fig. 30.2b.

Immediately after injection, the injection site should be gently massaged (Fig. 30.2c) until the filler has been evenly spread. The patient should make a fist of the newly injected hand while the physician manipulates the injected area to allow for more even distribution.

Posttreatment. Immediately post injection, photographs of the treated area may be taken after any directional markings have been removed. Patients are counseled NOT to massage the treated area on their own. Follow-up visits may be scheduled from 4 to 8 weeks post initial injection to document any adverse events and provide touch-up injection as necessary. Topical *Arnica Montana* may help reduce bruising and swelling. Vitamin K may be provided to the patient as well, for topical administration. Anecdotal reports have suggested that bromelain may have an obviating effect on bruising and swelling.

Adverse Events. Adverse events reported from injection of CaHA have typically been of short duration and low severity. They include, but are not limited to, edema,

Table 30.1 Procedure checklist for administration of soft tissue filler

☐ Informed consent obtained, patients screened for risk factors
☐ Pretreatment photograph obtained
☐ Areas to be treated marked for injection with washable marker
☐ Injection of CaHA and lidocaine mixture
☐ Postprocedure massage for several minutes
☐ Posttreatment photograph obtained usually after removal of markings
☐ Posttreatment instructions given (written and oral)
☐ Follow up appointment scheduled
☐ Treatment notes written into patient chart

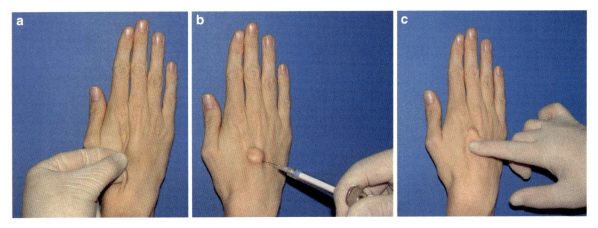

Fig. 30.2 Injection technique. This figure shows the tenting technique (Fig. 30.2a) when injecting a bolus of filler into the dorsal aspect of the hand (Fig. 30.2b). A massage of the treated area should follow injection of the bolus (Fig. 30.2c)

ecchymosis, temporary pain, and tissue soreness in the first days following injection. Patients taking blood thinners may experience more swelling and bruising than patients who are not taking these agents.

In addition, anecdotal reports to the authors have been noted concerning swelling of the hand post augmentation in a few patients. The swelling began immediately, post procedure in one case and as late as 3 weeks after injection in another. Risk factors in these few cases may have included the patient being greater than 60 years of age and injection with more than one CaHA syringe into each hand. Treatment consisted of watchful waiting, hand elevation, and perhaps oral steroids. In each of these anecdotal cases, the swelling resolved without sequelae.

CaHA in Other Nonfacial Areas

While nonfacial areas have traditionally not been treated with injectable filling agents, there are anecdotal reports of collagens being used for traumatic and postsurgical defects off of the face. Additionally, these agents have been used for cosmetic augmentation of the nipples, labia, clitoris, and penis. While these uses have been acknowledged, they are not typically widely performed. With the exception of postsurgical (mastectomy) or inverted/asymmetric nipple reconstruction and augmentation,[8,9] and the more recently described hand rejuvenation (Fig. 30.2c), other body areas generally have not been treated with fillers. Rather, fat trans-

fer has been the treatment of choice for most nonfacial augmentation procedures.

Moving beyond hands, certainly feet are an area of cosmetic concern for many aesthetically minded patients. With the increasing attention to grooming of the skin and nails of the feet associated with footwear fashion that exposes the tops of the feet, many patients would conceivably be candidates for dorsal subdermal injections of filling agents to address many of the same appearance factors that affect the backs of hands. The age associated thinning of the dermis combined with photo damage serves to expose the architectural anatomy of the dorsal foot. As can be seen with the before and after photos of the feet of a 42-year-old woman treated with CaHA (Fig. 30.3a, b), the aesthetically enhanced appearance rivals that of hand rejuvenation with CaHA (Fig. 30.4a, b).

The technique guidelines, administration, and mixing of CAHA with lidocaine are unchanged from hand augmentation. Additionally, foot augmentation patients are requested to refrain from wearing any tight-fitting footwear (especially over the instep portion of foot) for 2 weeks post injection. Those patients who have compromised circulation, diabetes, active infection, or any other type of medical condition that could impair healing and/or predispose to infection, ulceration or skin compromise are currently not recommended for this procedure.

Because no overcorrection is needed, the treatment provides real-time results as soon as the treatment is completed. The addition of anesthetic into the soft tissue compound allows deposition in areas traditionally

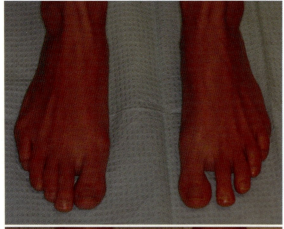

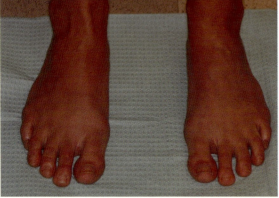

Fig. 30.3 Before and after photos of the feet of a 42-year-old female. Patient received 1.3 mL of CaHA in the left foot and 1.3mL of CaHA in the right foot

considered painful to treat, for example, the hands and feet. Within several weeks, the gel will dissipate, leaving the microspheres to form a cellular matrix in the tissue. Before and after results of the injection of the combined mixture of anesthetic and Radiesse are shown in Fig. 30.4.

Conclusion

Soft tissue fillers have been the mainstay of facial aesthetic correction for some time now. Some of these fillers have a versatility that lends them to new applications to other areas of the face. Both CaHA and PLA, for example, have approvals for facial correction; some clinicians may prefer the immediate correction property of CaHA over the accrued correction of PLA. We have found that both are good candidates for nonfacial applications too. In particular, CaHA has broad potential for treatment of both the aging hand and foot. As the elderly population inevitably expands, the call for viable treatment of the hand, with attenuation of attendant pain, will likely increase along with it. CaHA carries a favorable profile in terms of safety and efficacy in treatment of the face. We see no obvious reason why its use in nonfacial areas should be viewed with skepticism.

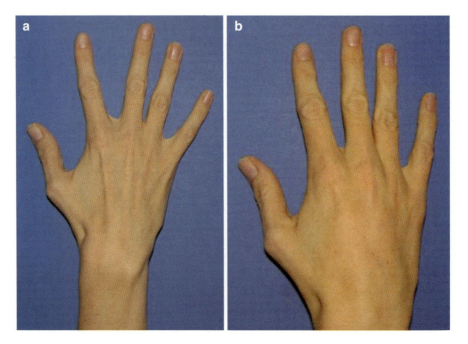

Fig. 30.4 Patient before and after hand augmentation. This figure shows a 38-year-old patient before (**a**) and immediately after injection of 1.3 mL of CaHA for augmentation of the hands (**b**)

Acknowledgements The authors express appreciation to BioForm Medical researcher staff members Robert Voigts, Dale DeVore, PhD, Michelle Johnson, and Xanthi Merlo for their studies on the properties of CaHA. The authors also thank the editors of the *Journal of Dermatologic Therapy* for permission to use images and some text that appeared earlier in their journal. Finally, the authors value the editorial assistance provided by David J. Howell, PhD, San Francisco, CA.

Disclosures. Dr. Werschler is an advisory board member, clinical investigator, consultant, investor, and/or speaker for Allergan, Inc, Artes, BioForm Medical, Inc, DermAvance Pharmaceuticals, Inc, Johnson & Johnson, MyoScience Inc, Medicis Pharmaceutical Corporation, Revance Therapeutics, and Sanofi-Aventis.

Dr. Busso has been an investigator for Radiesse and ArteFill clinical trials; he is a member of the BioForm Medical Education Faculty. He is also on advisory boards for Dermik and Allergan.

References

1. Graivier MH, Bass LS, Busso M, et al. Calcium hydroxylapatite (Radiesse®) for correction of the mid- and lower face: consensus recommendations. *Plast Recon Surg*. 2007;120(Suppl): 55S-66S.
2. Tzikas TL. Evaluation of Radiance™ FN soft tissue filler for facial soft tissue augmentation. *Arch Facial Plast Surg*. 2004;6: 234-239.
3. Felderman LI. CaHA for facial rejuvenation. *Cosmetic Dermatol*. 2005;18(22):823-826.
4. Becker H. Nasal augmentation with calcium hydroyxylaptite in a carrier-based gel. *Plast Recon Surg*. 2008;121(6):2142-2147.
5. Werschler WP. Treating the aging face: a multidisciplinary approach with calcium hydroxylapatite and other fillers, part 2. *Cosmetic Dermatol*. 2007;20(12):791-796.
6. Busso M, Applebaum D. Hand augmentation with Radiesse® (calcium hydroxylapatite). *J Dermatol Ther*. 2007;20(6): 315-317.
7. Busso M, Voigts R. An investigation of changes in physical properties of injectable calcium hydroxylapatite in a carrier gel (Radiesse®) when mixed with lidocaine and with lidocaine-epinephrine. *Dermatol Surg*. 2008;34(Suppl 1):S16-23.
8. Jacovella P. Calcium Hydroxylapatite Facial Filler (Radiesse™): indications, technique, and results. *Clin Plast Surg*. 2006;33(4): 511-523.
9. Evans KK, Rasko Y, Lenert J, et al. The use of calcium hydroxylapatite for nipple projection after failed nipple-areolar reconstruction: early results. *Ann Plast Surg*. 2005;55: 25-29. [discussion 29].

Chapter 31
Cosmeceuticals Off the Face

Zoe Diana Draelos

Introduction

Cosmeceuticals are a category of topical agents designed to improve the appearance of the skin. Traditionally, the cosmeceutical market has focused on products designed for facial application, yet the use of these topicals for body appearance improvement is rapidly increasing. Cosmeceuticals are substances found in both the over-the-counter (OTC) and prescription arena that can be effectively used by dermatologists to maintain or improve the results obtained with other rejuvenative procedures. Cosmeceuticals must be distinguished from colored cosmetics, designed only to adorn the body using pigments. The intent is that cosmeceuticals will produce an improvement in skin functioning by modifying texture, roughness, pigmentation, erythema, and desquamation. This chapter discusses how to use cosmeceuticals off the face.

Cosmeceuticals represent a broad category of products including cleansers, exfoliants, moisturizers, sunscreens, skin lightening agents, and antiaging therapies. Each of these areas will be evaluated for their utility off the face (Table 31.1). Facial application has been the main target area for the use of these products for many years. This is because the thinner facial skin is more amenable to visible change and possesses unique anatomic characteristics. The abundant sebaceous glands create the need for frequent facial washing, yet aggressive over removal of sebum induces flaky dry skin and increased wrinkles of dehydration. Wrinkles of dehydration do not occur on the body, but problems with dry skin are common requiring careful cleanser selection. Moisturizers are used more for improving skin feel than for wrinkle reduction. Exfoliants are used gently on the face for removal of desquamating corneocytes, but aggressively on the body for the reduction of calluses. Photoprotection remains important both on the face and the body, but clothing provides the bulk of the daily sun protection on the body while sunscreens play an important role during recreation. Finally, skin lightening and antiaging therapies are increasing in popularity on the body; however, efficacy is reduced due to the increased skin thickness off the face.

This discussion has focused on the differences between the well-established facial cosmeceutical market and the emerging body cosmeceutical market. Our next topic of discussion is the implementation of cosmeceuticals as a complement to minimally invasive cosmetic treatments.

Clinical Examination

All patients undergoing minimally invasive cosmetic treatments require the use of some cosmeceuticals for basic hygiene and the posttherapy maintenance phase. These products include cleansers and moisturizers with the addition of sunscreens. Other patients will require the use of cosmeceuticals for augmentation of the results obtained postprocedure. These cosmeceuticals include exfoliants, skin lightening agents, and antiaging moisturizers. Table 31.2 presents the ingredients and mechanism of action for these cosmeceutical categories. The art of cosmeceutical use is selecting the proper agents for the unique need of a specific patient. The rest of the discussion focuses on those cosmeceuticals available for treatment plan customization as outlined in Table 31.3.

M. Alam and M. Pongprutthipan (eds.), *Body Rejuvenation*,
DOI 10.1007/978-1-4419-1093-6_31, © Springer Science+Business Media, LLC 2010

Table 31.1 Function and attributes of body cosmeceutical categories

Product category	Function	Body use unique attributes
Cleansers	Removes environmental dirt, sebum, bacteria, and fungus to maintain skin hygiene	Must remove surface sebum without damaging intercellular lipids, must provide odor control in axilla and on genitalia
Exfoliants	Prevents and minimizes the build up of corneocytes	Callus formation in areas of body trauma (elbows, knees, heels, etc.) can be treated and controlled
Moisturizers	Creates an environment for optimal for barrier repair while creating tactile skin smoothness and pruritus reduction	Itch reduction, especially on sebum poor areas such as the hands, feet, lower arms, lower legs, and upper back, assumes importance
Sunscreens	Provides a thin covering over the skin surface to absorb and reflect UV radiation	Large body surface area application with copious sweating and frequent rubbing necessitates frequent application and reduces efficacy
Skin lightening agents	Decreases the production of melanin	Thick body skin creates challenges for pigment reduction and reduces efficacy
Antiaging therapies	Modifies skin functioning to create the appearance of younger skin	Body skin is less amenable to topical antiaging therapies, but photoaging is proportionately less on the body

Table 31.2 Composition of body cosmeceuticals

Product category	Main functional ingredients	Mechanism of action
Cleansers	Surfactants consisting of soaps and synthetic detergents (sodium lauryl sulfate, sodium laureth sulfate)	Oily sebum and oil soluble environmental dirt is emulsified by surfactant and water soluble environmental dirt are rinsed from body
Exfoliants	Physical exfoliants (polyethylene beads, ground nut pits, dissolving granules) possibly alone or combined with chemical exfoliants (salicylic acid, glycolic acid)	Desquamating skin cells are physically removed by abrasive particles and/or chemically removed by low pH substances intended to dissolve intercellular bridges
Moisturizers	Oily occlusive substances (petrolatum, mineral oil, dimethicone) are combined with humectants (glycerin, propylene glycol, sorbitol) to increase skin hydration	Occlusive substances create a water impermeable barrier over the skin surface and humectants attract water from the dermis to the epidermis and stratum corneum
Sunscreens	Organic (octyl methoxycinnamate, homosalate, octocrylene, oxybenzone, avobenzone, ecamsule) and inorganic (zinc oxide, titanium dioxide)	Organic substances absorb UV radiation converting it to heat while inorganic substances reflect UV radiation from skin surface
Skin lightening agents	Hydroquinone, kojic acid, deoxyarbutin, azelaic acid	Modulation of tyrosinase leads to decreased melanin production coupled with reduced exposure to UVA
Antiaging therapies	Retinoids (tretinoin, retinol, retinaldehyde, retinyl esters), botanicals extracts	Retinoids modulate keratinocytes differentiation, most botanicals function as antioxidants

Table 31.3 Problem oriented approach to cosmeceutical selection

Skin attribute	Cosmeceutical category	Mechanism of action for cutaneous improvement
Texture	Occlusive moisturizer, retinoid moisturizer, film-forming moisturizer	Increase skin hydration with petrolatum and dimethicone, normalize keratinocyte differentiation with tretinoin or retinol, create thin protein film over skin surface
Smoothness	Moisturizing body wash, emollient moisturizer	Minimize skin dryness with petrolatum depositing body wash, use emollient moisturizer with dimethicone to fill intercellular keratinocytes spaces
Desquamation	Exfoliant cleanser and moisturizer	Speed removal of desquamating corneocytes with polyethylene beads, Continue corneocyte removal process with urea and lactic acid moisturizer
Erythema	Antioxidant botanical moisturizer	Decrease erythema with anti-inflammatory botanical moisturizer (feverfew, bisabolol, licorice extract, etc)
Pigmentation	Sunscreen, skin lightening agent	Select inorganic sunscreen with zinc oxide to decrease pigment production, Inhibit pigmentation with hydroquinone

Body Cosmeceutical Treatment Application

Cleansers

Cleansers for the body must be selected to maintain hygiene while preserving the intercellular lipids, which form the skin barrier. The three major chemical categories of cleansers are soaps, syndets, and combars, which can be placed on a variety of cleansing implements from the hands to a washcloth to a disposable face cloth (Table 31.4). True soap is a specific type of cleanser with an alkaline pH of 9–10 created by chemically reacting a fat and an alkali to create a fatty acid salt with detergent properties. Soap efficiently removes both sebum and intercellular lipids making it an excellent general skin cleanser for wounded skin requiring debridement, but a poor choice for dry, sensitive body skin. Milder cleansing for normal to dry body skin is found in the syndet cleansers, which contain sodium cocoyl isethionate formulated at a neutral pH of 5.5–7. This more neutral pH removes fewer intercellular lipids preventing further barrier damage during body cleansing. Where infection or odor control is an issue, combar body cleansers at a pH of 7–9, containing soap and syndet combinations, along with the antibacterial triclosan should be selected. If the patient has extremely dry body skin or tendencies toward eczematous skin conditions, a moisturizing body wash that leaves behind a thin layer of petrolatum, dimethicone, or vegetable oils should be selected.

Exfoliants

Body skin cleansing may increase the amount of desquamating corneocytes. This may be due to excessive of removal of intercellular lipids, in which case a moisturizer should be used to improve skin texture and feel. However, in mature individuals, an increase in skin scaling may result from a desquamatory failure. This can be visualized as coarse skin scale on the anterior shins, thickened skin over the elbows or knees, and calluses of the feet. Moisturizers will temporarily smooth the skin scale, but the "dryness" will soon return requiring the use of an exfoliant. Exfoliants can physically or chemically dislodge the scale from the skin surface (Table 31.2). Physical exfoliants, such as polyethylene beads or ground fruit pits, can be placed in cleansers to scrub away the skin scale while chemical exfoliant moisturizers, containing urea or lactic acid, can dissolve the intercellular bridges allowing the skin scale to slough revealing healthy skin. Exfoliants can be used to rejuvenate the appearance of dry, aged body skin.

Moisturizers

Moisturizers form the largest category of cosmeceuticals and are applied to the body following cleansing to minimize transepidermal water loss (TEWL) thus creating an environment optimal for healing following a minimally invasive cosmetic procedure. Body moisturizers are also used to improve skin aesthetics and reduce itching. Moisturizers may also be a delivery vehicle for other cosmeceutical ingredients, discussed later in this chapter. There are three categories of substances that can be combined to enhance the water content of the skin include occlusives, humectants, and hydrocolloids (Table 31.5). Occlusives are oily substances that retard TEWL by placing an oil slick over the skin surface, while humectants are substances that attract water to the skin, not from the environment,

Table 31.4 Body cosmeceutical cleansers

Body cleanser category	Formulation	Appropriate patient selection
Soap (Ivory, P&G; Pure and Natural, Jergens)	Fatty acid salt, pH 9–10	Normal to oily skin, postprocedure wound debridment
Syndet (Dove, Unilever; Olay Bar, P&G)	Synthetic detergent (sodium cocoyl isethionate), pH 5.5–7	Normal to dry skin, general body cleansing
Combar (Dial, Dial Corporation; Irish Spring, Coast, Colgate-Palmolive)	Soap and syndet combined, pH 7–9	Triclosan antibacterial useful in patient with wound infection, bacterial colonization, or body odor
Moisturizing body wash (Olay Ribbons, P&G; Dove Nutrium, Unilever)	Synthetic detergent combined with petrolatum, dimethicone, and/or vegetable oils	Extremely dry skin, similar to conditioning shampoo, leaves behind a thin film of occlusive moisturizers to minimize skin scaling and roughness

Table 31.5 Body cosmeceutical moisturizers

Moisturizer category	Ingredients	Skin effect
Occlusive	Petrolatum, mineral oil, cetyl alcohol, dimethicone, cyclomethicone, soybean oil, lanolin, shea butter, cocoa butter, sesame oil, borage oil, all vegetable oils	Prevent water evaporation from skin, smooth desquamating corneocytes, place protective film over nerve endings to alleviate itch, add skin shine
Humectant	Glycerin, hyaluronic acid, sodium PCA, sorbitol, propylene glycol, vitamins, gelatin	Act as a sponge to hold water within the skin enabling hydration
Hydrocolloid	Proteins, hyaluronic acid, colloidal oatmeal	Create a physical barrier to water evaporation from the skin

unless the ambient humidity is 70%, but rather from the inner layers of the skin. Humectants draw water from the viable dermis into the viable epidermis and then from the nonviable epidermis into the stratum corneum. Lastly, hydrocolloids are physically large substances, which cover the skin thus retarding TEWL. Body moisturizers are typically more occlusive than those designed for the face, since the sebaceous glands are reduced on the body, yet they are formulated for better spreadability over large surface areas.

Sunscreens

Sunscreens are an important body cosmeceutical to prevent postprocedure pigmentation and to provide photoprotection. Sunscreens contain a careful combination of organic and inorganic ingredients designed to provide full UV spectrum protection (Table 31.6). Organic sunscreens contain filters, such as octyl methoxy cinnamate, octocrylene, and octyl salicylate, which undergo a chemical transformation, known as resonance delocalization, absorbing UV and radiating the energy from the body as heat. This reaction occurs within the phenol ring, which contains an electron-releasing group in the ortho- and/or para- position. This chemical reaction is irreversible rendering the filter inactive once it has absorbed the UV radiation. This has led to the recognition that photostable sunscreens are important to prevent the need for frequent reapplication. Photostability can be achieved by combining sunscreens, such as oxybenzone and octocrylene and avobenzone, or by selecting inorganic filters. Inorganic filters are ground particulates that reflect or scatter UV radiation, absorbing relatively little of the energy. They do not undergo a chemical reaction and are thus inherently photostable. Zinc oxide is an example of an inorganic filter that does not whiten skin, yet provides excellent protection from postprocedure body pigmentation. Sunscreens are

Table 31.6 Cosmeceutical sunscreens

Sunscreen categories	Spectrum of protection	Ingredients
Organic UVB filters	290–320 nm	Octyl methoxy cinnamate, ocytocrylene, octyl salicylate
Organic UVA filters	320–360 nm	Ecamsule, avobenzone, oxybenzone, menthyl anthranilate
Inorganic UVB/UVA filters	Total reflection of all radiation	Zinc oxide, titanium dioxide

probably most important following minimally invasive resurfacing on the hands, neck, and décolleté where it is difficult to achieve photoprotection with clothing.

Skin Lightening Agents

Skin lightening agents function to decrease the activity of tyrosinase, the key enzyme in melanin synthesis (Table 31.7), when used in combination with the previously discussed sunscreens. Hydroquinone, available in prescription strengths of 4% or higher and nonprescription strengths of 2% or less, represents the gold standard for skin lightening agents. Hydroquinone inhibits tyrosinase likely by interfering with copper binding, thereby reducing the conversion of dihydroxyphenylalanine (DOPA) to melanin, but it is also cytotoxic to melanocytes. Recent debate over possible carcinogenicity by damaging DNA in rodent models and cell cultures has caused the FDA to question its safety. This has led to the search for other cosmeceutical botanically derived pigment lightening agents, such as azelaic acid, kojic acid, arbutin, licorice extract, and vitamin C.

Azelaic acid is a 9-carbon dicarboxylic acid obtained from cultures of *Pityrosporum ovale* that may be a treatment alternative for individuals allergic to hydroquinone. Although its lightening effects are mild, several large studies done with a diverse ethnic background population

Chapter 32
Special Considerations in Asian Patients

Sherry Shieh and Henry H.L. Chan

Introduction

The approach to rejuvenation of the Asian neck and body requires a thorough understanding of key anatomic and physiologic traits and familiarity with the intrinsic and extrinsic aging process. As a group, Asians have a smaller frame and body weight, shorter stature, and short, muscular legs. Cutaneous racial differences include: decreased terminal body hair, reduced sweating, fewer leg veins, increased incidence of keloid formation, and higher epidermal melanin content that predisposes to postinflammatory hyperpigmentation (PIH). Histologically, the dermis of Asian skin is thicker, and wrinkling is delayed by approximately 10 years as compared to age matched Caucasian counterparts.[1] Photoaging in Asians is frequently characterized by pigmentary disorders such as solar lentigines and seborrheic keratoses on the head and neck.[2] The neck also ages differently in Asians compared to Caucasians. Poikiloderma of Civatte is uncommon, and platysmal neck bands in Asians are less problematic. Finally, differences in cultural aesthetic goals also exist. In Asians, there is a greater focus on toning and tightening of the body rather than performing procedures such as breast augmentation, liposuction, and abdominoplasty. Below, we will review various minimally-invasive rejuvenation methods and highlight special considerations when treating the Asian patient.

Treatment Applications

Botulinum Toxin A (Botox®)

According to the 2006 Survey of American Society of Plastic Surgeons, Botox® is the most common nonsurgical cosmetic procedure performed in Asians. While the forehead, glabella, and periorbital rhytides are the most commonly treated areas, treatment of nonfacial areas, such as the neck and gastrocnemius, are sometimes requested. Horizontal neck rhytids rather than platysmal bands are more problematic in Asian patients, and selection of patients can be improved with 30–40 units. Caution must be taken when injecting the neck with Botox® as muscle weakness and dysphagia are potential side effects. Masseter hypertrophy can be treated with Botox injection (50–65 units per jaw). As alluded to earlier, Asians have muscular calves, and this is often considered undesirable. Botox® is an acceptable nonsurgical alternative that can be used to reduce enlarged medial gastrocnemius muscles and create a more slender shape. Lee et al. have shown that doses of 72 units can be used with no functional impairment and a durability of 6 months.[3,4] The author has used doses of up to 100 units per leg safely with results lasting 9–12 months (Fig. 32.1). Appropriate consultation prior to injection is essential as the clinical outcome depends not only on the doses of injection but also the amount of exercise the patients perform. For example, the outcome would be suboptimal among regular runners. The technique involves six injections into the medial and lateral gastrocnemius muscle using a 27 G 1¼ in. needle.

Laser and Radiofrequency Skin Rejuvenation

Laser Considerations in Asian Skin

Skin types vary greatly amongst Asiatic races, and it is important to note that the Fitzpatrick skin typing system

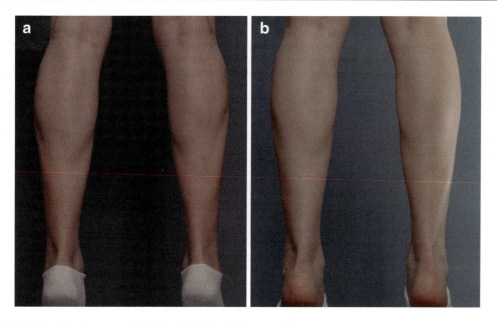

Fig. 32.1 (a) Enlarged gastrocnemius. (b) After 100 units of Botox per calf

is not directly applicable to the Asian population. Careful attention should be given to ethnic background and skin type when selecting laser parameters given the higher risk of PIH in this group. Means to reduce the PIH include: selecting longer wavelengths, ensuring adequate cooling, and increasing pulse duration. Strict sun avoidance and application of skin preparations containing sunblock, medium potency steroids, hydroquinone 4–6% and azelaic acid 20%, tretinoin, glycolic acid or kojic acid for 2 weeks before and after treatment are strongly advocated.

Neck Rejuvenation

The primary goal of laser neck rejuvenation in Asians is to address skin laxity and improve textural changes. Radiofrequency devices and fractional resurfacing can both be used safely on the neck in Asians with minimal downtime. Fraxel (Fraxel re:store, Solta Medical Inc., Hayward, CA) utilizes a 1,540 nm laser to create zones of microscopic thermal injury that are surrounded by normal tissue, which allows rapid re-epithelialization of the epidermis.[5] In Asian patients, cooling is critical to reduce bulk tissue heating and diminish the risk of PIH. Recently, it has been observed that decreasing density

levels can also reduce the risk of PIH in Asians.[6,7] *The typical parameters used for the neck are 40–50 mJ, treatment level 4–6, and 8 passes.* Radiofrequency tissue tightening with Thermage Thermacool TC (Solta Medical Inc., Hayward, CA, USA) causes dermal and subdermal tissue heating through the conduction of electric current with subsequent collagen remodeling and skin tightening. Patient satisfaction is high, especially when the upper neck is treated. With the use of effective cooling, lower fluences, and multiple passes, PIH is uncommon in Asians.

Body Contouring

Cellulite, central adiposity, abdominal laxity, and striae after childbirth are frequent complaints in Asian patients. Nonsurgical techniques are preferred and several radiofrequency and infrared devices show promise for treatment in Asian patients since their effect is independent of skin type. Velasmooth (Syneron Medical Ltd), is FDA approved for the treatment of cellulite and combines bipolar radiofrequency, infrared, and mechanical massage to improve cellulite. Sadick et al. showed an average decrease in 0.53 cm of the upper thigh and 0.44 cm of the lower thigh after 6 weeks of bi-weekly treatments.[8] Thermage with a deep contouring (DC™) tip can also be used for cellulite treatment (Fig. 32.2). Ultrashape (UltraShape Ltd, Tel Aviv, Israel) is a new focused ultrasound device that causes selective lipolysis (Fig. 32.3). In a multicenter study of 137 patients[9], a mean circumference reduction of 2 cm of treated areas was noted in the second week and sustained for 12 weeks. However, for Asians with a smaller body size, the results were much less impressive. A smaller transducer is necessary to improve outcomes.[10] For the

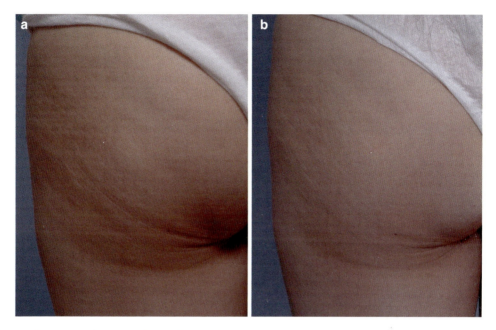

Fig. 32.2 (**a**) Cellulite of the buttock and thigh. (**b**) Cellulite reduction after Thermage deep tip

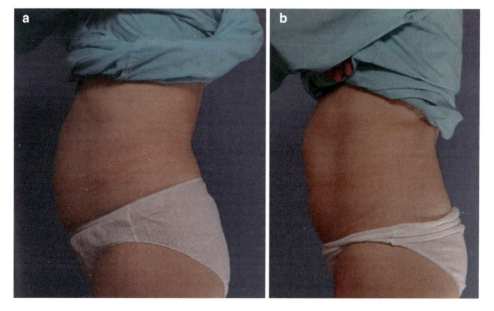

Fig. 32.3 (**a**) Abdominal pannus. (**b**) Ultrashape abdomen

treatment of abdominal striae, Thermage combined with the 585 nm pulsed dye laser (PDL) was reported to be successful in 37 Asian patients. After 1 session of Thermage and two PDL treatments 1 month apart, 89% of patients showed clinical improvement with histologic increase in elastin and collagen.[11] Thermage and other infrared devices, such as the Titan (Cutera, Brisbane, CA), and infrared handpiece (Starlux, Palomar, Burlington, MA), can also be used to tighten the abdomen. Further studies are needed to determine the optimal treatment parameters and long-term efficacy of these relatively new devices.

Hypertrophic and Keloid Scars

Hypertrophic and keloid scars resulting from acne or traumatic injury are commonly seen in the Asian population and may cause functional impairment, pruritus, and pain. The 585 nm PDL has been used at doses of 3.5–5.5 J/cm^2 with a 10 mm spot size to improve the appearance and symptoms of hypertrophic scars by selective destruction of blood vessels and decrease in collagenesis.[12,13] Manuskiatti showed that there was no significant difference between fluences of 3, 5, and, 7 J/cm^2 with a 5 mm spot size, but noted a trend towards improvement with lower fluences.[14] Lower subpurpuric doses avoid thermal injury and further scar induction. In Asians, a lower fluence should be used since melanin acts as a competing chromophore to hemoglobin and epidermal injury may occur. Our current approach is to perform a series of monthly intralesional injections of triamcinolone +/- 5-FU

followed by 595 nm PDL at subpurpuric doses (0.45 ms, 10 mm spot size, and 4–5 J/cm^2). Fraxel is also an effective treatment for hypertrophic scars on the body (Fig. 32.4). High energies and densities are necessary to improve hypertrophic scars (70 mJ, treatment level 8–11, 8–10 passes).

Hair Removal

Several lasers can be used safely for hair removal in Asians, including the long pulsed Alexandrite, Diode, and Nd:YAG.[15,16] A retrospective analysis of 805 patient comparing these systems revealed a slightly greater efficacy with the long-pulsed Alexandrite and long-pulsed diode laser compared to the long pulsed Nd:YAG.[17] Due to the increased epidermal melanin content in Asians which competes with the pigment in the hair follicle, lasers with longer wavelengths, longer pulse widths, and adequate cooling are necessary to avoid adverse effects. Intense Pulsed Light with a filter of 645–950 nm is also effective and safe in Asians.[18]

Conclusion

Noninvasive rejuvenation procedures amongst Asians are increasingly common. Knowledge of inherent differences in Asian skin types, variable treatment parameters, and an appreciation for cultural aesthetic goals allows safe and effective treatment of this growing population.

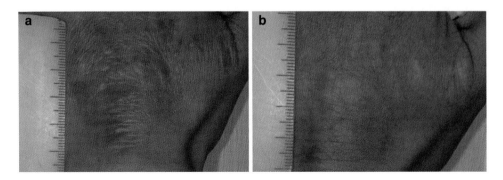

Fig. 32.4 (**a**) Burn scar. (**b**) After five full fraxel treatments

References

1. Yu S, Grekin R. Aesthetic analysis of Asian skin. *Facial Plast Surg Clin North Am*. 2007;15(3):361-365.
2. Chung JH. Photoaging in Asians. *Photodermatol Photoimmunol Photomed*. 2003;19:109-121.
3. Han KH, Joo YH, Moon SE, et al. Botulinum toxin A treatment for contouring of the lower leg. *J Dermatol Treat*. 2006; 17(4):250-254.
4. Lee JH, Huh CH, Yoon HJ, et al. Photoepilation results of axillary hair in dark-skinned patients by IPL: a comparison between different wavelength and pulse width. *Derm Surg* 2006;32(2):234-240.
5. Manstein D, Herron GS, Sink RK. Fractional photothermolysis: a new concept for cutaneous remodeling using microscopic patterns of thermal injury. *Lasers Surg Med*. 2004;34:426-438.
6. Chan HH, Manstein D, Yu CS, et al. The prevalence and risk factors of post-inflammatory hyperpigmentation after fractional resurfacing in Asians. *Lasers Surg Med*. 2007;39(5): 381-385.
7. Kono T, Chan HH, Groff WF, et al. Prospective direct comparison study of fractional resurfacing using different fluences and densities for skin rejuvenation in Asians. *Lasers Surg Med*. 2007;39(4):311-314.
8. Sadick N, Magro C. A study evaluating the safety and efficacy of the VelaSmooth system in the treatment of cellulite. *J Cosmet Laser Ther*. 2007;9(1):15-20.
9. Teitelbaum SA, Burns JL, Kubota J, et al. Noninvasive body contouring by focused ultrasound: safety and efficacy of the Contour I device in a multicenter, controlled, clinical study. *Plast Reconstr Surg*. 2007;120(3):779-89. [discussion 790].
10. Shek SY, Yu CS, Yeung CK, et al. Non-invasive body contouring with focused ultrasound technology. *Lasers Surg Med*. 2007;S20:60.
11. Suh DH, Chang KY, Son HC, et al. Radiofrequency and 585-nm pulsed dye laser treatment of striae distensae: a report of 37 Asian patients. *Dermatol Surg*. 2007;33(1):29-34.
12. Alster TS. Improvement of erythematous and hypertrophic scars by the 585nm flashlamp-pumped pulsed dye laser. *Ann Plast Surg*. 1994;32:186-189.
13. Nouri K, Jimenez GP, Harrison-Balestra C. 585nm pulsed dye laser in the treatment of surgical scars on the suture removal day. *Dermatol Surg*. 2003;29:65-73.
14. Manuskiatti W, Fitzpatrick RE, Goldman MP. Energy density and number of treatments affect respone of keloidal and hypertrophic sternotomy scars to the 585nm flashlamp-pumped pulsed-dye laser. *J Am Acad Dermatol*. 2001;45: 557-565.
15. Chan HH, Ying Y, Ho WS, et al. An in vivo study comparing the efficacy and complications of diode laser and long-pulsed Nd:YAG laser in hair removal in Chinese patients. *Dermatol Surg*. 2001;27(11):950-954.
16. Hussain M, Polnikorn N, Goldberg DJ. Laser assisted hair removal in Asian skin: efficacy, complication, and the effect of single versus multiple treatments. *Dermatol Surg*. 2003;29(3): 249-254.
17. Bouzari N, Tabatabai H, Abbasi Z, et al. Laser hair removal: comparison of long-pulsed Nd:YAG, long-pulsed alexandrite, and long-pulsed diode lasers. *Dermatol Surg*. 2004;30(4 Pt 1):498-502.
18. Lee HJ, Lee DW, Park YH, et al. Botulinum toxin A for aesthetic contouring of enlarged edial gastrocnemius muscle. *Dermatol Surg*. 2004;30(6):867-871.

Chapter 33
Treatment and Prevention of Dyspigmentation in Patients with Ethnic Skin

Smita S. Joshi and Roopal V. Kundu

Introduction

Ethnic skin, also referred to as skin of color, is primarily composed of Fitzpatrick skin types IV–VI and encompasses many racial and ethnic groups, including African–Americans, Asians, and Hispanics. Body rejuvenation can be successfully completed for these patients, but it requires knowledge of adverse reactions in darker skin. The increased melanin in richly pigmented skin can lead to greater susceptibility to postinflammatory hyperpigmentation (PIH), particularly from an underlying inflammatory cutaneous disorder or secondary to an irritation from therapeutic interventions (Fig. 33.1). Prevention of inciting inflammation, sun avoidance, and topical depigmenting agents are the mainstay of therapy for dyspigmentation in ethnic skin.

Clinical Examination and Patient History

The physician must elicit a careful history prior to performing any body rejuvenation procedure in a patient with ethnic skin. Inquiry into a history of PIH or hypopigmentation, dermatologic reactions to previous procedures or skin trauma, delayed wound healing, and hypertrophic scar or keloid formation should be initiated (Fig. 33.2).[1] Sunscreen use, tanning, and recent sun exposure should also be reviewed. A medication history should be obtained with particular attention to photosensitizing agents such as tetracyclines, retinoids, nonsteroidal anti-inflammatory drugs, and oral contraceptives.[1] The patient's Fitzpatrick skin type must be determined, however, the practitioner must also ask about the patient's ethnicity as patients with lighter phenotypes may exhibit skin characteristics of type IV–VI individuals.[1] Important screening questions for darkly pigmented patients are summarized in Table 33.1.

An important goal in the treatment of patients with darker skin is the prevention of PIH. Prior to initiating any body rejuvenation procedure on sun-exposed sites, counseling on sun avoidance is mandatory. It is essential to educate persons of skin of color about the association of sun and dyschromia. Most people of color do not feel it is necessary for them to wear sun protection because of their innate pigment and lower risk of skin cancer; however, daily sun protection with a minimum of SPF 15 should be strongly encouraged to help limit and prevent uneven skin color and PIH. Patients should avoid sun exposure for 4 weeks prior to body rejuvenation. A body rejuvenation procedure should be delayed on an actively sunburned or tanned area of skin.

Outside of sun avoidance techniques, pretreatment with depigmenting agents has been used adjunctively to prevent PIH. Hydroquinone is the mainstay of therapy. Hydroquinone 4% twice daily can be added 2 weeks prior to and 2 weeks post any intervention that has potential to lead to PIH. Other adjunctive therapies include azelaic acid cream used twice daily in either the 15% gel or 20% cream formulation.

It is advisable to stop use of topical retinoids or cosmeceuticals containing any retinoid derivatives at least 1 week prior to a procedure. These can be resumed after their postprocedure visit, typically 1–2 weeks after intervention. Photosensitizing medications may be discontinued for the preprocedural period after consulting with the patient's primary physician.[1]

M. Alam and M. Pongprutthipan (eds.), *Body Rejuvenation*, DOI 10.1007/978-1-4419-1093-6_33, © Springer Science+Business Media, LLC 2010

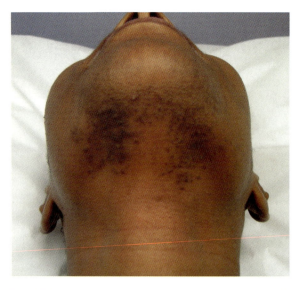

Fig. 33.1 Postinflammatory hyperpigmentation (PIH). PIH secondary to pseudofolliculitis barbae and years of daily plucking to treat ingrown hairs

Table 33.1 Important screening questions for darkly pigmented patients

How often do you…
    Apply sunscreen? What strength of sunscreen do you use? Tan?
Do you have…
    A recent tan? How much sun exposure have you had over the last month?
    Any upcoming trips or outings planned that will involve significant sun exposure?
    A history of abnormal darkening or lightening of the skin, abnormal scarring, or skin reactions?
    A history of wound healing problems?
    A history of hypertrophic scars or keloid scars?
Do you wear long-sleeved shirts, pants, wide-brim hats, or any other garments to protect your skin from the sun?
What is your ethnic/racial background?
Does anyone in your family have a history of abnormal scarring or skin reactions?
What medications do you take? (Specifically note any photosensitizing agents)

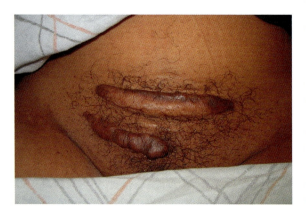

Fig. 33.2 Keloid Scar. Keloid formation subsequent to ingrown hairs and attempts at physical epilation along lower abdomen and suprapubic region

Treatment Application of Dyspigmentation in Ethnic Skin

Topical hydroquinone is the gold standard for treating PIH. Other treatment modalities include cosmetic cover-up, topical retinoids, azelaic acid, and chemical peels.[1,2] There are also several cosmetic skin brightening agents (non-FDA approved) commercially available in the United States including arbutin, kojic acid, and licorice extract.[2] Table 33.2 summarizes the most commonly used topical treatments for PIH in dark skin. Prior to using any topical agent, a small test spot should be applied to an inconspicuous part of the body (i.e., upper inner portion of arm) and any irritation or allergic response should be noted.

Postinflammatory hypopigmentation is less common but more difficult to treat, typically requiring passage of time to allow for any potential melanocytes to resume producing melanin. Repigmentation, if to occur, can be expected 1–3 months postprocedure. Along with sun protective measures, avoidance of topical bleaching agents or any treatment regimens which may further irritate the skin is essential.

Pigmentary, or melanin, incontinence is a unique form of PIH that is not amenable to topical depigmenting agents.

Discontinuation of isotretinoin for at least 6 months prior to a procedure is also recommended.

For patients with active dyschromia, guidance on cosmetic camouflage options to use prior to and posttreatment, such as CoverFX© and Dermablend®, which have a large palate of colors to help closely match skin tone, may also be offered.

Table 33.2 Topical treatments for post-inflammatory hyperpigmentation in dark skin

Treatment	Dose
Hydroquinone	<2% formula over the counter, 3–4% prescription formulations, 5–10% compounded formulations
Azelaic acid	15% gel, 20% cream
α-Hydroxy acid (glycolic acid)	Start at 20–30% solution, gradually increase
β-Hydroxy acid (salicylic acid)	20% solution, 30% solution
Kojic acid	1–4% formula
Arbutin	3% formula
Licorice extract	Various concentrations
Topical retinoids	Multiple formulations ranging from 0.02 to 0.1% creams and gels

Histologically, it is seen as an accumulation of melanin and melanophages in the upper dermis and treatment modalities such as Q-switched laser therapy have been used with limited success.[3]

Hydroquinone

Hydroquinone is a hydroxyphenolic compound that inhibits the tyrosinase enzyme, reducing melanin production.

Dose Selection

Hydroquinone is available in over the counter concentrations (<2%) and prescription formulations (3 and 4%). There are no evidence based recommendations for treating the body as opposed to the face; however 4% hydroquinone is often suitable for mild to moderate PIH. Higher concentrations (5–10%) may be necessary to treat severe PIH but may be unstable and irritating.[2]

Treatment Technique

Hydroquinone 4% may be used prophylactically 2 weeks prior to and 2 weeks post any body rejuvenation procedure that has the potential to lead to PIH. Hydroquinone 4% may also be used to treat any existing area of PIH. Hydroquinone should be applied twice daily (morning and night) and may be used for months, resulting in gradual depigmentation. Patients should be advised to use broad spectrum sunscreens during and after treatment. Hydroquinone will bleach both lentigines and freckles, but will spare café-au-lait spots and pigmented nevi.

Alternative Treatment Methods

Antioxidants, such as vitamin C, retinoids, and alpha-hydroxy acids, may be used as additives to increase penetration and enhance efficacy in the treatment of PIH.[2] Hydroquinone has also been combined with both topical retinoids and glucocorticoids to enhance efficacy.

Management of Adverse Effects

Adverse reactions include nail discoloration and irritant or allergic contact dermatitis; however, the latter may be avoided by performing a test spot of the agent prior to regular use. Paradoxically, PIH may occur from the contact dermatitis. Reversible hypopigmentation in the form of a halo around the treated area of hyperpigmentation is often seen in skin of color patients.[2] Individuals must be carefully counseled to use hydroquinone products only twice daily and to limit treatment only to affected areas to prevent this adverse effect. Fortunately, these side effects usually resolve spontaneously with the discontinuation of hydroquinone.

The most serious side effect of hydroquinone is development of ochronosis with prolonged use of high concentrations over large body surface areas. It is more common in South African women and is infrequently reported in the United States.[2] However, products with high concentrations of hydroquinone can be obtained illegally and may result in an increase in the incidence of hydroquinone-induced ochronosis in the United States. Ochronosis is often considered permanent. Treatment is difficult, but may respond to use of topical retinoids and topical corticosteroids and/or combined with a series of superficial salicylic acid chemical peels.[4]

Azelaic Acid

Azelaic acid is a naturally occurring nonphenolic dicarboxylic acid isolated from cultures of *Pityrosporum Ovale*.

Dose Selection and Treatment Techniques

Azelaic acid is available as a 15% gel (Finacea™) and a 20% cream (Azelex®) formulation. It should be applied twice daily (morning and night) to hyperpigmented macules. Azelaic acid has no depigmenting effect on normally pigmented skin, freckles, lentigines, or nevi due to its selective effects on abnormal melanocytes.[2]

Management of Adverse Effects

Azelaic acid is generally very well tolerated but may cause local irritation such as tingling and stinging sensations.

Keratolytic Agents (α-Hydroxy Acids and β-Hydroxy Acid)

Hydroxy acids agents reduce the thickness of hyperkeratotic stratum corneum by reducing corneocyte adhesion.

Dose Selection and Treatment Technique

α-Hydroxy acids (lactic acid, glycolic acid, citric acid, glucuronic acid, and pyruvic acid) are found in a variety of natural products including cane sugar, fruits, and yogurt as well as in cleansers, moisturizers, and chemical peeling agents.[1] Therapy should begin at low concentrations (20–30%) with a gradual increase in the concentration and frequency of use to limit side effects. Salicylic acid, the most commonly used β-hydroxy acid, is available commercially as a superficial peeling agent in solution form at concentrations of 20 and 30% (B-Liftx®). Salicylic acid acts synergistically with 4% hydroquinone to reduce hyperpigmentation.[5]

Management of Adverse Effects

Local irritation is common, but can be minimized if the keratolytic agent is introduced at lower concentrations. Paradoxically, PIH may occur if keratolytic agents are started at too high concentrations. Sunscreen must be used judiciously before and after treatment to minimize the risk of PIH. Salicylic acid chemical peels have been found to be safe in darker-skinned patients and most effective when combined with 4% hydroquinone.[5] Salicylism has been reported with widespread and prolonged use of salicylic acid, however it is extremely rare.

Topical Glucocorticoids

If there is a brisk inflammatory reaction after a procedure, a low-potency topical glucocorticosteroid (i.e., classes V–VII) can be added to the postprocedure regimen to not only reduce erythema and dermatitis, but also possibly elicit the well-recognized side effect of hypopigmentation from topical corticosteroid use. High and super-potent topical steroids are not advisable because of their known depigmenting effects, however repigmentation of affected skin usually occurs if the topical steroid is removed promptly.

Examples of Class V–VII Glucocorticoids

0.05% Desonide
0.025% Triamcinolone acetonide
0.1% Hydrocortisone butyrate
0.01–0.025% Fluocinolone acetonide
0.2% Hydrocortisone valerate

Laser Therapy

Lasers may be used cautiously in darkly complexioned individuals when utilized for hair removal, tattoo pigment removal, skin resurfacing, and vascular lesions. The increased epidermal melanin in richly pigmented skin may interfere with the absorption of laser energy aimed at another target. Postinflammatory hyperpigmentation is a frequently reported side effect of laser therapy and sunscreen should be initiated several weeks prior to and continued after therapy to reduce this risk.

Q-swtiched ruby laser has been used to treat PIH, but with little success.[3] No other studies to the authors' knowledge have specifically investigated laser treatment of PIH in darker individuals. However, laser therapy has been demonstrated to successfully treat other dyschromias. In Asians, the Q-switched alexandrite laser has been found to be effective for freckles and intense pulsed light for lentigines.[3]

Conclusion

With the consideration of prevention of potential PIH and working knowledge of available treatment modalities of dyspigmentation, body rejuvenation can be safely performed in persons of richly pigmented skin. While hydroquinone is the gold standard for treating PIH, with rapidly advancing innovation in laser technology and increased research in ethnic skin, it is likely that laser therapy may be a preferred treatment modality of the future.

References

1. Roberts WE. Chemical peeling in ethnic/dark skin. *Dermatol Ther*. 2004;17(2):196-205.
2. Halder RM, Richards GM. Management of dyschromias in ethnic skin. *Dermatol Ther*. 2004;17(2):151-157.
3. Bhatt N, Alster TS. Laser surgery in dark skin. *Dermatol Surg*. 2008;34(2):184-194. discussion 94–95.
4. Levin CY, Maibach H. Exogenous ochronosis. An update on clinical features, causative agents and treatment options. *Am J Clin Dermatol*. 2001;2(4):213-217.
5. Grimes PE. The safety and efficacy of salicylic acid chemical peels in darker racial-ethnic groups. *Dermatol Surg*. 1999;25(1): 18-22.

Index

Printed in the United States of America